Orthopaedic Radiology

Pattern recognition and differential diagnosis

To my late father,
Alfred Reichenbaum

Orthopaedic Radiology

Pattern recognition and differential diagnosis

Peter Renton

FRCR, DMRD

Consultant Radiologist, Royal
National Orthopaedic
Hospital, London and
Stanmore, and University
College Hospital, London

Honorary Senior Lecturer,
Institute of Orthopaedics and
Dental School, University
College, London

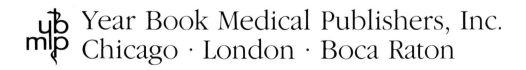
Year Book Medical Publishers, Inc.
Chicago · London · Boca Raton

First published in the United Kingdom in 1990
by Martin Dunitz Ltd, London

Distributed in the United States of America and Canada by Year Book
Medical Publishers, Inc., 200 North LaSalle Street, Chicago, IL

Library of Congress Cataloging-in-Publication Data

Renton, Peter, F.R.C.R.
  Orthopaedic radiology : pattern recognition and differential diagnosis /
  Peter Renton.
    p. cm.
  Includes bibliographies and index.
  ISBN 0–8151–7231–1
  1. Radiography in orthopedics. 2. Diagnosis, Differential.
I. Title. II. Title: Pattern recognition and differential diagnosis.
  [DNLM: 1. Bone Diseases–radiography. 2. Diagnosis, Differential. 3.
Pattern Recognition.   WE 225 R422o]
RD734.5.R33R46   1990
617.3–dc20
DNLM/DLC
for Library of Congress   89-8910
                                                                CIP

Laserset by Scribe Design, Gillingham, Kent
Colour separation by Adroit Photo Litho Ltd, Birmingham
Printed and bound in England by Butler & Tanner Ltd, Frome, Somerset

Contents

Acknowledgments

This book was written at the suggestion of Professor Leslie Klenerman, now of Liverpool University and formerly of Northwick Park Hospital. I am grateful for his encouragement.

Many of the illustrations have been taken from the files of the Radiology Museum of the Institute of Orthopaedics, London, with permission. I am conscious of my debt to my colleagues and indeed, to all those who have sent us films over the years. The illustrations have been provided by the Medical Photographic Department of the Institute of Orthopaedics and I am especially grateful to Mr Dirk de Camp for the care he has taken over them.

This book could not have been undertaken without the constant help of the Radiology Museum secretary, Veronika Aurens, BA, who also typed and arranged the manuscript. I am most grateful to her and to the late Sally Jones, and Mary Banks of the publishers, Martin Dunitz Ltd.

Peter Renton 1990

Preface

The aim of this short text is to provide an easy to read system of orthopaedic radiology for trainees in both orthopaedics and radiology. The approach is based on pattern recognition, first popularized by that great teacher Dr George Simon in his book *Principles of bone X-ray diagnosis*, which is now out of print. Diseases are described according to their predominant radiological features, rather than their pathological groups. These features form the basis of individual chapters. Using this method of instruc-

tion, it is inevitable that some conditions are described in more than one chapter. This is desirable as it reinforces information and also reduces the need for cross-referencing. The emphasis of each chapter, however, alters the way in which each disease is described.

The author hopes that the text will provide an understanding of radiological change and differential diagnosis, comprehensive lists of which are interspersed throughout. Suggestions for further reading are given at the end of the book.

1 | Decrease in bone density

Loss of bone density may be:

1 generalized;
2 regional, affecting many but not all bones, often in continuity, for example, a whole limb;
3 focal. Focal lesions may be multiple and separated by normal bone.

A bone which shows a decrease in density can be described as osteopenic. This term does not imply a particular pathology and avoids labelling a patient with a specific disease entity which may not be present. It is used to describe a subjective radiological appearance of bone which may be due to different causes and is also subject to observer variation. Osteopenia may also be mimicked by faulty radiographic technique, especially by the use of a high kV.

Normal bone consists of cortex and medulla, which vary in thickness at different sites. Typically, the cortex is thick in the midshaft of the femur and thin at the distal femoral metaphysis. Medullary trabeculae often reflect local stresses, which are well demonstrated in the femoral neck and vertebral bodies. The overall radiographic image of a bone is largely due to the anterior and posterior cortices overlain. At the margin, particularly of a round bone, the curved cortex has sufficient depth to be radiologically visible end on. Therefore cortical bone loss is the most significant factor in the reduction of bone density.

The major causes of generalized osteopenia are:

1 Osteoporosis
2 Osteomalacia
3 Hyperparathyroidism
4 Diffuse malignant disease.

Osteoporosis

Most osteopenic patients are osteoporotic; however, the terms are not interchangeable. Osteoporosis may be defined as an absolute quantitative deficiency of bone substance. The bone which remains is qualitatively normal. Therefore, there is a decrease in bone mass per unit volume.

Methods of assessing osteoporosis

Radiographic photodensitometry

Comparison is made between the subject's metacarpal and a normal metacarpal embedded in perspex and radiographed on the same film (Figure 1.1), or an aluminium step wedge. This is an adequate, simple and fairly reproducible technique which requires an accurate light densitometer.

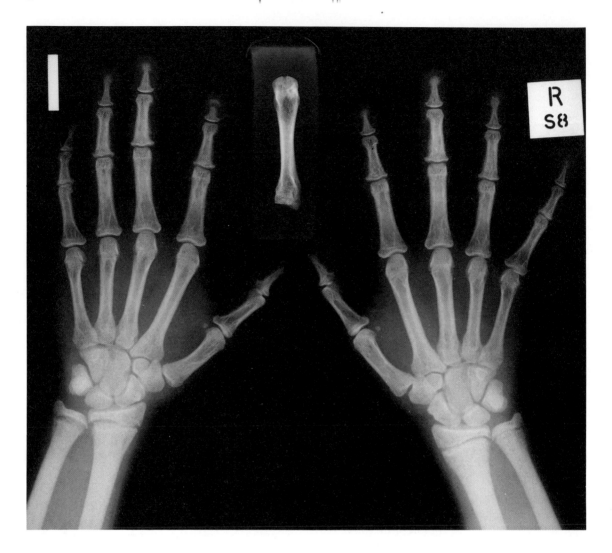

Figure 1.1

In radiographic densitometry, a
normal metacarpal is imaged
with the patient's hand. In this
case, there is evidence of
hyperparathyroidism, shown by
subperiosteal bone resorption,
distal tuft resorption and
resorption of bone at the distal
radial and ulnar metaphyses.

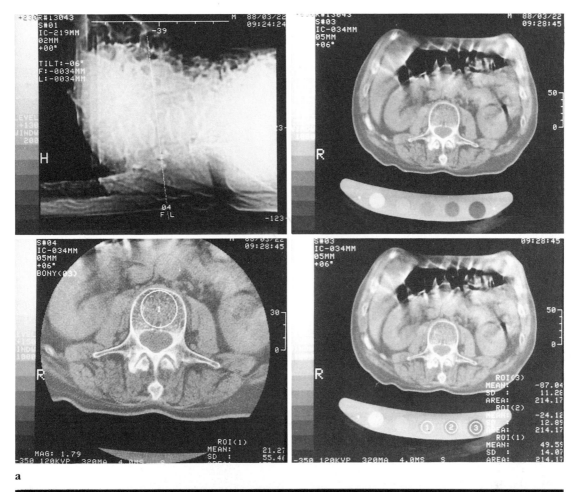

a

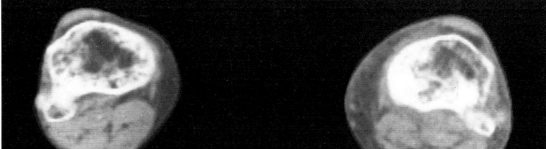

b

Figure 1.2

(**a**) Density readings obtained on the CT scanner are compared with the standard readings obtained on phantoms. (**b**) CT scan showing osteoporosis in the upper tibiae, and loss of trabeculae.

Photondensitometry

A low-energy source of monochromatic gamma radiation is scanned across part of the body and the attenuated beam is recorded by a collimated scintillation scanner. The loss of radiation through bone is compared with the loss through an equivalent amount of the adjacent soft tissue. The technique can be made more sophisticated by using two sources of different energies. The apparatus is expensive but the findings are accurate and reproducible.

Computerized tomography (CT) of the spine

Cortical and medullary densities are simply and accurately assessed by this technique which is easily reproduced (Figure 1.2).

Radiological quantitative morphometry

Using a standard radiographic technique, the thickness of the midshafts and medulla of the second, or second, third and fourth metacarpals are assessed at right angles to their midpoints. The measurements made with Vernier calipers can be used for various calculations to assess cortico-medullary ratios. There may be difficulties in visualizing the inner cortical margin, and, if the cortices are not homogeneous (as in hyperparathyroidism), the cortical width does not represent cortical bone mass. These techniques are often used in specialized units and are relatively simple to perform.

Qualitative visual assessment

Radiologically visualized bone density is the result of a balance between osteoblastic and osteoclastic activity, between bone formation and resorption. Therefore, if osteolysis exceeds osteogenesis, a loss of total bone mass occurs. Radiologically, osteoporosis becomes visible when approximately 50 per cent of bone mass is lost. Bone loss is seen at the cortex and the medulla.

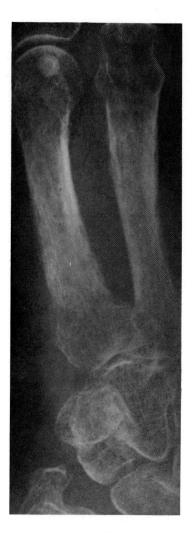

Figure 1.3

Bone resorption in Sudeck's atrophy appears as loss of definition of the metacarpal cortices with endosteal scalloping and accentuation of the cortical Haversian systems. The subperiosteal bone resorption resembles that seen in hyperparathyroidism. The carpal bones show loss of density centrally, with thin cortices sharply defined against the demineralized centra.

Cortical osteoporosis

There are three cortical sites of bone formation and loss—endosteum, periosteum and central cortex. Cortical changes are best visualized using a magnifying glass or macroradiography. Bone resorption within the cortex is seen as an increase in the number of cortical lucent striations (Figure 1.3), which are small cigar-shaped cortical lucencies aligned parallel to the long axis of the cortex. Normally none, or only one or two are seen within the midshaft of the metacarpal cortex. When easily visible, or if three or more are seen across the width of the cortex, excessive bone resorption is taking place (Table 1.1). These changes are not usually seen in conditions of decreased bone formation but occur especially in hyperparathyroidism, thyrotoxicosis, Sudeck's atrophy and following immobilization.

Resorption of cortical bone from its medullary border results in a thin pencil line of cortex around the affected bones (Figure 1.3). The width of the very sharply defined cortex may be less than 1 mm, and indicates that mineralization of the remaining bone is proceeding normally so that cortical margins remain distinct (Table 1.2). Areas of endosteal scalloping may be widespread. Local scalloping may be the result of a focal or aggressive process, such as a local tumour.

In the spine the cortices become progressively thinner but remain crisp (Figure 1.4). Eventually the thinned upper and lower end-plates become hairline in thickness. Vertebral margins should be assessed as well as the cortices around pedicles on the anteroposterior view, as these also become thinner and crisper with progressive osteoporosis. There are two major groups of medullary trabeculae: vertical, along the lines of stress, and horizontal, parallel to the end-plates. These are normally obscured by minor trabeculae and overlying soft tissues. The latter tend to obscure bone detail, especially if the patient is obese, or if the film is taken during expiration or prolonged breathing (which otherwise blurs out soft tissues). The film then looks grey. Trabecular detail is also lost if the kV used for the exposure is too high.

As osteoporosis increases, the randomly arranged trabeculae are lost, followed by the horizontal trabeculae, leaving only the vertical trabeculae along the lines of stress. Eventually these too may be lost so that the end stage has

Table 1.1   Causes of generalized osteoporosis in the adult.

Condition	Cause
Osteoporosis of the elderly Postmenopausal osteoporosis	?Oestrogen deficiency
Cushing's syndrome Steroid administration	Reduced osteoblastic activity
Heparin administration	Possible inhibition of bone formation
Thyrotoxicosis	Increased osteoclastic activity greater than increased osteoblastic activity
Hypogonadism Acromegaly	Related to hypopituitarism
Diabetes	Insulin dependent ? Related to protein breakdown
Liver disease and alcoholism	? Related to increased steroid levels
Weightlessness - space travel	Disuse
Osteogenesis imperfecta	Abnormal bone matrix
Hyperparathyroidism	Increased osteoclastic activity
Dietary deficiency	Vitamin C, calcium

Table 1.2   Regional osteoporosis.

Immobilization

Reflex sympathetic dystrophy syndrome

Transient osteoporosis of the hip

Regional migratory osteoporosis

Inflammatory joint disease

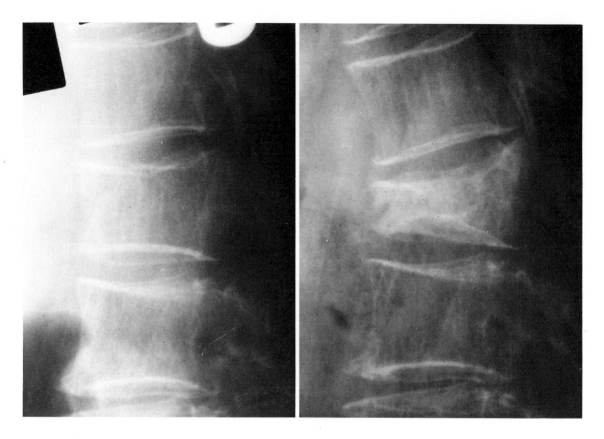

Figure 1.4

In this osteoporotic patient the initial film (*left*) was taken immediately after a fall which resulted in back pain. The cortices are thinned but sharply defined against the vertebral centra which contain only sparse, vertical weight-bearing trabeculae. There is an anterior fracture of a lumbar vertebral body. Six weeks later there is further collapse with sclerosis of the affected vertebral body (*right*). There is no expansion, and the weight-bearing trabeculae stand out in the adjacent intact vertebral bodies.

only thin, sharp vertebral margins and sharply pencilled pedicles in contrast to a grey, homogeneous and featureless vertebral centrum (Figure 1.4).

The pathological definition of osteoporosis has been expanded to include the clinical feature of fractures.

Changes in vertebral body shape

The normal vertebral body has essentially parallel end-plates, although there may be slight end-plate concavity with 1–2 mm of central depression. In the thoracic spine, the anterior height of the vertebral body may be 1–2 mm less than the posterior (Figure 1.5). This does not imply collapse and may be seen in contiguous vertebral bodies.

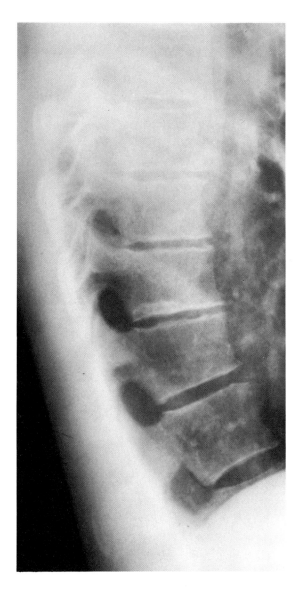

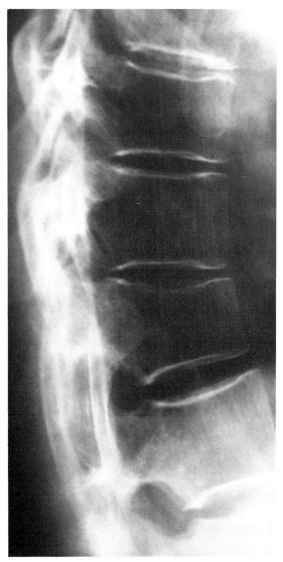

Figure 1.5

Wedging of thoracic vertebral
bodies may be a normal feature.

Figure 1.6

Osteoporotic wedging of a lower
thoracic vertebral body where
the deformity affects the upper
end-plate.

Osteoporosis may result in vertebral compression which can be acutely painful or pass
unnoticed by the patient. Wedging usually affects
the upper end-plate more than the lower, so that
the difference in height between anterior and
posterior surfaces of the vertebral bodies is over
2 mm (Figure 1.6). Flattening may occur, and the
flat-ended vertebral body usually does not
expand significantly either laterally or sagitally
(Figure 1.4). Expansion in collapse is a feature of
Paget's disease (Figure 1.7) and occasionally of
primary and secondary bone tumours. In most
cases, a collapsed, osteoporotic vertebral body is
said to implode, but callus formation is not
usually seen in collapsed osteoporotic vertebrae.
Collapse in osteoporosis is not generalized
throughout the spine and it is unusual to find
many vertebral bodies in contiguity affected by
collapse.

'Codfish' vertebrae resemble the fish vertebrae
in shape, with deep, smooth, biconcave end-plate
depressions. This feature is seen in any condition
associated with bone softening, including
osteomalacia (Table 1.3). In osteoporosis, the
end-plate depressions may be more marked on
the upper surfaces and affected bodies are not
always contiguous. In osteomalacia, the change
is seen more diffusely throughout the spine.

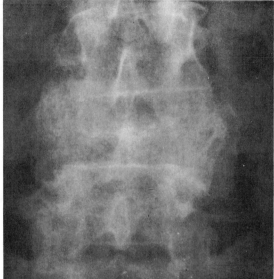
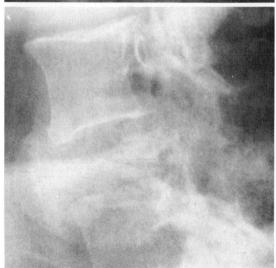

Table 1.3   Conditions associated with codfish vertebrae.

Normal in young adults

Osteomalacia and osteoporosis

Idiopathic juvenile osteoporosis

Osteogenesis imperfecta

Sickle-cell disease

Thalassaemia

Figure 1.7

In this example of compression
in Paget's disease, the vertebral
body of L4 shows abnormal
texture with loss of cortico–
medullary differentiation. There
is marked flattening of the
expanded body, which lies
beyond the adjacent vertebral
bodies.

In young athletic patients, a codfish type vertebral body may be seen, where the upper and lower end-plates are significantly depressed. This change occurs at the site of the discal nucleus, as can be seen at discography and usually occurs in the lumbar spine (Figure 1.8).

End-plate irregularities (Schmorl's nodes) occur in osteoporosis due to local discal herniations into weakened end-plates, and end-plate microfractures (Figure 1.9).

Osteoporotic patients generally seem to form less new bone as part of a degenerative osteoarthrosis and are probably more susceptible to fractures of the spine, for example, than those who are more normally mineralized.

Two main groups of trabeculae may be identified in the femoral neck: (1) A vertical compressive group ascending from the calcar to the femoral head; and (2) an arcuate tensile group extending from below the greater trochanter to the inferomedial portion of the femoral head (Figure 1.10). As with the spine, these trabeculae initially become more prominent with increasing osteoporosis, due to resorption of the normal, randomly arranged trabeculae. Further resorption progressively absorbs the tensile, and then compressive, group.

In the skull, generalized osteoporosis results in prominence of the sutures and surrounding bone which appears relatively sclerotic. The squamous temporal bone is naturally thin and shows early osteoporosis (Figure 1.11).

Generalized osteoporosis

This is most commonly seen in the elderly and in the postmenopausal female (Table 1.1). Maximal bone mass is reached between 20 and 40 years of age in both sexes, after which women lose bone more rapidly than men until 80 years of age, when the loss becomes equal.

The changes which occur have been described in the previous section. Cortical thinning and medullary trabecular loss affect the long bones, skull, metacarpals and phalanges, and particularly the vertebral bodies. Fractures of vertebral bodies produce wedging with loss of height, particularly at the superior end-plates, and end-plate irregularities with Schmorl's nodes. Compression fractures are randomly distributed in the lower thoracic and lumbar spine. They are

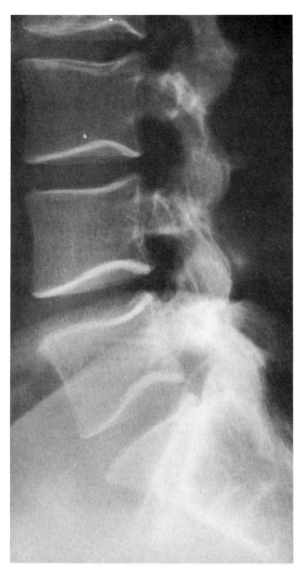

Figure 1.8

End-plate depressions are normal in the adult lumbar spine and correspond to the site of the turgid discal nucleus.

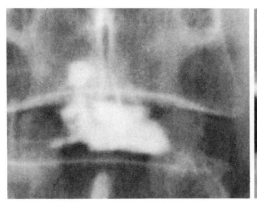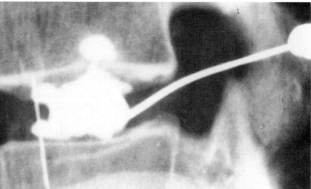

Figure 1.9

Schmörl's node. A defect in the cortical margin at the lower end-plate of a lumbar vertebral body is demonstrated to fill with contrast at lumbar discography, indicating a local discal herniation resulting in a Schmörl's node.

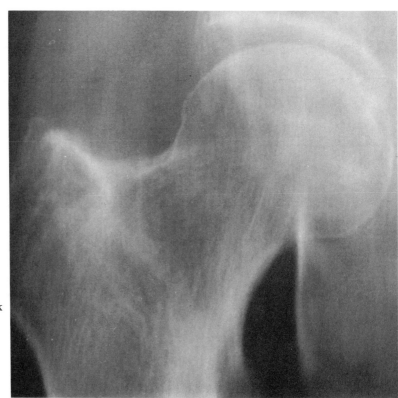

Figure 1.10

The two main groups of trabeculae in the femoral neck are demonstrated. There is a superior arcuate group and a more medial and vertically directed group of trabeculae extending upwards from the calcar.

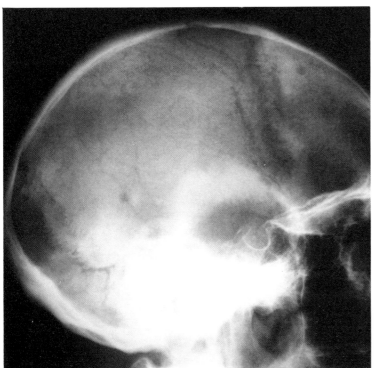

a

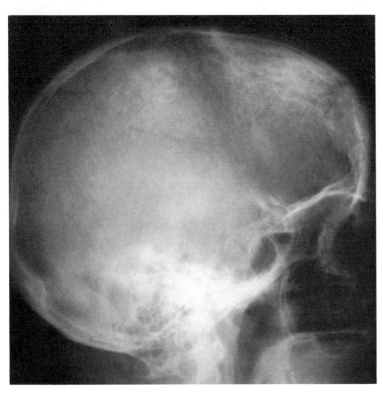

b

Figure 1.11

(**a**) Osteoporosis in the skull results in marked demineralization of the squamous temporal bone and accentuation of the adjacent suture. (**b**) Another osteoporotic patient in whom the changes are more diffuse. Even hyperostosis frontalis interna is poorly visualized.

not necessarily contiguous and do not heal with callus, which makes them difficult to date. Mild trauma may cause vertebral compression, which produces back pain, but neurological complications are unusual. Height loss may occur with an increased lumbar lordosis and high thoracic smooth kyphosis. Femoral neck, transcervical and Colles' fractures are also more common in patients with osteoporosis. Upper femoral fractures may be spontaneous through osteoporotic bone, or may follow only minor trauma. Patients with trochanteric fractures may be more porotic than those with transcervical fractures. Such patients often have little evidence of osteophytosis as part of a degenerative process around the affected hip, even if considerable hip joint space narrowing may be present.

Fractures through the distal radius and ulna, especially Colles' fractures, increase with age. These are related to local loss of bone mass. The older and more osteoporotic the patient, the greater the degree of comminution of fracture parts.

Cushing's syndrome

This may be due to adrenocortical disease or steroid therapy. Changes may be severe, particularly in the axial skeleton, where vertebral compression leads to end-plate sclerosis with local callus formation, a specific feature of this form of osteoporosis (Figure 1.12). The changes associated with high-dose steroid therapy also include avascular necrosis, particularly of the femoral head but also of the humeral head (Figure 1.13). Rib 'cough' fractures are also seen, particularly in patients receiving steroids for lung disease. A dose of 10–15 mg/day for three years is thought to be required to cause these changes.

Hyperthyroidism

This is a very infrequent cause of radiologically visible osteoporosis; however, the diagnosis will be clear as the clinical disease will be severe.

Heparin osteoporosis

Patients receiving treatment for ischaemic coronary and cerebrovascular disease for up to

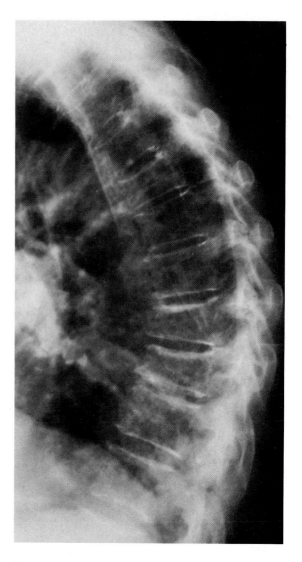

Figure 1.12

In this patient with Cushing's syndrome, osteopenia with a smooth kyphos is associated with wedging of thoracic vertebral bodies. In the mid-thoracic spine, wedging is associated with thickening of the upper end-plates due to hyperplastic callus. This is a feature unique to Cushing's syndrome, as vertebral collapse is not accompanied by callus formation in other conditions.

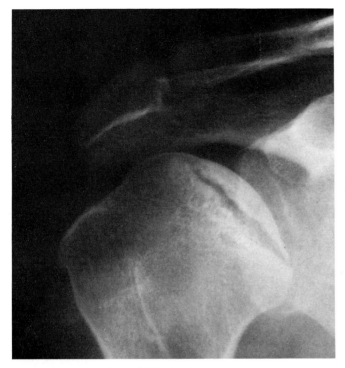

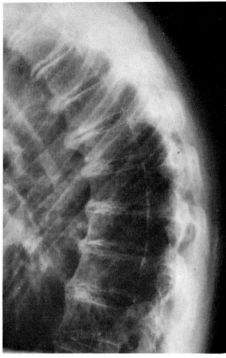

Figure 1.13

Cushing's syndrome. The humeral head is sclerotic, fissured and deformed, indicating avascular necrosis in a patient receiving steroids.

Figure 1.14

In acromegaly the bones are demineralized, indicated by the pencilling of the end-plate cortices, and a smooth thoracic kyphos is associated with new bone anteriorly on the vertebral bodies.

15 years, who have received over 15 000 units heparin daily, have been described with osteoporosis, rib and vertebral fractures; however, this is a rare condition. Female patients with a history of thromboembolism in pregnancy may also be on long-term heparin and develop osteoporosis.

Acromegaly

This is often associated with osteoporosis as a manifestation of concurrent hypopituitarism, but the bone and soft tissue changes of acromegaly predominate. Vertebral bodies are elongated in the sagittal plane as part of the general overgrowth of bone, and are osteoporotic (Figure 1.14).

Alcoholism

Alcoholism associated with osteoporosis is not always related to hepatic cirrhosis or malnutrition. Alcohol has been shown to elevate the

Figure 1.15

(a) (a) In osteogenesis imperfecta, there is generalized demineralization of bone, with bowing of the tibia and fibula. The fibula, in particular, is gracile. Transverse, pathological fractures are seen in both bones.

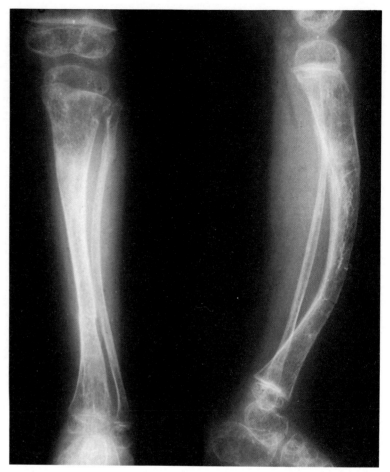

a

plasma cortisol levels so that the osteoporosis may be steroid-related.

Osteogenesis imperfecta

This generalized disorder of connective tissue is seen in two main forms—a severe form inherited recessively, which presents in utero or early in life, and a late, milder form inherited as a dominant condition (see also Chapter 6, page 328). The later form may not present until adult life.

Initially, the bones are often normal in shape but fracture repeatedly after minor, inappropriate trauma. Osteoporosis may not be marked in adults but the combination of osteoporosis with bone deformity is strongly suggestive of the disease. The fibula may be bowed (Figure 1.15a). This unusual combination also occurs in Still's disease (juvenile chronic arthritis) (Figure 1.15b), while in Paget's disease fibular bowing is associated with osteosclerosis (Figure 1.15c).

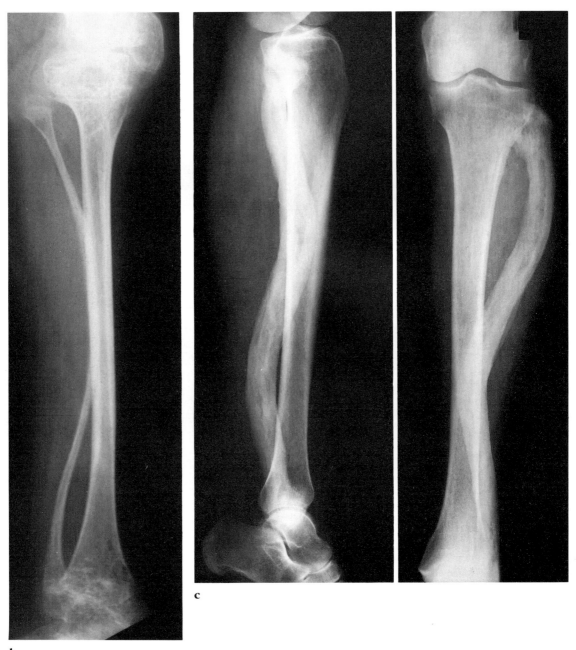

b

c

Figure 1.15 *continued*

(**b**) Juvenile chronic arthritis also results in fibular bowing. (**c**) Paget's disease of the fibula is seen with widening of the bone. The typical bony texture of Paget's disease extends to both articular surfaces with loss of cortico–medullary differentiation. Non-involvement of the tibia results in fibular overgrowth and bowing.

Figure 1.16

Upward concavity of the ribs in
osteogenesis imperfecta may be
the result of posterior fractures,
or muscle pull on softened
bones.

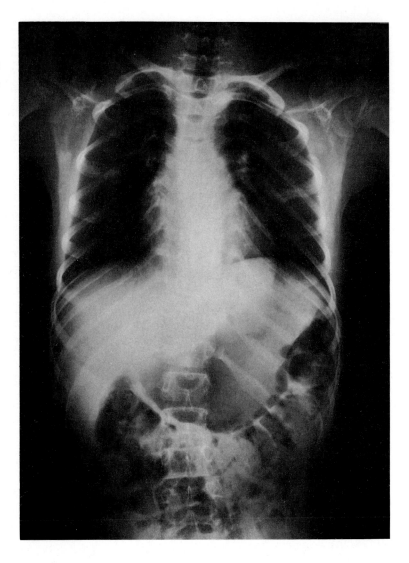

Ribs may be softened, resulting in upward
concavity (Figure 1.16). Protrusio acetabuli may
be seen (Figure 1.17a), as in rheumatoid arthritis
associated with osteoporosis (Figure 1.17b).
Osteoarthritis associated with protrusio will
often result in normal or increased bone density
(Figure 1.17c), similar to the idiopathic or
familial forms of protrusio (Figure 1.17d) (Table
1.4).

Fractures of the paired long bones (radius and
ulna, tibia and fibula) in osteogenesis imperfecta
may result in a pseudarthrosis which is also

**Table 1.4   Causes of protrusio
acetabuli.**

Osteogenesis imperfecta Rheumatoid arthritis	Associated with osteoporosis
Osteoarthritis Idiopathic	Associated with normal bone density
X-linked hypophosphataemic osteomalacia	Associated with increased bone density

found in neurofibromatosis and idiopathic juvenile osteoporosis (Figure 1.18). Fractures in osteogenesis imperfecta tend to heal with hypertrophic callus formation (Figure 1.19), occasionally resulting in cross fusion (Figure 1.20a). The phenomenon of cross fusion also occurs after Caffey's infantile cortical hyperostosis (Figure 1.20b), osteomyelitis (Figure 1.20c), trauma (Figure 1.20d) and, partly, in congenital fusions at the proximal radio-ulnar joint.

The main features of the severe recessive form of the disease, presenting in utero or childhood, are multiple fractures associated with osteoporosis (Figure 1.21). Fractures may be seen with broad, shortened limb bones, often with a cyst-like change in the shafts, or with thin, slender, bowed bones. Many of the fractures are classically diaphyseal, unlike those in idiopathic juvenile osteoporosis (Figure 1.22) which are metaphyseal and not associated with gross callus formation.

Osteogenesis imperfecta may occur at any age, while idiopathic juvenile osteoporosis only occurs around puberty. The skull changes of osteogenesis imperfecta—osteoporosis and thinned calvarial bones and Wormian bones—are not seen in idiopathic juvenile osteoporosis (Figure 1.23) (Table 1.5).

Table 1.5 Differential signs between osteogenesis imperfecta and idiopathic juvenile osteoporosis

Signs	Osteogenesis imperfecta	Idiopathic juvenile osteoporosis
Age	Infants, adults	Around puberty
Shaft fractures	Diaphyseal	Metaphyseal
Vertebral changes	Collapse	Collapse
Skull changes	Wormian bones Osteoporosis Dentinogenesis imperfecta	—
Modelling abnormalities	Can be gross	Minimal

Battered baby syndrome

Fractures are almost inevitably part of this syndrome; however, these children are seldom generally osteoporotic. Deformity is localized to fracture sites and the fractures, of different generations, are diaphyseal and metaphyseal (Figure 1.24). Fractures are the only visible skull changes (Figure 1.25).

Scurvy

This rare disease is currently seen mainly in infants or in elderly, often mentally defective patients. It is caused by a vitamin C deficiency which results in defective collagen synthesis. Patients may present with bleeding due to capillary fragility and, in the elderly, scurvy may also contribute to the overall development of osteoporosis. Bleeding beneath the periosteum results in the formation of a lamellar periostitis which incorporates into the shaft after treatment (Figure 1.26).

In infants with scurvy, osteoporosis produces marked cortical thinning, especially at ring epiphyses, such as those at the knee, where sharp, thin, cortical outlines surround featureless centra (Wimburger's sign). However, rachitic epiphyses and metaphyses are poorly defined and without sharply demarcated cortical margins. The well-defined, thin band of provisional calcification in scurvy also contrasts with the subjacent metaphyseal bone which shows a local accentuated band of osteoporosis crossing the entire metaphysis (see also Chapter 5, page 267). This zone of osteoporosis may fracture, giving marginal metaphyseal spurring known as Pelkan's spur. A lack of focal destructive osteoporotic lesions elsewhere distinguishes the metaphyseal bands of lucency in scurvy from those seen in leukaemia and neuroblastoma (see page 267).

Immobilization

This also causes osteoporosis and metaphyseal lucency not usually generalized to all four limbs (see page 266). Osteoporosis after immobilization is most commonly seen following fractures, but may also result from enforced bed rest or paralysis, and has also been described following

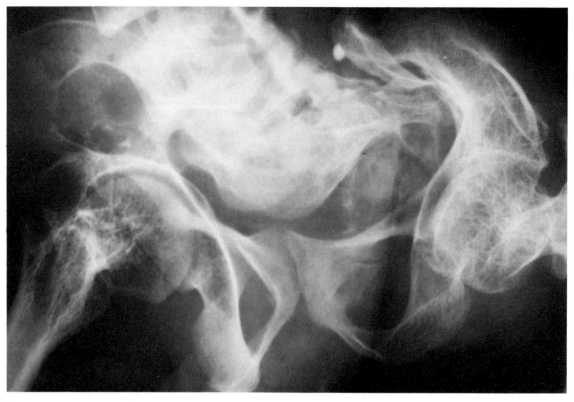

a

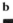
b

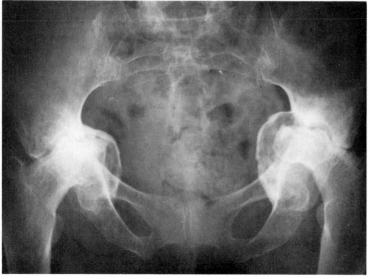

Figure 1.17

(**a**) In this case of osteogenesis imperfecta, demineralization of bone has produced a gross scoliosis and protrusio of both hips. The bones around the obturator foramina are also thin, gracile and distorted. (**b**) With protrusio in rheumatoid arthritis, the medial walls of the acetabula are grossly displaced internally and vary in thickness. The joint spaces are narrowed superiorly but widened medially, and the articular surfaces of the femoral heads are irregular and sclerotic. This patient had severe

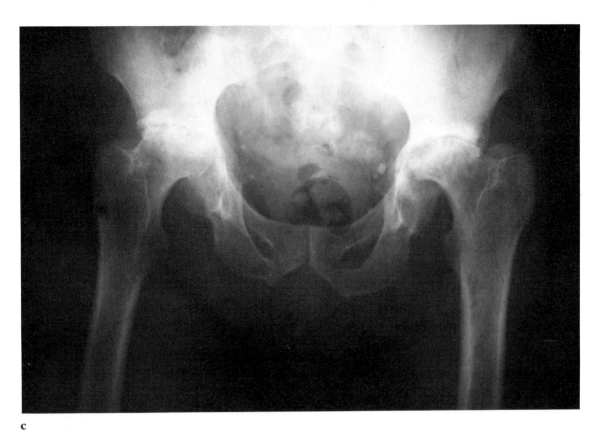

c

d

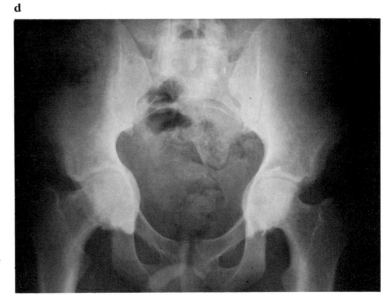

rheumatoid deformities of the hands. (**c**) The appearances in this case of protrusio in osteoarthritis differ very little from the previous case. This patient does not have rheumatoid arthritis, and the degree of protrusio is less. Both femoral heads have lost bone in the weight-bearing regions, and the joint spaces are narrowed superiorly as well as medially. The acetabular roofs also show deepening and reactive sclerosis. (**d**) This young patient with congenital protrusio has no underlying arthritis. Bone density is normal.

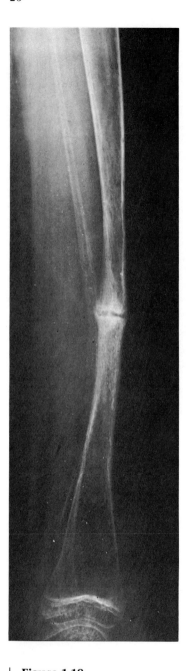

Figure 1.18

In this case of osteogenesis
imperfecta, bones are decreased
in density. The fibula is thin and
bowed, and a transverse fracture
across the midshaft of the tibia is
associated with sclerosis at a
pseudarthrosis.

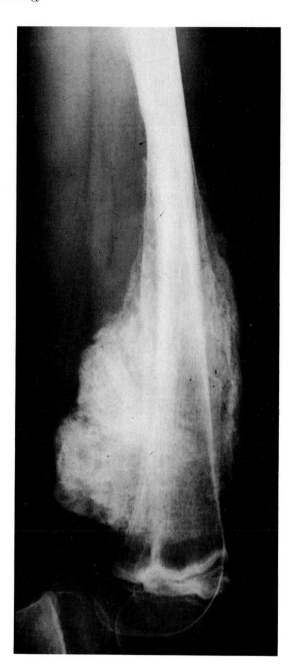

Figure 1.19

A previous fracture is present at
the midshaft of the femur, while
distally a more recent fracture is
healing with hypertrophic callus
in this patient with osteogenesis
imperfecta.

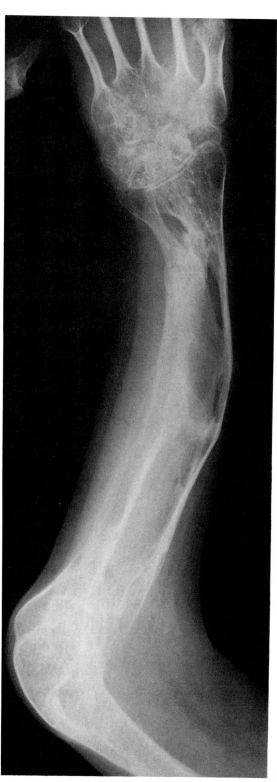

a

Figure 1.20

(**a**) In this case of osteogenesis imperfecta, there is osteoporosis, the radius and ulna are thin and bowed, and they are connected by new bone across the interosseous membrane which is presumably the result of union of callus following fractures. Abnormal modelling of the carpal and metacarpal bones is also shown.

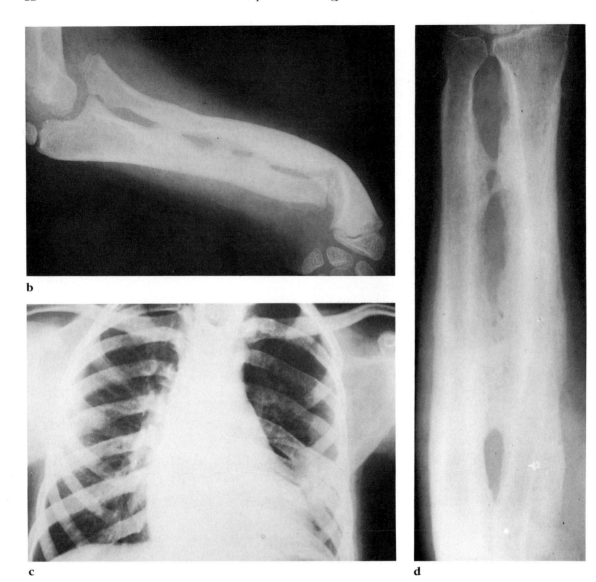

b

c   d

Figure 1.20 *continued*

(**b,c**) Caffey's infantile cortical hyperostosis has been severe in this patient. Cross-fusion and growth anomalies are present in the radius and ulna, and left ribs. (**d**) Cross-union in osteomyelitis. Following infection, the cloaking layers of periosteal new bone have united across the interosseous membrane.

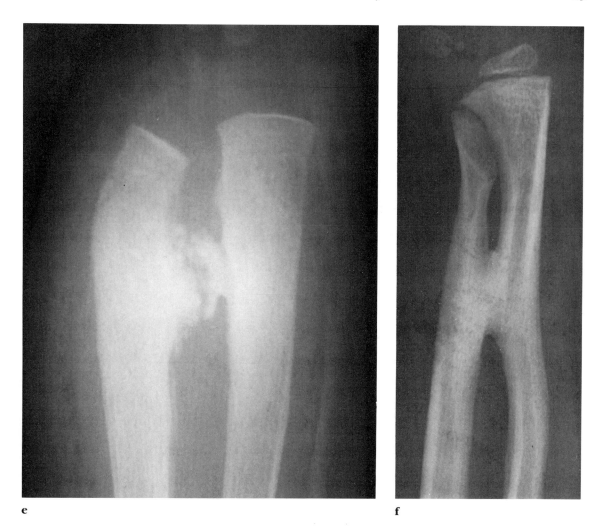

e

f

Figure 1.20 *continued*

(**e**,**f**) Cross-fusion following trauma between the radius and ulna after non-accidental injury.

Figure 1.21

The severe recessive form of
osteogenesis imperfecta often
presents at birth with multiple
fractures. This child was stillborn.
Fractures in utero have resulted
in shortening and broadening of
all the long bones, as well as
gross platyspondyly and rib
fractures.

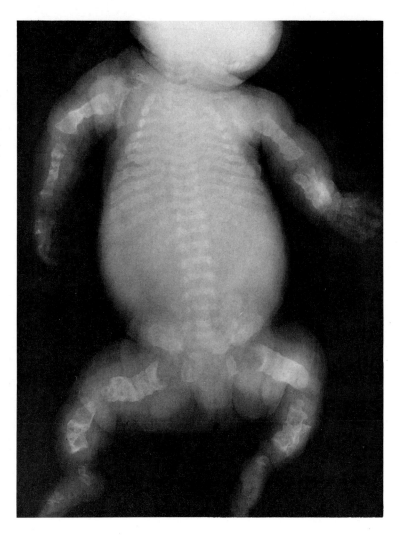

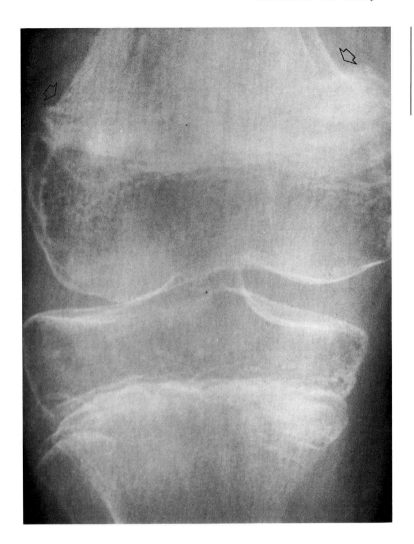

Figure 1.22

This case of idiopathic juvenile osteoporosis shows classical metaphyseal fractures (arrows); the bones are generally demineralized.

Figure 1.23

Skull changes in osteogenesis imperfecta usually involve Wormian bone formation and bony softening at the base resulting in a 'tam-o-shanter' deformity.

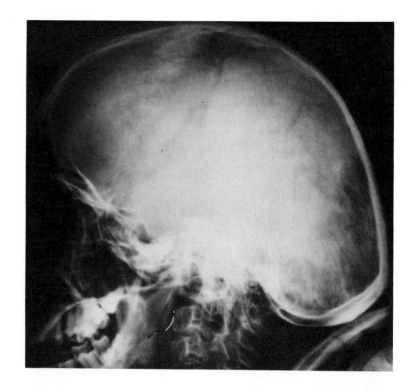

Figure 1.24

This radiograph of a battered baby shows multiple rib fractures with hyperplastic callus. The fractures are aligned, presumably as a result of one local blow.

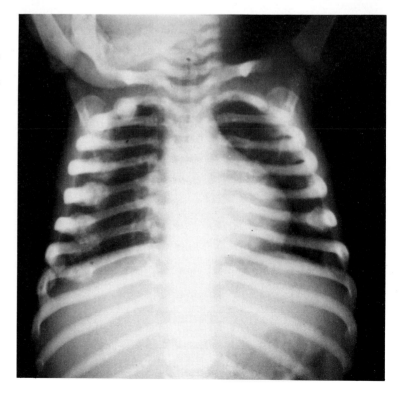

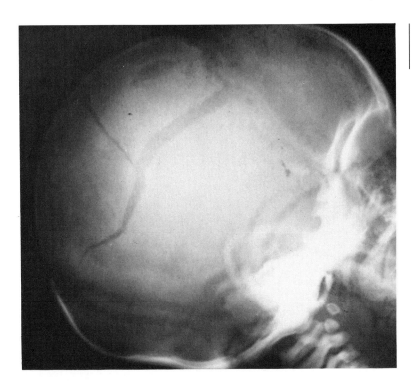

Figure 1.25

This battered baby has fractures of the skull.

weightlessness in space travel. Skeletal immobilization is followed by early loss of bone and hypercalcuria.

Bone loss after a fracture is most marked distal to the fracture, even if the joints above and below are immobilized. The young and old exhibit this change earlier than middle-aged patients. Histologically, there is intense osteoclastic and decreased osteoblastic activity. If the fracture is through bone affected by Paget's disease or hyperparathyroidism, the distal osteoporosis is even more marked (Figure 1.27).

Acute or subacute osteoporosis following a fracture is usually only seen in the limbs, and may be uniform with cortical thinning and medullary trabecular loss. In younger patients other forms may be seen. Cortical striations may become more prominent so that three or four cigar-shaped lucencies may be seen across the cortex (Figure 1.28). Subcortical bone is resorbed in the articular regions, producing pronounced osteoporosis beneath pencilled cortices. Immobilization in children causes bands of lucency extending across the entire metaphysis, and endosteal scalloping may occur (see Chapter 5, page 266). The carpal and tarsal bones are especially affected. Bone loss is not always uniform but may also be patchy or spotty in both the cortex and medulla, the latter change being superimposed upon the overall loss of bone density. This change can be alarming and so pronounced that the fracture line may not be

Figure 1.26

Scurvy. (**a**) There is overall loss
of bone density with sharply
demarcated cortices. This is
especially prominent at the
epiphyses. Metaphyseal
fractures giving marginal
metaphyseal spurring are
shown. The loss of bone
density is uniform. (**b**) Two
weeks later, the same patient has
formed new bone beneath the
elevated periosteum.
Metaphyseal fractures are still
prominent.

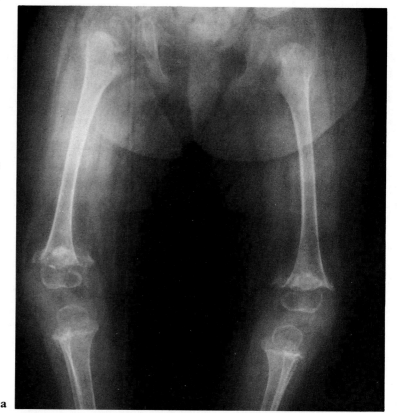

a

b

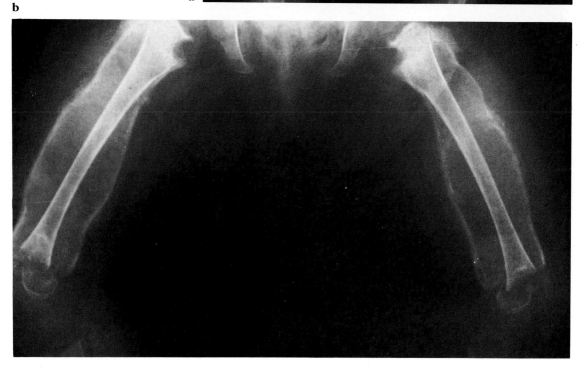

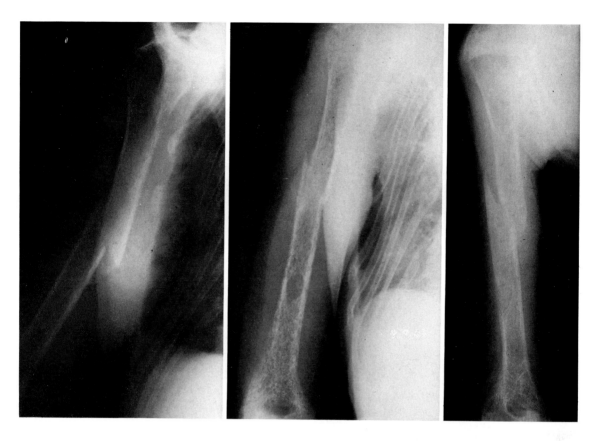

Figure 1.27

Fracture in hyperparathyroidism. The initial bone density was reduced at the time of the fracture (*left*). After a short interval and immobilization, intense spotty osteoporosis is seen affecting both the cortex and medulla, and brown tumours are rendered more prominent (*centre*). The last film shows some recovery of bone density on mobilization, but also shows the resultant soft tissue wasting (*right*).

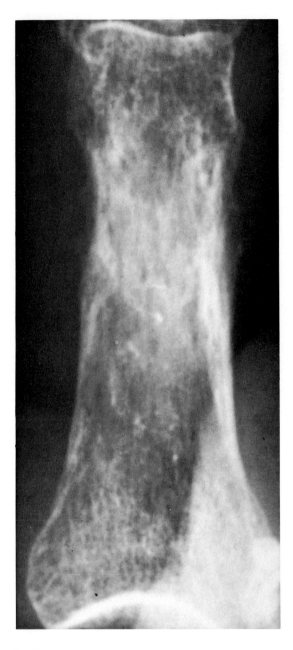

Figure 1.28

In this osteoporotic patient
cortical striations are prominent
and cortico–medullary
differentiation is lost.
Osteoporosis is accentuated in
the subarticular regions.

clearly visible. With resumption of function and
weight-bearing, remineralization occurs but
often not to the levels seen in the contralateral
normal limb (Figure 1.29).

Polio and other forms of muscular paralysis

When presenting in childhood, these are associated with diffuse chronic osteoporosis and hypoplasia of bone. In addition to cortical thinning
and a loss of medullary trabeculation, there is a
loss of bone length and width. Foramina, such as
those in the pelvis, are smaller on the affected
side. Muscle bulk is diminished and subcutaneous and perimuscular fat increased (Figure
1.30) (see Chapter 7, page 349).

Reflex sympathetic dystrophy syndrome (RSDS)

This is also known as Sudeck's atrophy or
osteodystrophy. Changes are usually seen in the
extremities following trauma; however, they may
follow compartmental soft tissue infection or
limb surgery. Radioisotope bone scans of the
affected limb demonstrate increase in both
perfusion and bone uptake around all the joints
of the affected limb (Figure 1.31), as well as in
the contralateral limb in many cases. The diagnosis is based on the history of the injury, the
examination of the limb, which may be swollen,
painful and tender, and the radiological findings.
Osteoporosis is widespread and extreme. The
cortices are extremely thin, scalloped, and show
excessive Haversian trabeculation, especially in
the ring-like bones of the carpus and tarsus. The
cortex may even be defective in places and
subcortical and metaphyseal bone is hypertran-
sradiant. Medullary bone appears to be patchily
resorbed, since it is absent in certain areas and
relatively dense elsewhere. Joint spaces are
preserved unless another pathology is present,
and this preservation can exclude local infective
processes. Thus, the radiology is that of a severe
form of immobilization, with soft tissue swelling
and pain, but no joint narrowing (Figure 1.32).

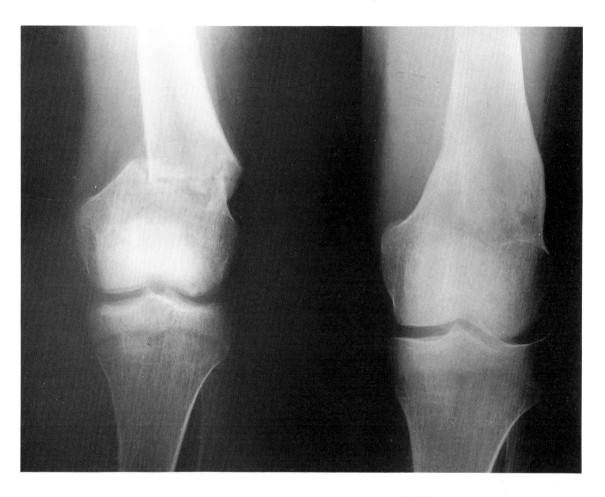

Figure 1.29

The initial radiograph, taken shortly after a distal femoral fracture, shows quite marked subarticular and metaphyseal radiolucency. A radiograph taken five years later shows good fracture healing and some restoration of bony density. The submetaphyseal lucency can still be seen in the proximal tibia. Growth arrest lines are also demonstrated.

Figure 1.30

Progressive osteoporosis and
bony hypoplasia result from the
muscle atrophy of polio.

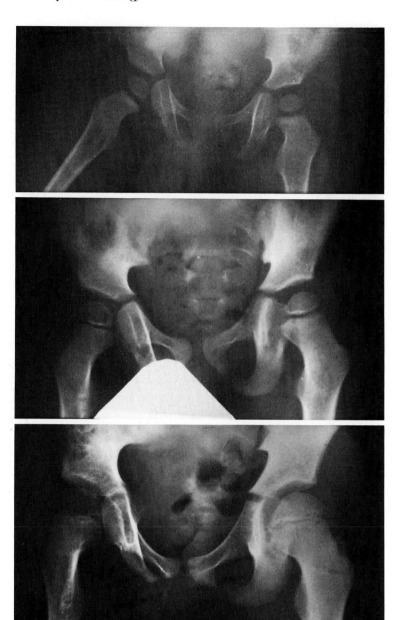

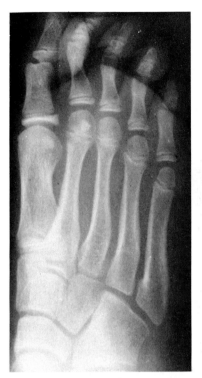
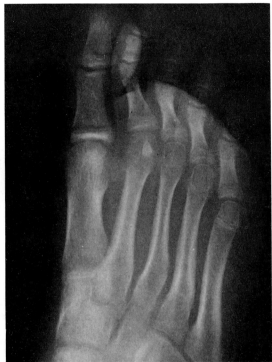

a

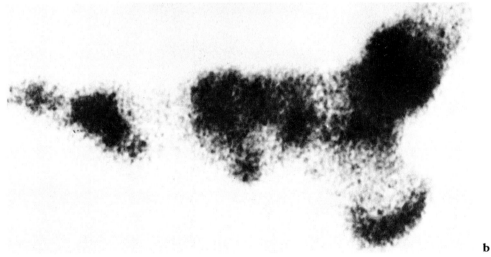

b

Figure 1.31

Reflex sympathetic dystrophy syndrome. (**a**) The initial radiograph shows normal appearances at the time of a proximal injury (*left*). The subsequent radiograph shows marked demineralization, accentuated in the metaphyses of the phalanges (*right*). Bone density in the tarsus is also markedly reduced. (**b**) The radioisotope bone scan shows a marked increase in uptake throughout the foot, but especially in the periarticular regions.

Figure 1.32

This patient with reflex sympathetic dystrophy syndrome had sustained a fracture of the left leg which was put in plaster and immobilized. The right lower limb retains a normal density throughout, but the gross osteoporosis of the left limb with associated soft tissue swelling is part of this syndrome, which was so painful that the patient had to have her foot amputated.

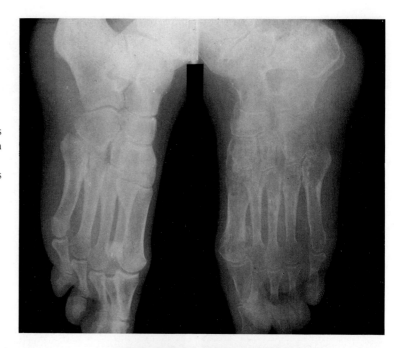

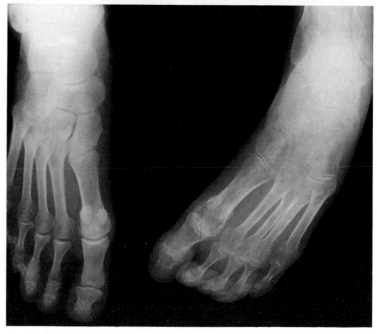

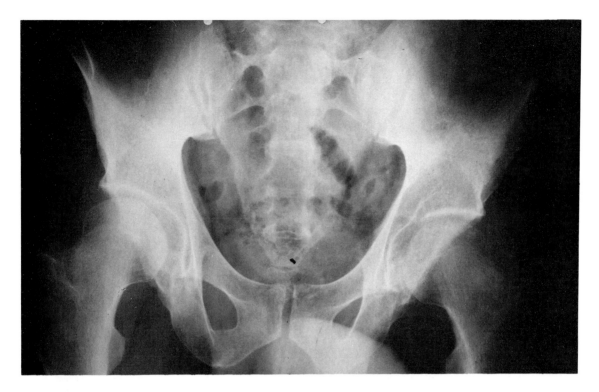

Figure 1.33

In this male patient with transient osteoporosis, the left hip shows quite marked loss of bony density. The cortex of the femoral head is poorly defined, and the joint space is minimally narrowed.

Transient osteoporosis

This painful condition affects the hip in both sexes, but usually only the left hip in females, often during pregnancy. Bone loss is progressive in the femoral head and acetabulum with cortical thinning and medullary bone loss, as in infection, but the joint space remains intact. The condition is self-limiting (Figure 1.33). Another form of this disease is migratory, so that different joints are transiently and serially affected.

Rickets and osteomalacia

This condition is characterized by an increase in the proportion of non-mineralized osteoid in bone. Rickets in children primarily affects the chondro-osseous complex at the epiphysis which is the area of linear growth. After epiphyseal fusion, osteomalacia affects lamellar bone, resulting in different radiological appearances of two diseases with the same aetiology.

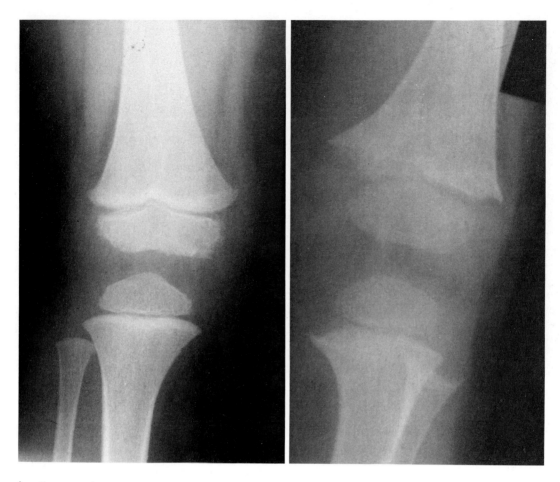

Figure 1.34

Comparison between rachitic
and normal bone. The abnormal
joint shows metaphyseal
irregularity and splaying, with an
increased width of the epiphyseal
plate. Bone density generally is
reduced.

Worldwide, the commonest cause of rickets
and osteomalacia is vitamin D deficiency. In the
UK this is still seen frequently in vegetarian
immigrants from Africa and Asia who, in addition,
do not receive as much sunlight as in their native
lands. Sunlight is needed for the conversion of
cholesterol to 1-hydroxycholecalciferol, which is
an inactive precursor of vitamin D. If a patient of
Indian origin who is a vegetarian presents with
local or general bone pain, osteomalacia must be
excluded (as incidentally must tuberculous disease, especially in the spine). Among Western
populations, the commonest causes of rickets
and osteomalacia are congenital or acquired
abnormalities of mineral metabolism which are
usually resistant to the normal therapeutic doses

of vitamin D. These diseases are uncommon in comparison with osteoporosis.

The clinical profile of osteomalacia is one of bone pain and tenderness, with muscular weakness. Back and limb pain may result from fractures and there may be joint pain and deformities. In children, there is bulging of the limbs and ribs at chondro-osseous junctions (rickety rosary).

Radiology of rickets

Characteristic radiological changes are seen initially and are most prominent at areas of maximum growth and stress. At the wrist, around the knee, and at the anterior ends of the ribs, the epiphysis loses its sharp outline and becomes fuzzy, as does the adjacent metaphyseal sclerotic line representing the provisional zone of calcification (Figure 1.34). Eventually the metaphysis becomes irregular, radiolucent and broad. This broadening is appreciable clinically and is probably a stress reaction at softened bone. The epiphyseal plate appears widened (over 3 mm) due to defective mineralization of the epiphysis and the adjacent metaphysis.

All the epiphyses may be affected and the apophyses also show these changes. Elsewhere, lack of mineralization of subchondral bone causes irregularity at the sacroiliac joints and symphysis pubis, so that these joints can become more difficult to visualize than usual in children.

There is an increase in osteoid on the trabeculae, which consequently are proportionally less mineralized. This leads to radiological blurring of cortical and medullary bone, resulting in a fuzzy or hazy appearance, sometimes with an apparent decrease in radiological density. However, occasionally trabecular coarsening suggests an increase in density.

Softening of the bone may result in bowing in the lower limbs, which may be associated with protrusio acetabuli, and is especially associated with X-linked hypophosphataemic rickets and osteomalacia (Figure 1.35).

In children, the metaphyseal region is normally the site of increased uptake on the radioisotope bone scan. This change is also seen at the anterior ends of the ribs and at the apophyses. In rickets, this uptake is further

increased at these characteristic sites. Pathological fractures may also be seen radiologically and on scintigraphy (Figure 1.36).

Radiology of osteomalacia

The characteristic, diagnostic radiological feature of osteomalacia is the Looser's zone, although this occurs only in a minority of biochemically-diagnosed cases. Looser's zones are short, transverse bands of radiolucency extending inwards from the cortex, particularly at sites of major stress, including the lateral margin of the scapula, ribs, proximal femora medially and around the obturator rings (Figure 1.37). At some sites they may be related to local vascular channels. They consist of osteoid seams and are surrounded by bands of sclerosis, representing healing. The more sclerosis present, the easier the Looser's zone is visualized. They are rarely present in childhood.

With progressive deformity from bone softening, true transverse fractures occur in osteomalacia (Figure 1.38).

In children the synchondrosis at the ischium remains open until around seven years of age. Looser's zones in osteomalacia arise at the same site but should not be confused with it after the age of ten years (Figure 1.37).

Looser's zones may also be diagnosed on the isotope bone scan which may be preferable to the radiographic skeletal survey. The distribution of foci of increased uptake ('hot spots') is symmetrical and at the expected sites for Looser's zones, but increase in uptake is seen particularly at the anterior rib ends. Malignant metastatic disease, however, has a totally random distribution in the axial skeleton (Figure 1.39). Changes in osteomalacia reflect:

1   bone softening with multiple levels of vertebral collapse, often contiguous and codfish in type, as well as limb deformity;

2   multiple areas of non-mineralized osteoid deposition in cortex and medulla, giving streaky lucency and demineralization;

3   poorly-defined trabeculae producing fuzziness due to excessive non-mineralized osteoid on the trabeculae;

4   changes of secondary hyperparathyroidism particularly in the hands (see below).

Figure 1.35

In this patient with X-linked
rickets, there is bowing with an
increase in bony density.

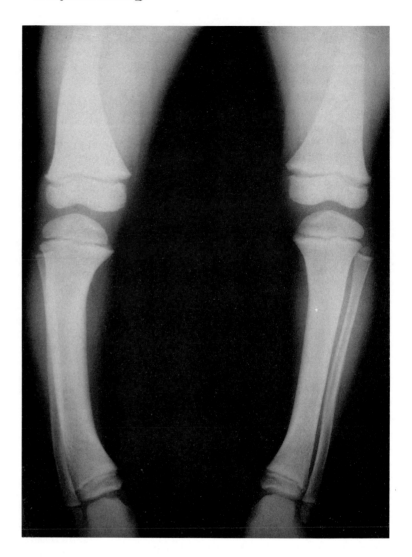

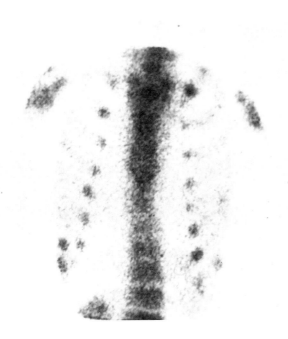

Figure 1.36

Radionuclide scan in osteomalacia. The foci of increased uptake are at costochondral junctions, which are abnormal in rickets (the rickety rosary). The distribution is not random, as in metastatic disease, and is too widespread to suggest trauma.

Figure 1.37

Characteristic sites for Looser's zones include the obturator ring and the shafts of long bones. The ulna in particular shows diminished bone density. The Looser's zones are healing.

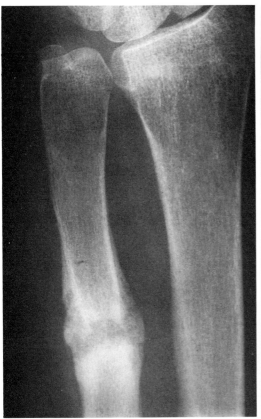

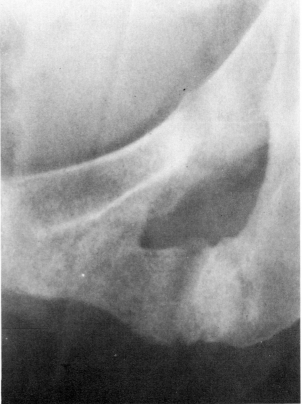

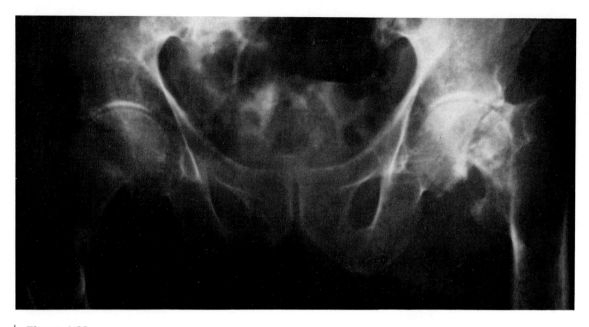

Figure 1.38

True transverse fractures are
seen in the left femoral neck and
in the pertrochanteric region on
the right, in this osteomalacic
patient.

Figure 1.39

Radioisotope bone scan showing
metastatic disease, with a random
distribution of the foci of
increased uptake.

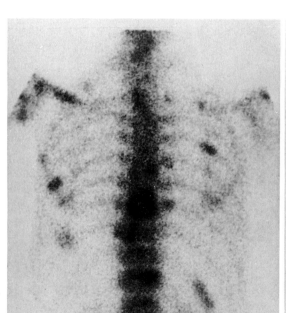

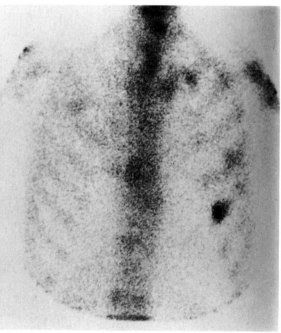

Differential signs in rickets and osteomalacia

Metaphyseal irregularity

Metaphyseal irregularity with demineralization has a number of causes (Table 1.6) (see also Chapter 5).

Table 1.6 Causes of metaphyseal irregularity.

Rickets

Hypophosphatasia

Enchondromatosis

Metaphyseal dysostosis (see also page 286)

Rickets

The changes are widespread in distribution and extend across the entire metaphysis. The epiphyseal plate is widened and the epiphysis poorly corticated.

Hypophosphatasia

This is a rare condition transmitted as an autosomal recessive disease of varying severity, with bone changes prominent in infants. The metaphyseal changes are similar to those of rickets, but are more severe, and associated with gross loss of mineralization. Generalized metaphyseal irregularity is marked and extends far inwards towards the diaphysis, giving a broad, scraggy and poorly mineralized metaphysis in severe cases (Figure 1.40). As well as demineralization, bowing and fractures are found, resulting

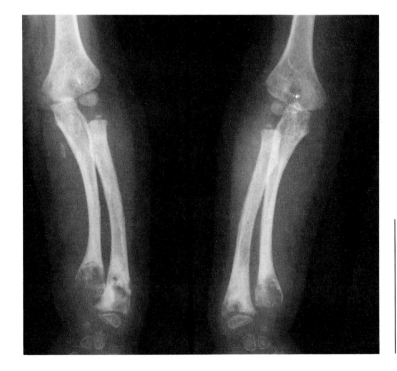

Figure 1.40

Demineralization is seen in this patient with hypophosphatasia. The ring epiphyses of the wrist are normal. However, there is marked deformity with irregularity of the metaphyses at the wrist (see also Chapter 5, page 291).

Figure 1.41

Hypophosphatasia. The sutures are not visualized and the skull vault is poorly mineralized.

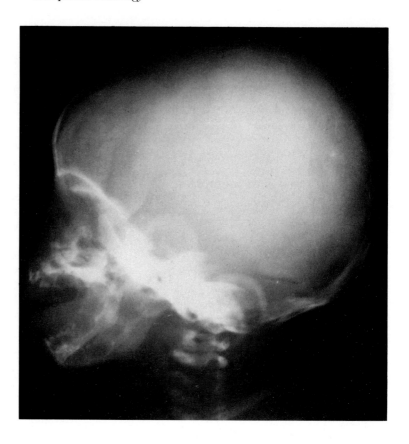

in shortening and periostitis. Loss of density in the skull is severe and the bones may scarcely be visible. Craniostenosis or Wormian bones may also be seen (Figure 1.41).

Osteogenesis imperfecta

Skull demineralization is accompanied by wide sutures and Wormian bones (Figure 1.23). Craniostenosis does not occur. Fractures are seen in osteogenesis imperfecta and hypophosphatasia but the zone of provisional calcification at the metaphysis is not irregular in osteogenesis imperfecta and the epiphysis is corticated.

Enchondromatosis (Ollier's disease)

This exists in various radiological forms. In one type, long streaky radiolucent islands of irregu-

larly calcified cartilage stream backwards from the zone of provisional calcification so that the metaphysis becomes irregular and broadened in appearance (Figure 1.42). Deformities often coexist, especially in the distal radius and ulna (hypoplastic broad ulna, curved broad radius). Similar changes also occur in diaphyseal aclasia (see Chapter 7, page 366). Overall, however, bone density is normal and the epiphysis well defined.

Metaphyseal dysostosis

The most common form of this rare disease is the Type Schmid. Metaphyseal changes are similar to, but less severe than, those seen in rickets. There is mild splaying and irregularity of the metaphyses in childhood (Figure 1.43). Bone density is normal or even increased, Looser's zones do not appear and the skull is normal.

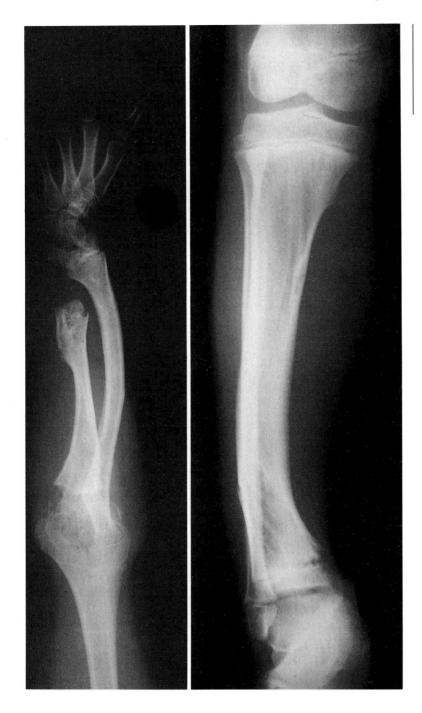

Figure 1.42

Ollier's disease. Irregular strands of lucency extend backwards into the shaft of the bone from the epiphyseal plate (see also Chapter 7)

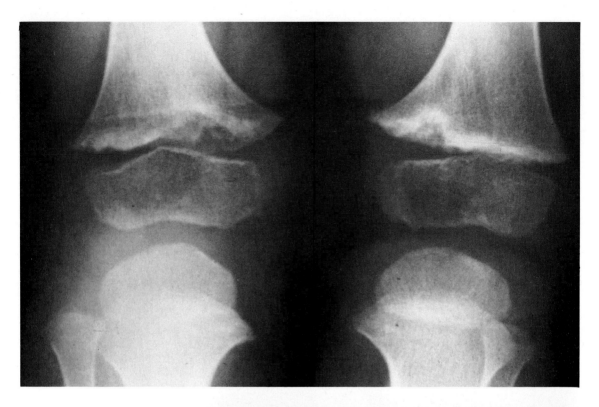

Figure 1.43

In metaphyseal dysostosis, Type Schmid, bone density is preserved. There is slight irregularity of the distal femoral metaphyses.

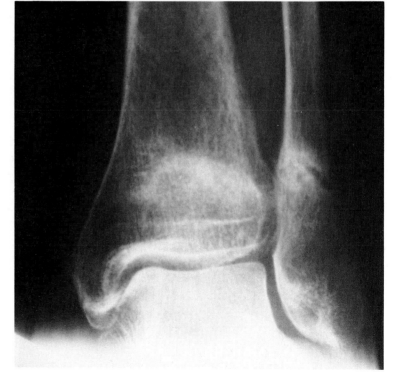

Figure 1.44

Stress fractures are present at the distal tibia and fibula.

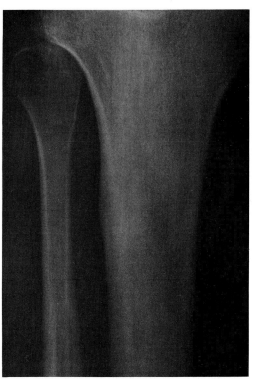

a

Figure 1.45

Stress fracture. (**a**) Localized
thickening of the cortex and
some increase in density of the
underlying medulla can be seen.
(**b**) The radioisotope bone scan
shows a local area with increased
uptake corresponding to the
abnormality seen on (**a**).

b

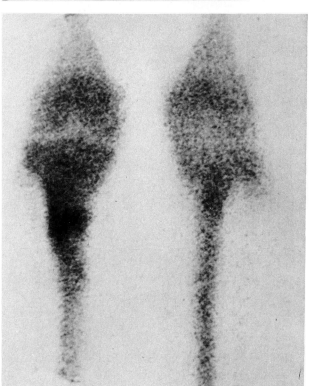

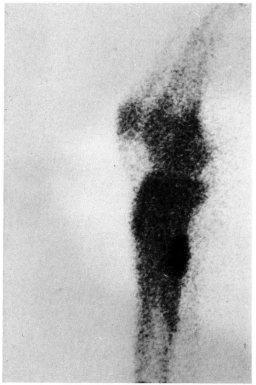

Orthopaedic radiology

Table 1.7 Location of stress fracture by activity.

Location	Activity
Sesamoids of metatarsals	Prolonged standing
Metatarsal shaft	Marching; ground stamping Prolonged standing Ballet Postoperative bunionectomy
Navicular	Marching; ground stamping Long distance running
Calcaneus	Jumping; parachuting Prolonged standing Recent immobilization
Tibia—mid and distal shaft	Ballet Long distance running
Tibid—proximal shaft (children)	Running
Fibula—distal shaft	Long distance running
Fibula—proximal shaft	Jumping; parachuting
Patella	Hurdling
Femur—shaft	Ballet Long distance running
Femur—neck	Ballet Marching Long distance running Gymnastics
Pelvis—obturator ring	Stooping Bowling Gymnastics
Lumbar vertebra (pars interarticularis)	Ballet Heavy lifting Scrubbing floors
Lower cervical, upper thoracic spinous process	Clay shovelling
Ribs	Carrying heavy pack Golf Coughing
Clavicle	Postoperative radical neck dissection
Coracoid of scapula	Trap shooting
Humerus—distal shaft	Throwing a ball
Ulna—coronoid	Pitching a ball
Ulna—shaft	Pitchfork work Propelling wheelchair
Hook of hamate*	Holding golf club, tennis racquet, baseball bat

● Speculative stress fracture.
Adapted from Daffner RH, Stress fractures, *Skeletal Radiol* (1978) **2**: 221–9, with permission.

Looser's zones and similar lesions

Looser's zones

These are usually widespread in distribution and often at classical sites (Figure 1.37). Several lesions resemble Looser's zones.

Stress fractures

Stress fractures are transverse bands of lucency (the fracture) surrounded by sclerosis (callus) (Figures 1.44 and 1.45a). Pain is the presenting symptom and the lesion can be seen on an isotope bone scan before it becomes visible on the plain film (Figure 1.45b). Characteristic activities give stress fractures at characteristic sites (Table 1.7). The lesions are often symmetrical but not widespread.

Osteoid osteoma, osteoblastoma and Brodie's abscess

These may have a similar appearance and present as painful, focal, often osteolytic lesions with a central lucency in which calcification may or may not be present (Figure 1.46). They are

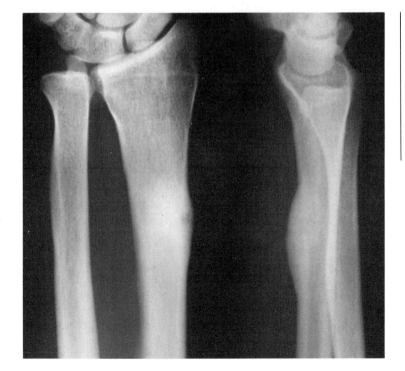

Figure 1.46

There is 'heaping up' of cortex and periosteal new bone at the site of a tumour, with an associated radiolucency, within which is a fleck of ossification. These appearances are typical of a cortical osteoid osteoma.

almost inevitably solitary and surrounded by reactive sclerosis which may be so marked that it obscures the underlying lesion (see Chapter 3, page 144).

Other forms of osteomalacia

X-linked hypophosphataemic rickets and osteomalacia

In this condition, which is vitamin D resistant, rachitic changes in infancy and osteomalacic changes in the adult are associated with gross bowing of the long bones, especially in the lower limbs, and an increase in bony density which becomes more pronounced with age (Figure 1.35). The bowed, dense, long bones are increased in width and show gross cortical thickening. In the adult, these features co-exist with changes which suggest seronegative spon-

dylarthritides, such as ankylosing spondylitis or Reiter's syndrome. There is sacroiliac irregularity and fusion, paravertebral ossification, and ossification at musculo-tendonous insertions (see Chapter 4, page 233). Patients have hypophosphataemia and hyperphosphaturia. Articular erosions are not present and the dense and bowed bones rule out an arthropathy.

Tumoural rickets and osteomalacia

Patients presenting with these conditions are also hypophosphataemic and hyperphosphaturic, but do not show bowing or sclerosis of bone. The changes are due to a number of bone and soft tissue tumours which secrete a hormone which inhibits renal tubular phosphate resorption. These tumours include haemangiopericytoma, often of the maxillary antra (Figure 1.47), fibrous dysplasia, neurofibromatosis and giant-cell

Figure 1.47

Haemangiopericytoma of the antrum (same patient as in Figure 1.37). A large soft tissue mass erodes the left antrum, destroying its wall and extending into the infratemporal fossa as well as the nasal passage.

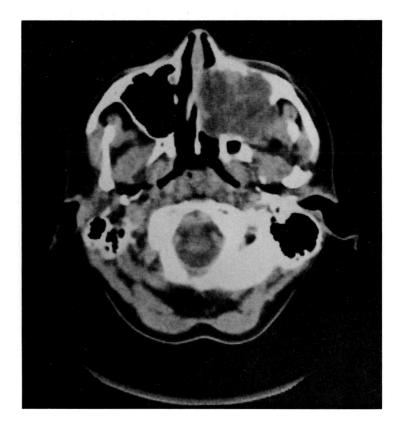

tumour. In patients with characteristic biochemical changes, the bone scan will demonstrate the typical distribution of osteomalacic change, and may also demonstrate the tumour. Otherwise the radiological changes do not differ from those seen in rickets or osteomalacia. The tumour must be totally removed for treatment to be effective.

Hyperparathyroidism

Most cases of hyperparathyroidism are due to solitary functioning thyroid adenomas. The disease classically occurs in middle-aged or elderly females whose bones may already be osteopenic. Parathormone has an anabolic effect which is said to occur if low doses are administered over a long period, while high doses administered over a short period promote a catabolic effect. Catabolism involves the resorption of bone by osteoclasts and osteocytes under parathormone stimulation.

Radiological changes in hyperparathyroidism

Demineralization

Overall, osteoporosis is the commonest radiological finding in hyperparathyroidism, but unfortunately it is not specific. Moreover, the disease often occurs with a background of post-menopausal or senile osteoporosis, so that even after satisfactory treatment the bones never return to normal density.

Subperiosteal bone resorption

This change is almost pathognomonic for hyperparathyroidism and is inevitably present in hyperparathyroid patients with bone disease. It occurs earliest and in its most gross form at the radial aspects of the middle phalanges of the ring and little fingers (Figure 1.48). The cortex loses definition and becomes less dense due to enlargement of the cigar-shaped Haversian systems, as in RSDS. Spiculation occurs externally and the distal phalangeal tufts become eroded (Figure 1.49). Subperiosteal bone resorption follows, most commonly at the proximal tibial metaphysis medially (Figure 1.50), along the

radial and ulnar shafts, around the acromio-clavicular and sterno-clavicular joints and at the musculo-tendinous insertions around the pelvis. The iliac crests, iliac spines and ischia are eroded, as in ankylosing spondylitis (Figure 1.51). Even the sacroiliac joints may be eroded by subarticular osteoclasis. Very occasionally, paraspinal and paradiscal new bone has been described (Table 1.8).

There is erosion of the superior aspects of the upper ribs (Figure 1.52), which also occurs in conditions associated with muscle wasting (Table 1.9).

Skull changes were very common in patients with bone changes in hyperparathyroidism, with 50 per cent of patients with bone disease having changes in the skull alone. The incidence of skull change in the UK is currently low.

Table 1.8 Causes of paraspinal ossification.

Ankylosing spondylitis
Psoriasis
Reiter's disease
Hyperparathyroidism
Pseudohypoparathyroidism
X-linked hypophosphataemic osteomalacia

Table 1.9 Causes of superior rib erosion.

Hyperparathyroidism
Rheumatoid arthritis
Other collagen diseases
Polio
Muscle wasting in old age

Figure 1.48

This hyperparathyroid patient has subperiosteal bone resorption, particularly on the radial aspect of the middle phalanges. There is also erosive change at the joints, which is best seen at the distal interphalangeal joint of the little finger. Distal tuft erosion is also present.

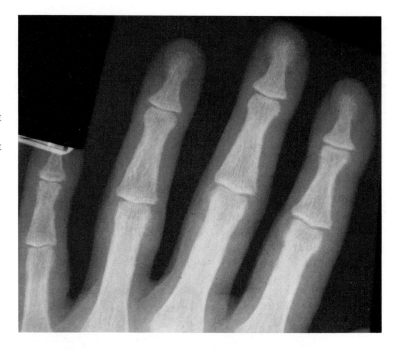

Figure 1.49

Hyperparathyroidism. This macroradiograph shows resorption of the distal phalanx with associated pseudoclubbing. The cortex has been resorbed by subperiosteal and endosteal bone resorption.

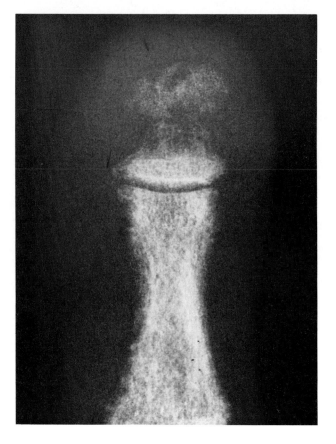

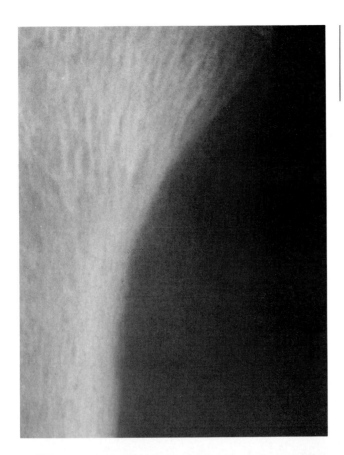

Figure 1.50

Resorption of the medial cortex of the proximal tibial metaphysis has occurred in this hyperparathyroid patient.

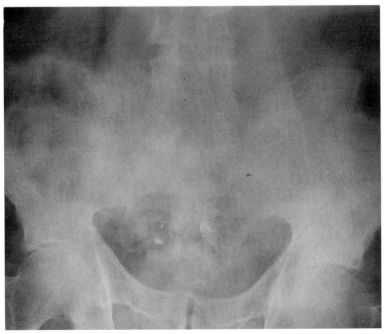

Figure 1.51

Hyperparathyroidism. Erosions occur at the iliac crests, ischial spines and around the sacroiliac joints.

Figure 1.52

Hyperparathyroidism.
Resorption is seen around the
acromio-clavicular joint, on the
inferior surface of the medial
clavicle and on the upper aspects
of thoracic ribs.

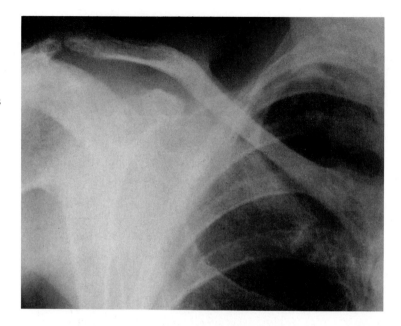

Figure 1.53

The skull in
hyperparathyroidism. (**a**)
Punctate radiolucencies give a
pepper pot appearance. The
grooves for the meningeal
vessels are ill defined because of
local bone resorption.

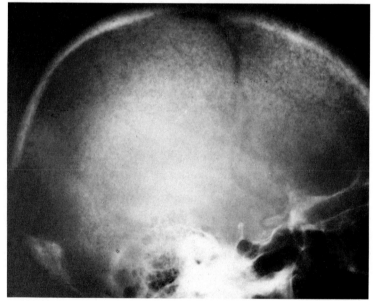

a

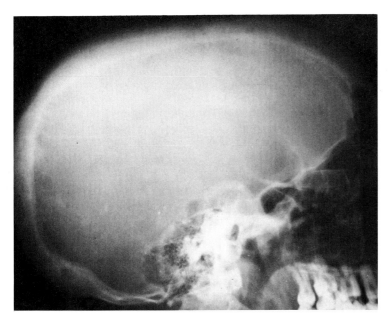

b

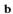

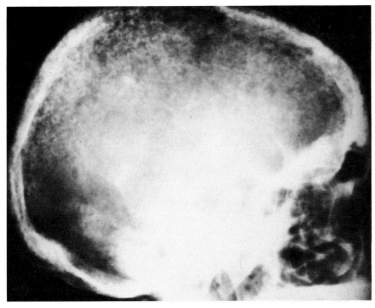

c

Figure 1.53 *continued*

(**b**) In this patient the skull vault is actually thickened and there is a loss of tabular differentiation, giving a pseudo-Paget appearance. (**c**) In this patient there is a mixture of osteolysis and sclerosis.

Changes in the skull include:

1 widespread focal areas of osteolysis, producing a poorly defined 'pepper pot' appearance (Figure 1.53a);
2 loss of definition of tables and meningeal groove markings giving a 'pseudo-Paget' appearance (Figure 1.53b);
3 bone sclerosis in primary hyperparathyroidism, presumably due to calcification in fibrous tissue. Increased density is unusual outside the skull in primary disease (Figure 1.53c).

The purely lytic or mixed sclerotic and lytic pattern must be distinguished from malignant metastatic disease or myeloma, since both sets of conditions may be associated with elevation of the serum calcium level. Patients with skull changes in hyperparathyroidism will inevitably have the hand changes of subperiosteal bone resorption, whereas those with malignant disease do not. Isotope bone scanning is necessary in either case and further lesions should be examined radiologically.

Subperiosteal bone resorption is also seen in the jaws as loss of the lamina dura, which is the hard cortical line of the socket surrounding the teeth (Figure 1.54). However, this is not as commonly seen as the change in the phalanges. Loss of the lamina dura also occurs with lytic infections, eosinophilic granuloma, dental cysts, metastatic disease and ameloblastoma, and with sclerotic lesions such as Paget's disease and cementoma.

Tumours

Brown tumours are related to osteoclastic overactivity, and are generally multiple and often well corticated (Figure 1.55). They may be subarticular or in the shaft. Multiple, fairly well-demarcated lytic lesions which are not significantly expansile and do not contain calcific flecks always suggest the possibility of hyperparathyroidism. Similar lesions may be seen in fibrous dysplasia (Figure 1.56), but these tend to be unilateral and are not associated with subperiosteal bone resorption. Eosinophilic granuloma also gives multiple lytic lesions in bone but

Figure 1.54

This hyperparathyroid patient demonstrates resorption of the lamina dura around the mandibular dentition. In addition, there is a cyst around the root of the right upper canine tooth.

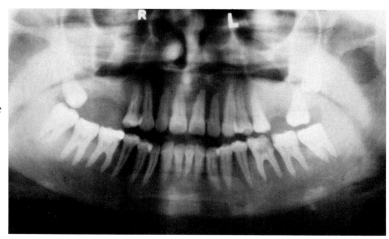

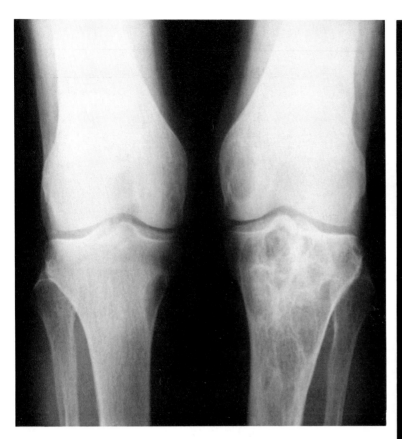

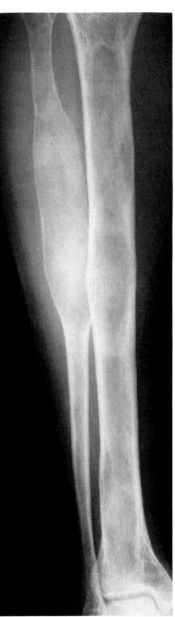

Figure 1.55

Multiple brown tumours in hyperparathyroidism are seen bilaterally in subarticular and metaphyseal locations. Chondrocalcinosis is also present.

Figure 1.56

Expansile lesions of the upper tibia and fibula are present in this patient with fibrous dysplasia. The cortex is thinned but preserved and sharp. The lesions are widespread throughout both long bones and, in places, show the typical ground-glass appearance of fibrous dysplasia. Bony definition, particularly at the cortices in areas not affected by the lesions, is much more normal than in hyperparathyroidism where there is usually a degree of demineralization and cortical erosion.

Figure 1.57

Hyperparathyroidism. The initial
radiograph shows a brown
tumour in the distal phalanx of
the left ring finger and another in
the proximal phalanx of the right
index finger (*top*). Following
parathyroidectomy, the lesion in
the left hand heals with sclerosis,
while the right-sided lesion
becomes dense at its margin
(*bottom*).

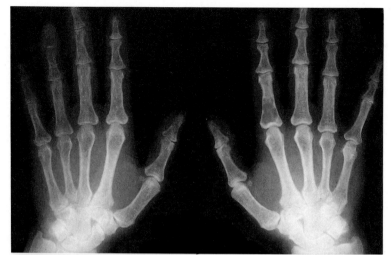

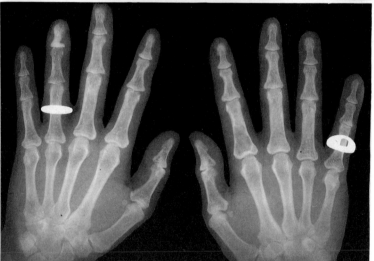

should not be diagnosed over the age of 35 years.
Fibrous dysplasia can occur at all ages but lesions
tend to calcify with age.

After treatment, lytic lesions in hyperparathyroidism may become dense or remain lytic with
increased density only at the margins (Figure
1.57) and the cyst-like lesions may suffer pathological fracture. Tumours do not occur in the
absence of subperiosteal bone resorption.

At the present time, primary hyperparathyroidism is not a significant cause of bone disease. The
disease is often diagnosed biochemically on
routine screening, and patients may not have any
bone changes. If they do, they will have subperiosteal bone resorption at the phalanges
which is best seen using macroradiography or a
magnifying glass. An X-ray of the hands is always
indicated in those with suggestive biochemistry.

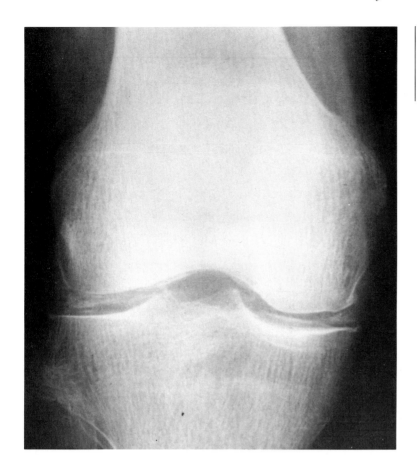

Figure 1.58

Chondrocalcinosis in hyperparathyroidism. Both the articular and meniscal cartilages are affected.

An isotope bone scan will exclude tumoural lesions, while an abdominal X-ray or ultrasound examination excludes renal calcification.

Chondrocalcinosis

Calcification, especially at the menisci in the knees and wrist, but also at articular cartilages elsewhere, occurs in the elderly as part of the aging process. Hyperparathyroidism should be excluded in patients of 55 years of age and below who exhibit multiple joint involvement with chondrocalcinosis (Figure 1.58). Pseudogout and gout also give chondrocalcinosis and are painful (Table 1.10). Gout is associated with

large erosions and soft tissue swelling, but overall bone density is usually preserved.

Table 1.10 Causes of cartilage calcification.

Old age
Hyperparathyroidism
Gout
Pseudogout
Ochronosis
Wilson's disease
Haemochromatosis
Oxalosis

Erosions

These occur in hyperparathyroidism due to subcortical osteoclastic resorption of bone in subarticular regions. In patients with an overall loss of bone density, the lesions are poorly defined and occur at the sacroiliac and acromio-clavicular joints and symphysis pubis. The carpus, metacarpo- and metatarsophalangeal joints are affected specifically and the appearances may resemble those seen in rheumatoid arthritis, but always occur in the presence of subperiosteal bone resorption (Figure 1.59).

Secondary hyperparathyroidism

Hyperparathyroidism may also be seen in patients with pre-existing osteomalacia. Parathyroid hyperplasia arises to compensate for high serum phosphate and low serum calcium levels.

Renal osteodystrophy

The term describes the bone changes in patients with chronic renal failure. The changes of osteomalacia or rickets arise as the diseased kidneys are unable to hydroxylate 25-hydroxycholecalciferol. Secondary hyperparathyroidism then occurs, with some differences possibly due to the catabolic effects of parathor-mone (see Chapter 2, page 110).

Periostitis on long bone shafts is generally absent in primary hyperparathyroidism but occurs in renal osteodystrophy (Figure 1.60). Brown tumours, osteoclast aggregates and chondrocalcinosis are less common in renal osteodystrophy. Visceral, periarticular and vascular soft tissue calcification occur more commonly in renal osteodystrophy than in primary hyperparathyroidism.

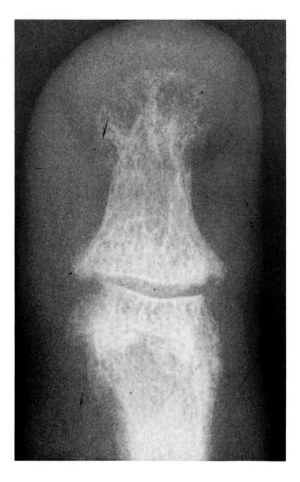

Figure 1.59

Hyperparathyroidism. There is resorption of the distal tuft with para-articular erosions. Subperiosteal bone resorption is also seen along the shaft of the middle phalanx.

Widespread osteoporosis due to marrow infiltration

Sickle-cell disease and thalassaemia

These are haemolytic anaemias, to which the body responds by marrow hyperplasia. The degree of hyperplasia depends on the severity of the disease. Sickle-cell disease occurs in patients of African descent, thalassaemia in those of Mediterranean descent (particularly Cypriots in the UK), while Gaucher's disease is said to be more common in Jews of European origin. Changes predominate in the areas of the body containing red marrow. In severe disease the

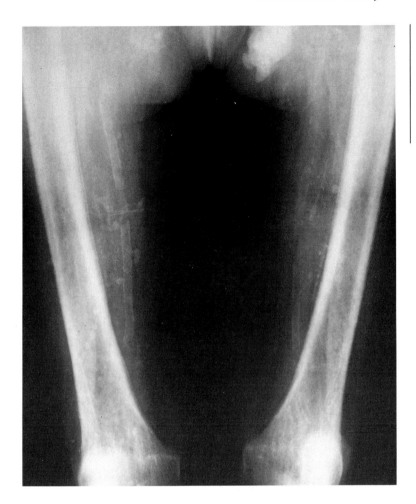

Figure 1.60

Periostitis is uncommon in primary hyperparathyroidism but does occur in renal osteodystrophy. There is also gross vascular and soft tissue calcification in this osteodystrophic patient.

entire skeleton may be affected and extramedullary haemopoiesis may occur (Figure 1.61), with thoracic and abdominal soft tissue masses, as well as splenomegaly. Thalassaemia, which causes more severe anaemia, may have the most pronounced bone change. In sickle-cell disease, thalassaemia and Gaucher's disease, marrow hypertrophy causes loss of medullary trabecula-tion and cortical thinning. The number of residual weight-bearing trabeculae are reduced but are rendered prominent. In thalassaemia particularly, marrow hypertrophy leads to bone expansion. In the skull, changes include thickening of the vault bones which spares the basi-occiput, and obliteration of the facial sinuses by blood-producing marrow, sparing the ethmoids,

Figure 1.61

In thalassaemia, extramedullary haemopoiesis results in a paraspinal soft tissue mass. The vertebral bodies are expanded and demineralized, and the cortices are thinned. There is also a loss of medullary trabeculation.

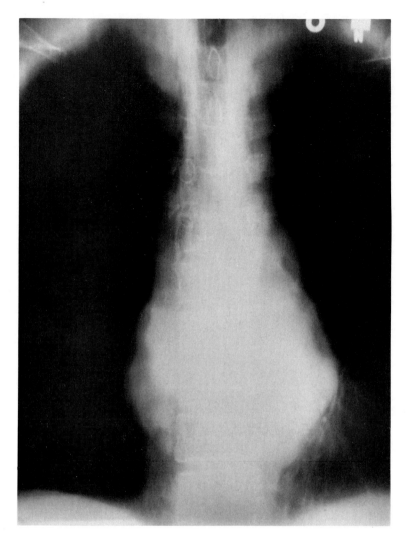

which is said to be due to a local lack of marrow. A 'hair-on-end' appearance is associated with frontal bossing in thalassaemia (Figure 1.62). Vertebrae and ribs are expanded by marrow hypertrophy. However, generalized malignant infiltration does not expand bone. In thalassaemia, expansion of vertebral bodies is associated with multiple levels of collapse, often of the codfish type. Expansion of long bones leads to a rectangular appearance of the osteoporotic metacarpals, metatarsals and phalanges (Figure 1.63) and an 'Erlenmeyer flask' appearance at the ends of the major long bones (Figure 1.64) (see Chapter 5, page 280 and Chapter 7, page 350). Expansion of ribs with cortical thinning is associated with notching of the undersurface due to locally increased circulation (Figure 1.65) (Table 1.11).

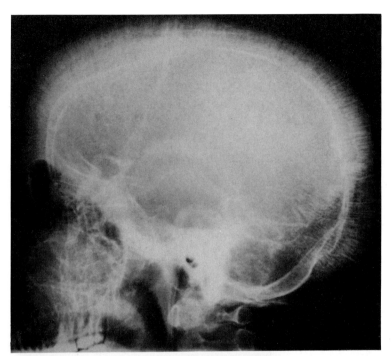

Figure 1.62

Thalassaemia. The skull shows a marked hair-on-end appearance affecting the entire vault, but sparing the basi-occiput. The maxillary antra are obliterated by being filled with trabecular bone, and similar changes occur in the sphenoid. The squamous temporal bone, however, shows a simple loss of bone density.

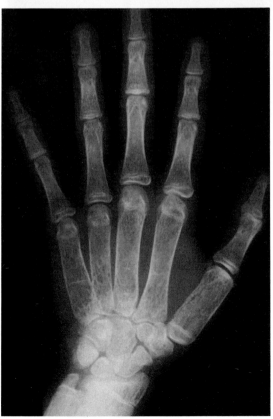

Figure 1.63

In this thalassaemic patient there is undertubulation with gross diaphyseal expansion in the metacarpals. The cortices are thinned and medullary trabeculation diminished. The nutrient foramina are increased in size, particularly in the middle phalanges.

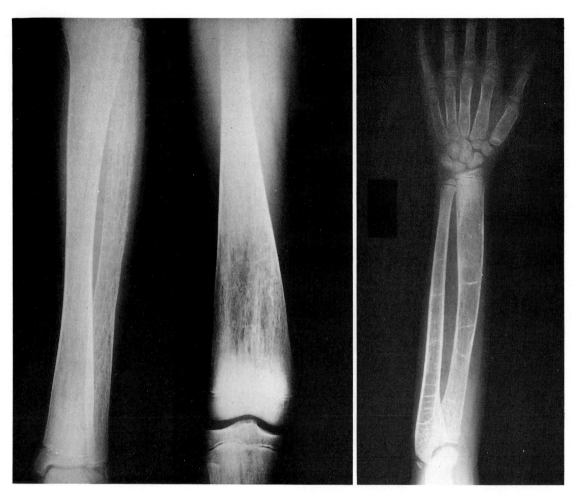

Figure 1.64

Thalassaemia. Expansion of the
tubular long bones, particularly
at the metaphyses, results in an
Erlenmeyer flask appearance.
The cortices are thinned and the
medullary trabeculation is
deficient. The fibula is expanded
and the cortex on its lateral
aspect has been broken through,
presumably by marrow
hyperplasia, and a hair-on-end
appearance has resulted.

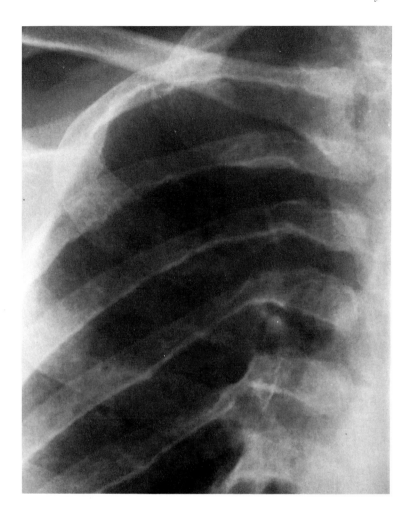

Figure 1.65

This thalassaemic patient has rib notching due to a local increase in vascularity.

Table 1.11   Causes of notching on the undersurfaces of ribs.

Arterial

Aortic obstruction:
  Coarctation
Subclavian obstruction:
  Taussig–Blalock operation
  Obstructive arteritis
Pulmonary oligaemia:
  Pulmonary artery atresia
  Pulmonary stenosis
  Fallot and Ebstein's anomalies
Thalassaemia

Venous

Superior vena caval obstruction
Inferior vena caval obstruction

Arteriovenous

Arteriovenous fistulae (pulmonary and/or parietal)

Neurogenic

Neurofibromatosis

Idiopathic

Unknown cause

Adapted from Sutton D (ed.), *Textbook of radiology*, 1st edn., (E & S Livingstone: Edinburgh 1969), with permission.

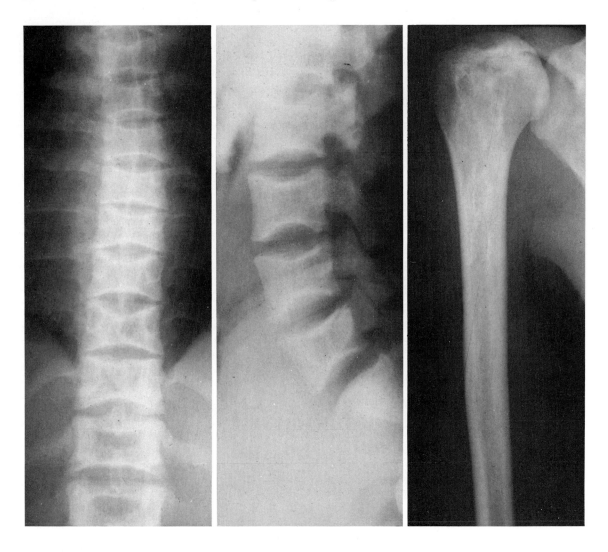

Figure 1.66

Sickle-cell disease. There are
deformities of the vertebral end-
plates with both a codfish
appearance in the lumbar spine
and step deformities due to end-
plate infarcts in the thoracic
region. The proximal humerus
shows avascular necrosis.

Heart failure and cardiac enlargement are also
seen in thalassaemia and the enlarged liver may
show an increased density, particularly on the CT
scan, due to increased iron deposition following
haemolysis. Areas of functioning marrow hyperplasia may be shown using bone-marrow-seeking
isotopes.

Marrow hypertrophy is the predominant
radiological pattern in thalassaemia. However,
sickle-cell disease has infarction as the predominant feature, combined with marrow hypertrophy, which is not as pronounced, so that bone

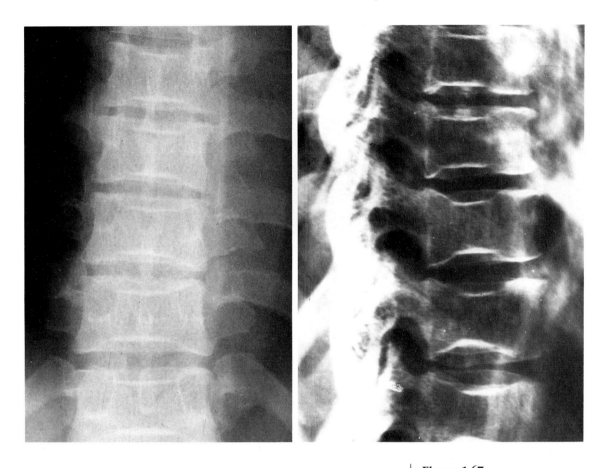

Figure 1.67

Sickle-cell disease. Cortical infarcts at the vertebral end-plates have resulted in failure of growth in the affected areas, while growth proceeds normally in the remainder of the vertebral body.

expansion is not a prominent feature and may even be absent. Any osteoporosis due to marrow expansion may be obscured by the widespread infarction which results in osteosclerosis.

In sickle-cell disease, there is trabecular loss, cortical thinning and collapse in the vertebral column (Figure 1.66) and sharply right-angled step defects in the end-plates, probably due to local infarcts (Figure 1.67). Similar changes occur in Gaucher's disease.

Avascular necrosis of articular surfaces is seen (Figure 1.68) and cortical infarcts cause a 'split

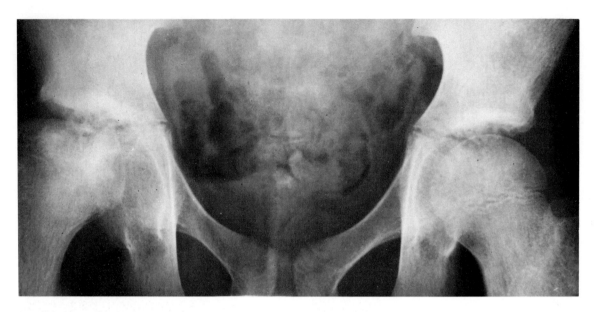

Figure 1.68

Avascular necrosis in sickle-cell
disease. The right femoral head
shows reactive sclerosis around
an area of structural failure of the
articular cortex following
infarction. The left femoral head
is quite markedly demineralized
but not yet collapsed.

cortex' (Figure 1.69). This 'bone-within-a-bone'
appearance is due to the 'tombstone' of the old
cortex lying within the new (Table 1.12).

Changes in sickle-cell disease can occur early
in life. Sickle-cell dactylitis occurs in babies,
when focal expansile lesions of phalanges are

Table 1.12   Causes of cortical splitting.

Osteomyelitis
Sickle-cell disease
Gaucher's disease

associated with soft tissue swelling, periostitis
and pathological features in the affected bone
(Figure 1.70), which may be compounded by
blood-borne infection by *Salmonella* or *Escher-
ichia coli*.

Involvement of affected epiphyses may lead to
premature fusion and local growth arrest. In the
chest, heart failure may follow anaemia, and
pulmonary infarcts may lead to pulmonary arterial hypertension.

The radioisotope bone scan shows the acute
infarction before plain radiographic changes and
can also be used to assess healing. In sickle-cell
disease, the spleen is usually small due to
repeated infarction.

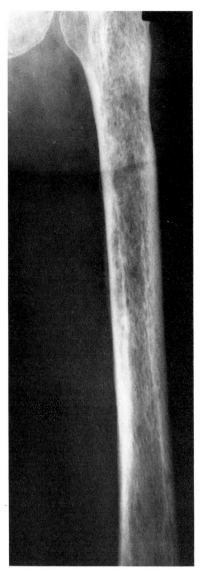

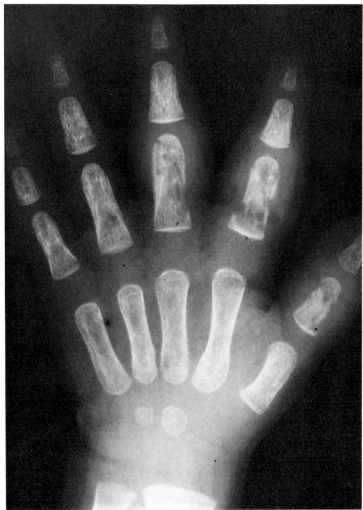

Figure 1.69

Cortical splitting in sickle-cell disease. The parallel lines lying within the new cortex represent the tombstones of the old necrotic cortex. In this patient there is a widespread abnormality of bone texture which is mainly lytic with some areas of reactive sclerosis, presumably in areas of dead bone.

Figure 1.70

Sickle-cell dactylitis involves soft tissue swelling over areas of bone destruction in many of the phalanges. The phalanges are expanded, bullet-shaped and demineralized. Split cortices can also be seen in many of the metacarpals. Pathological fractures occur throughout the areas of osteomyelitis.

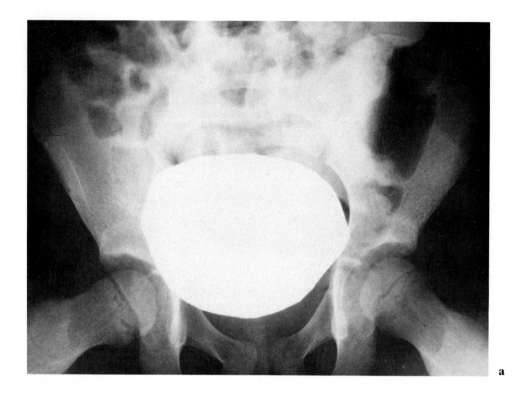

a

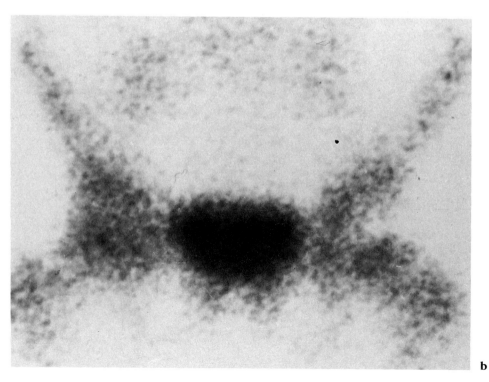

b

Gaucher's disease

There is an accumulation of abnormal lipid in the reticulo-endothelial cells (Gaucher cells), giving hepatosplenomegaly, marrow infiltration and hypertrophy. The infiltration of the marrow may be diffuse, producing cortical thinning, often with endosteal scalloping, and loss of medullary trabeculation, or focal, giving a more 'bubbly' change which may resemble myeloma. Infiltration gives bone expansion producing an Erlenmeyer flask appearance (see Chapters 2, 5 and 7) but the Gaucher cell infiltrate also causes occlusion of blood vessels in bone by extrinsic compression, resulting in some of the infarctive changes seen in sickle-cell disease (Figure 1.71).

Patients with Gaucher's disease may show avascular necrosis of articular surfaces, cortical infarcts giving split cortices and end-plate infarcts of vertebral bodies with general or focal lytic lesions, but sclerosis of infarcted bone is also seen (see Chapter 2, page 115). There may be bone infections and pathological fractures. Fibrosarcoma is a rare complication of infarction in both sickle-cell and Gaucher's diseases.

Malignant infiltrative disorders

In theory, widespread malignant disease causes extensive demineralization. In infants, leukaemia and neuroblastoma and, in the elderly, myeloma and metastatic cancer of the breast are the most common causes of this change. However, in practice, a purely generalized osteoporotic pattern is unusual. In infantile leukaemia and neuroblastoma, widespread bone destruction does occur, but there is usually metaphyseal accentuation of the destructive process (see Chapter 5, page 267). A 'raindrop' pattern of bone destruction emphasizes the malignant nature of the process which will not be present with other causes of childhood osteoporosis (Table 1.13).

Sutural diastasis due to hydrocephalus and tumour deposition in the sutures may also be found and should not be confused with Wormian bones. In addition neuroblastoma may be associated with spinal erosion and abdominal calcification.

In adults, breast malignancy and myeloma are probably the cause of most cases of widespread malignant infiltration resulting in osteopenia. These patients are usually elderly and will therefore already have a reduced bone density.

Table 1.13   Causes of generalized demineralization in children.

Leukaemia
Neuroblastoma
Scurvy
Rickets
Idiopathic juvenile osteoporosis
Osteogenesis imperfecta

Figure 1.71

Gaucher's disease. (**a**) There is early flattening of the left femoral head. The tip of the greatly enlarged spleen is seen in the left flank. (**b**) The radioisotope bone scan in the same patient shows a defect in the left femoral head region.

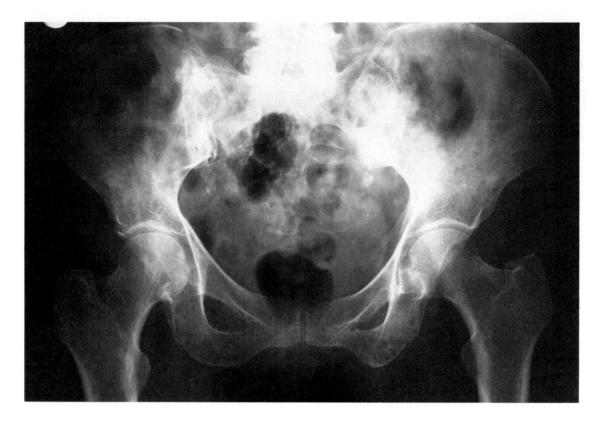

Figure 1.72

In myelomatosis there is
an overall loss of bone density
with a slight accentuation in the
upper femora and ischia. A
raindrop pattern of radiolucency
can be seen. These appearances
may be the sole manifestation of
myelomatosis.

Myeloma is thought not to cause destruction of
vertebral pedicles, although metastases do. It is
usual for widespread myelomatosis and carcino-
matosis to produce focal destruction of bone in
addition to generalized demineralization. Pedicular or cortical destruction may be difficult to
visualize in an already demineralized axial skeleton but must be investigated. The radioisotope
bone scan is invaluable in the detection of
metastases. Only rarely is malignant disease so
widespread and uniform that uptake on the scan
is uniformly increased, and therefore mistaken
for normal. Occasionally this change is seen with
widespread sclerotic metastases in both breast
and prostatic malignant disease.

Myeloma may produce diffuse osteoporosis,
but again focal lesions or a raindrop pattern of
destruction should be looked for. Cortices

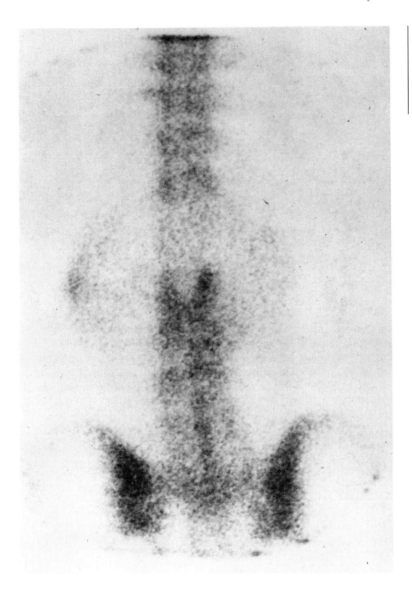

Figure 1.73

This radioisotope bone scan shows a total absence of uptake in the vertebral bodies of a lumbar spine affected by myelomatosis.

around the vertebral bodies, sacral formina and cortical lines on the pelvis or acetabula, should be assessed for integrity (Figure 1.72). The isotope scan is not always positive in myeloma as deposits may present with focal 'cold' areas of uptake as defects on the scan (Figure 1.73).

2 | Osteosclerosis

An increase in bone density may be generalized and diffuse, widespread but focal, or due to a solitary lesion. The diagnosis of osteosclerosis is perhaps more easily made than that of osteopenia, particularly if the changes are focal. Most of the radiographic image of a bone, and its density, is due to the cortex, therefore cortical thickening and periosteal new bone will cause an increase in radiological bony density. These changes may result from stress and hypertrophy, which occur,

Table 2.1 Causes of generalized or widespread increase in bony density.

Sclerotic metastases Myelosclerosis Mastocytosis Lymphoma Sickle-cell disease Leukaemia Myeloma	Leukaemia Myeloma } Rarely sclerotic if untreated	May be associated with splenomegaly	Diffuse osteosclerosis with normal modelling
Paget's disease Sickle-cell disease Renal osteodystrophy Fluorosis and other heavy metal poisoning Osteopetrosis Craniotubular dysplasias			Often or always associated with changes in bone contour
Osteopoikylosis Osteopathia striata	Mainly around joints with normal modelling	Congenital forms	

Table 2.2 Causes of focal multiple or solitary sclerotic lesions.

Paget's disease*

Infarcts*

Osteomyelitis*

Fibrous dysplasia*

Metastases*

Lymphoma*

Mastocytosis

Leukaemia

Myeloma*

Healing benign or malignant bone lesions*

Osteomas*

Bone islands*

Osteopathia striata

Osteopoikylosis

Melorheostosis

Tuberous sclerosis

*May be solitary.

for example, in athletes. However, Africans also seem to have denser bones, probably due to thicker cortices.

Focal medullary osteosclerosis is perhaps more easily recognized, because a focal lesion, such as a solitary bone island, is clearly seen against surrounding medullary bone. If the increased density is widespread, cortico–medullary differentiation may be lost. However, widespread sclerosis may be difficult to assess. Thick or bulky soft tissues, or an underexposed film, may cause bones to look diffusely dense. Even an isotope bone scan may show an increase in uptake which is so diffuse that differentiation from normal may be difficult.

Increase in bone density (Table 2.1 and Table 2.2) may be assessed by the same techniques used in the measurement of osteoporosis (see page 2).

Osteosclerosis with expansion

Osteitis deformans (Paget's disease)

This is a common disease in the elderly which is usually found incidentally, and is slightly more common in men. In both men and women, incidence at autopsy rises from 3 per cent at 40 to around 10 per cent at 85 years of age. It is more common in the UK and USA than in Scandinavia and is less common in Africa and Asia. This may be because populations in these continents are younger, and investigated less often.

The initial stage of the disease is one of active resorption of bone which is not usually seen radiologically in the weight-bearing skeleton. However, it is seen in the skull vault as an advancing front of osteolysis, known as osteoporosis circumscripta (Figure 2.1), and may also be seen in the anterior tibia (Figure 2.2a). In long bones the lytic process starts at an articular surface, extending in continuity to the other end of the bone behind a flame-shaped front of osteolysis (Figure 2.2a). This is associated with cortical resorption and loss of cortico-medullary differentiation so that only a few cortical trabeculae remain.

The resorptive phase is followed by the laying down of new bone with an abnormal pattern so that lucency is progressively replaced by a dense, woolly sclerosis with loss of normal cortico-medullary differentiation (Figures 2.2b and 2.3). In the spine, bone condenses beneath vertebral end-plates, giving a 'picture-frame' appearance. The newly laid down bone may show a mixed sclerotic and lytic pattern but, with time, the disease progresses towards total sclerosis and total involvement of a bone, particularly if small (Figure 2.4). Initially the bone scan shows increased uptake even if radiological changes are minimal (Figure 2.5); however, the end stage of total sclerosis may be quiescent on the scan, although bone expansion is present.

In the reparative stages of the disease, new bone is laid down beneath the periosteum on the cortex, producing an increase in the external diameter of the bone, and also endosteally, encroaching upon the medullary cavity. Cortico-medullary differentiation remains poor, the external contours of the bone remain smooth or

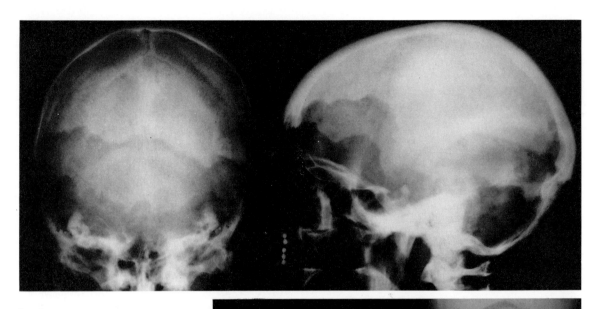

Figure 2.1

Osteoporosis circumscripta. An
unusual feature of Paget's disease
of the skull is gross loss of bone
density with a geographical
margin.

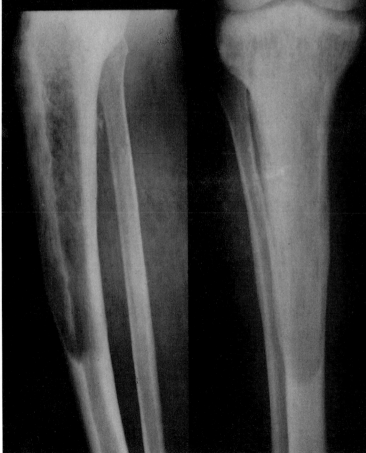

Figure 2.2

Paget's disease of the tibia. (**a**)
Quite marked radiolucency is
seen in the anterior tibia
extending to the proximal
articular surface and ending
inferiorly in a flame shape. This
precedes the osteosclerotic
phase and, in this patient, is
associated with expansion of the
bone and cortical thickening. **a**

slightly undulant, and occasionally a tendon 'pulls off' an exostosis at its insertion (Figure 2.6).

Paget's bone is soft, so that bowing (Figure 2.7), deformity and pathological transverse or increment fractures occur (Figure 2.8). In the spine, vertebral expansion in the sagittal and coronal planes is associated with vertebral col-lapse which may cause spinal cord compression, often in association with a picture-frame appearance (Figure 2.9) (Table 2.3).

After a fracture and immobilization, the bone distal to the fracture line becomes extremely demineralized. A similar phenomenon is seen in hyperparathyroidism. Callus shows all the features of Paget's disease.

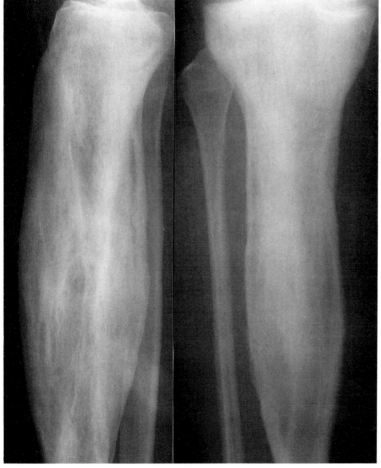

b

Figure 2.2 *continued*

(**b**) The later film shows further expansion of bone and subsequent sclerosis with an amorphous texture. The pathological process still ends inferiorly in a flame shape.

Figure 2.3

The progression of Paget's
disease is shown in two films
taken one year apart.

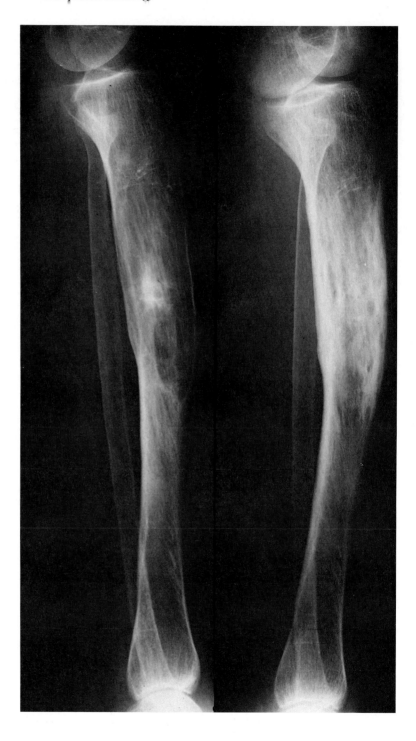

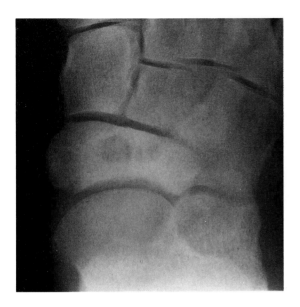

Figure 2.4

Paget's disease of the tarsal navicular. A characteristic end-stage of Paget's disease is shown by expansion of the bone with total sclerosis, cortical thickening and an almost uniform bone texture. The whole bone is affected.

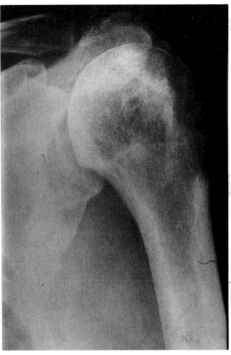

a

Figure 2.5

(**a**) In this patient with Paget's disease, the cortex is thickened, cortico–medullary differentiation is poor, and there is an increase in density in the medulla. There is a typically coarse trabecular pattern which extends to the proximal articular surface. (**b**) In the same patient, a radionuclide bone scan shows the gross increase of uptake in the affected area, extending to the articular surface.

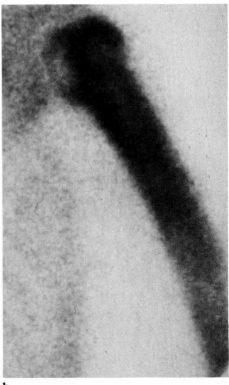

b

Figure 2.5 *continued*

(**c**) A bone scan shows a
diffuse increase in uptake in the
skull with vault thickening. (**d**)
The CT scan demonstrates the
thick vault and loss of cortico–
medullary differentiation.

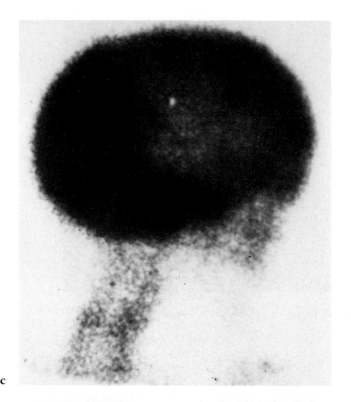

c

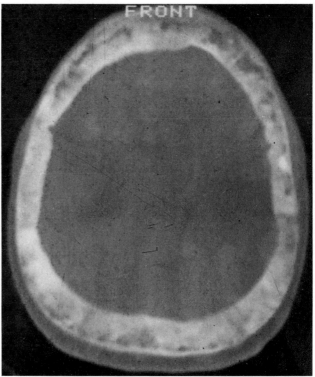

d

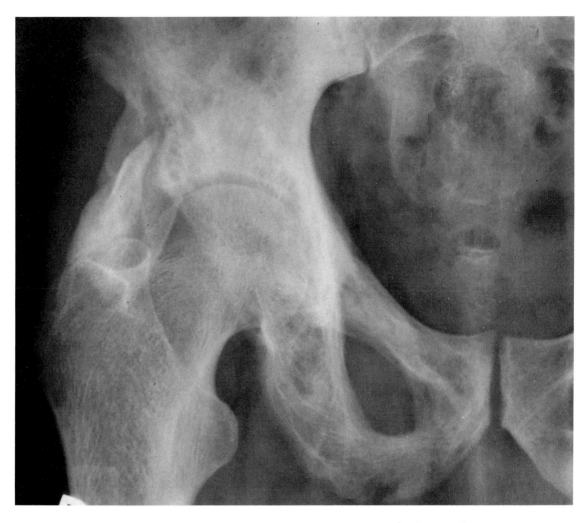

Figure 2.6

Paget's disease. The right innominate bone shows expansion, cortical thickening, loss of cortico–medullary differentiation and a coarsened medullary trabecular pattern. A large exostosis is shown in the region of the anterior inferior iliac spine, which has the same abnormal bone texture of Paget's disease and which may be compared with the normal proximal femur. This lesion follows tendinous avulsion of softened bone.

Figure 2.7

This patient with Paget's disease
has gross expansion of the tibia
with a typically coarsened
trabecular pattern and loss of
cortico–medullary
differentiation, initially extending
upwards to the proximal
midshaft with a flame shape, but
eventually reaching the upper
tibial articular surface. There is
bowing as a result of softening.
The fibula is rarely the site of
Paget's disease and is unaffected
in this patient.

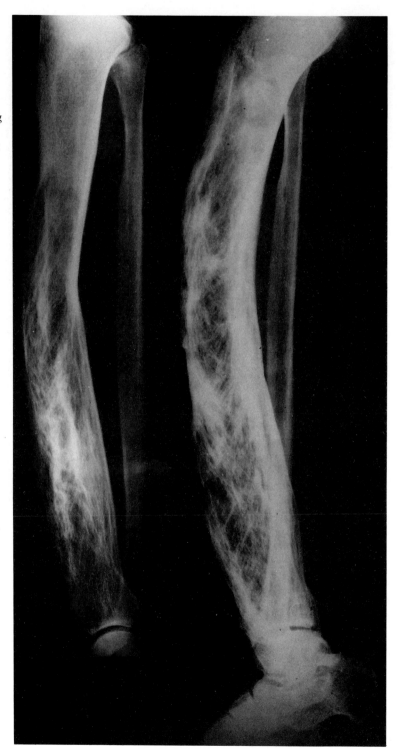

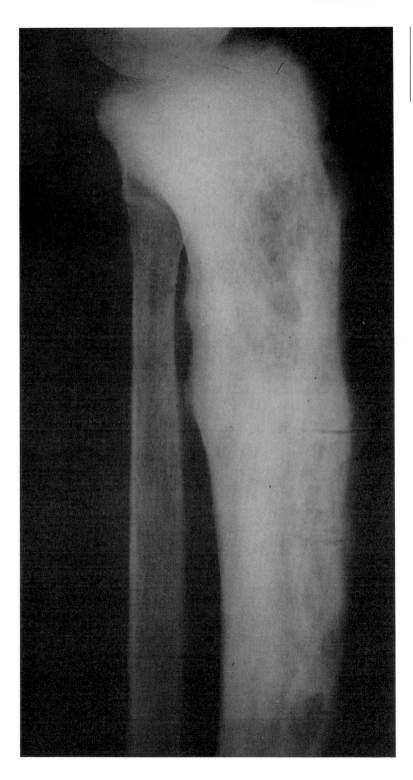

Figure 2.8

Transverse increment fractures are seen in Paget's disease extending to the anterior tibial cortex.

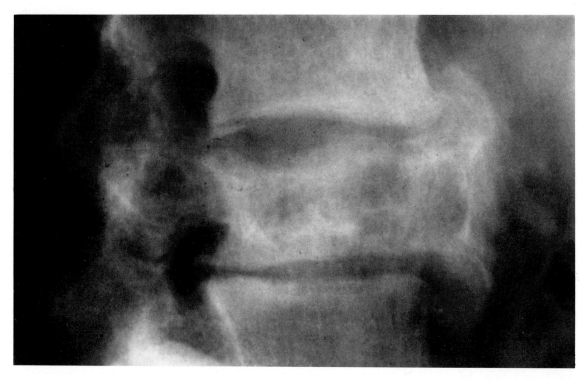

Figure 2.9

Paget's disease. On the lateral view there is collapse of a lumbar vertebral body, which is associated with expansion of the bone anteriorly, and a picture-frame appearance due to condensation of bone beneath the end-plates.

Table 2.3   Causes of bone softening and deformity.

Fibrous dysplasia

X-linked and other forms of osteomalacia

Osteogenesis imperfecta

Osteopetrosis

Still's disease (juvenile rheumatoid arthritis) in the paired long bones

Neurofibromatosis in the paired long bones

Protrusio acetabuli is seen in rheumatoid arthritis and osteoarthritis and as a congenital lesion

NB These are unusual changes in disorders other than Paget's disease.

Figure 2.10

Paget's sarcoma. (**a**) The body of L2 shows an increase in density and anterior expansion, as do the posterior elements. There is a large osseous mass arising from the vertebral body and spreading into the local soft tissues. There is obstruction to the flow of contrast at radiculography. The appearances are those of malignant degeneration in Paget's disease. (**b**) The radioisotope bone scan shows increase in uptake in the affected, expanded vertebral body, and also uptake in the soft tissue tumour mass to the left of the spine. There is also an obstructive uropathy on the right side.

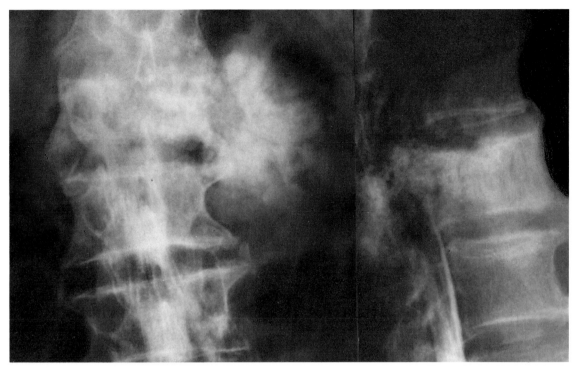

a

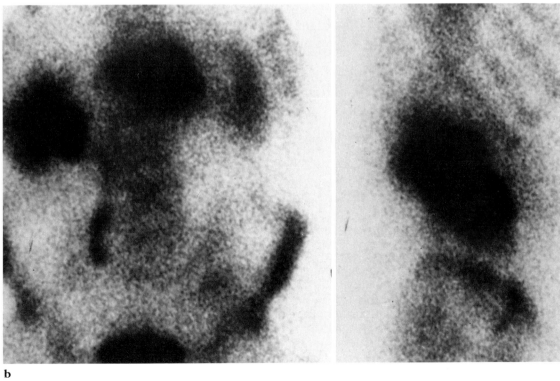

b

Figure 2.10 continued

(**c**) The CT scan shows the abnormal bone texture of the vertebral body and the sarcomatous mass on its left side.

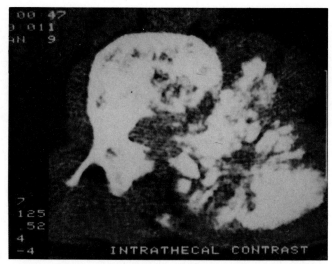

c

Pain in Paget's disease should alert the radiologist to the presence of a fracture or tumour. Associated tumours include osteogenic sarcoma (Figure 2.10), chondrosarcoma and fibrosarcoma, as well as giant-cell tumour.

Osteosclerosis without expansion

Sclerotic metastatic deposits in bone

As Paget's disease occurs primarily in the elderly, it is most likely to be radiologically confused with widespread sclerosing osseous metastases. The most common malignant tumours of bone are metastases, only 10 per cent of which are solitary. However, a solitary metastasis is more common than a solitary malignant primary bone tumour. Metastases usually occur after 45 years of age, whereas most primary bone tumours (benign and malignant) are seen in younger patients.

In an autopsy study (Galasko CSP 1986, see Appendix), 57 per cent of patients with breast malignancy and 55 per cent of those with prostatic malignancy developed bone metastases, while lung cancer metastasized to bone slightly less often (44 per cent).

Metastases are most commonly present in the vertebral column, ribs, skull and proximal long bones (Figure 2.11), but are unusual distal to the knee or elbow. They occur, therefore, in areas of red marrow formation which have a high local blood flow.

Metastatic spread from the pelvis (prostate, bladder, uterus) to the ribs, vertebral column, and pelvic bones is facilitated by the valveless system of paravertebral veins of Batson. Occasional metastases to the hand or foot often have their origin in the lung and usually are lytic.

The distribution of metastases within the axial skeleton is random, and is best seen using skeletal scintigraphy (Figure 2.11). As the sclerosing process spreads, the medulla becomes obliterated and the bone may become uniformly sclerotic, with loss of cortico-medullary differentiation and visible trabeculation (Figure 2.12).

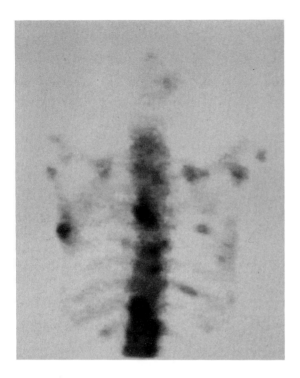

Figure 2.11

A radioisotope bone scan shows
the widespread and random
distribution of skeletal
metastases.

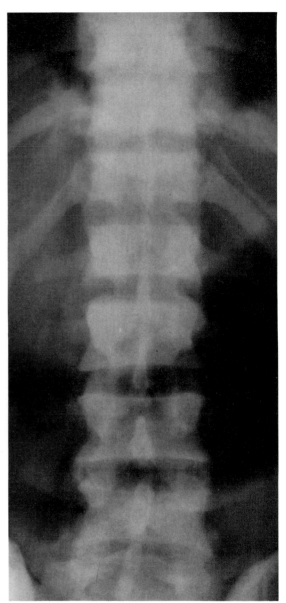

Sclerotic metastases arise mainly from primary
malignancy in the breast, prostate and gastroin-
testinal tract. These primary sites may also result
in lytic or mixed sclerotic and lytic metastases,
but most lesions in bone due to prostatic
metastases are sclerotic.

New bone formation in metastases develops:

1   in the fibrous stroma associated with cer-
    tain metastases, particularly prostatic,
    where the stroma ossifies in the presence
    of osteoprogenitor cells;

Figure 2.12

Secondary deposits from
carcinoma of the prostate can be
seen. There is widespread
osteosclerosis with no expansion
of the vertebral bodies. The
pedicles and the spinous
processes are affected. Cortico-
medullary differentiation is
diminished or lost.

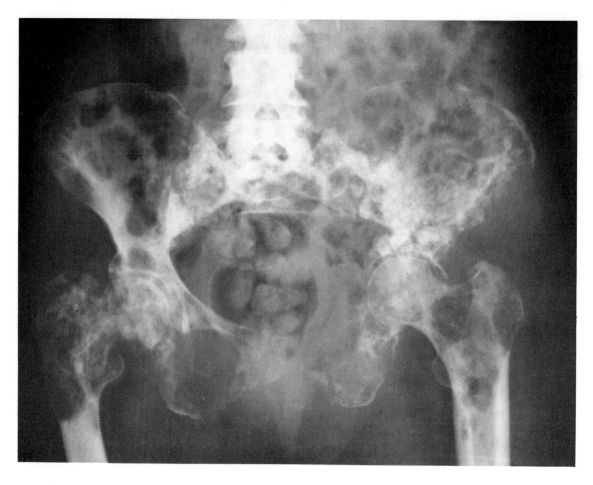

Figure 2.13

This patient has metastatic disease from carcinoma of the breast, with widespread areas of osteolysis throughout the pelvis and in the proximal femora. There is also some reactive sclerosis. The patient therefore has a mixed pattern of disease which is predominantly lytic.

2   as a reactive phenomenon secondary to bone destruction. Destruction by a tumour on one side of a trabeculum may be associated with woven bone deposition on the other side.

This phenomenon occurs in almost all metastases, with the exception of myeloma, lymphoma, leukaemia and highly anaplastic and aggressive lytic metastases, where destruction occurs more rapidly than any sclerosing reaction.

In normal adult vertebral bodies, less than 1 per cent of bone is woven; however, in most metastases, with the exceptions mentioned above, there is often up to 40 per cent, which implies active repair.

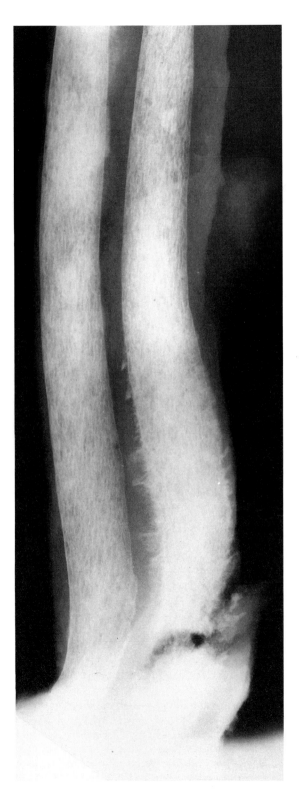

In malignant sclerotic metastatic disease from breast, and particularly prostate, the initial site of change in the axial skeleton is medullary. In the vertebral body, the pedicles are involved. Progression of the lesions leads to developing obliteration of the medullary cavity with loss of cortico-medullary differentiation and trabecular architecture (Figure 2.12), while lytic areas of bone destruction cause cortical scalloping. Medullary lucency may infrequently be present in prostatic metastases but is more common with breast metastases (Figure 2.13). Areas of preserved bone density remain, so that changes are not uniform.

Periostitis and expansion of bone is unusual in metastatic disease. The degree of expansion which occurs in Paget's disease is not seen. Occasionally a periosteal reaction may produce an undulant outer margin. Malignant sunray spiculation, which occasionally occurs with malignant deposits (Figure 2.14), only occurs in Paget's disease if it undergoes malignant degeneration.

In the axial skeleton, the ribs are less generally involved in Paget's disease than in prostatic disease, so that widespread rib sclerosis is more likely to be due to prostatic metastases (Figure 2.15). Softening and bowing do not occur with malignancy but pathological fractures do.

The skull is not expanded by prostatic metastases and the disease tends to be less uniform than the changes in Paget's disease although tabular differentiation may be lost.

Figure 2.14

Metastatic disease. Sunray spiculation with bone expansion in sclerotic metastatic deposits from carcinoma of the bladder.

Figure 2.15

This patient with metastatic disease from carcinoma of the prostate has widespread osteosclerosis in the ribs which makes Paget's disease less likely. In addition, the bones are not expanded.

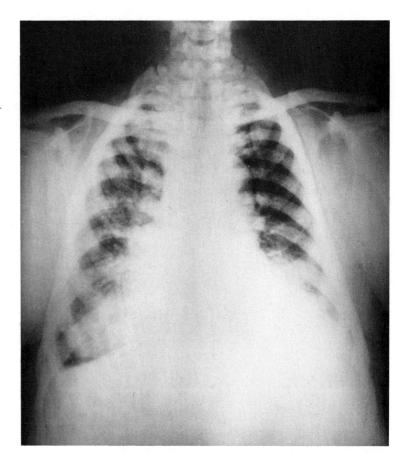

Other organs are affected in malignant disease. Pulmonary metastases and lymph node enlargement may be present, as well as splenomegaly (Table 2.4).

Table 2.4   Causes of diffuse sclerosis in malignant disease.

Sclerotic metastases—prostate, lung, bladder, breast, carcinoid, uterus

Following therapy for malignant disease

Myelosclerosis
Mastocytosis } Osteosclerosis with splenomegaly
Lymphoma
Leukaemia

Osteosclerosis with splenomegaly

Myelosclerosis

This is a disease of unknown aetiology in which the marrow is initially replaced by a fibrous ground substance (myelofibrosis), which becomes progressively ossified. Dense bone may finally occupy up to 70 per cent of the marrow as calcium is deposited in the fibrous matrix.

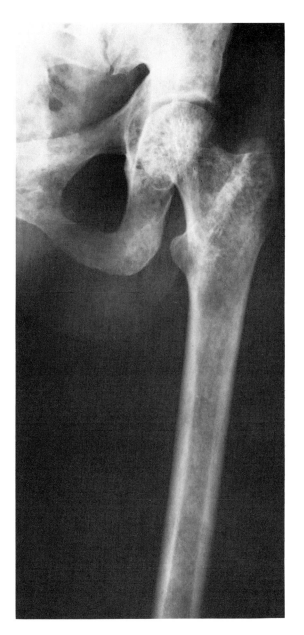

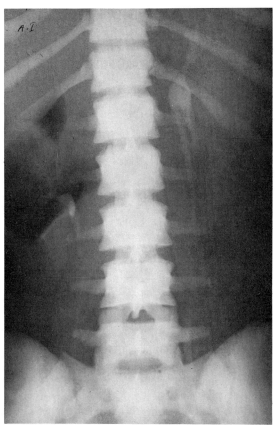

Figure 2.17

In this patient with myelosclerosis there is widespread diffuse uniform osteosclerosis without bone expansion. Massive splenomegaly displaces the left kidney and ureter towards the midline.

Figure 2.16

Myelosclerosis. A diffuse increase in density is seen in the medullary cavity of the femur and pelvic bones. In places, there is resorption of the cortex with endosteal scalloping.

In the myelofibrotic stage, the skeleton is of
normal density, but with progressive ossification
the thoraco-lumbar spine, ribs and pelvis show
an increase in medullary density which is often
uniform, though foci of extra sclerosis may be
present (Figure 2.16). Cortico-medullary differentiation and trabecular detail are lost. The
peripheral skeleton and skull are less frequently
involved and may even show signs of marrow
hyperplasia. The long bones of the axial skeleton
are not abnormally modelled as periostitis is
absent.

Massive splenomegaly and, to a lesser extent,
hepatomegaly are inevitable (Figure 2.17). Soft
tissue masses elsewhere are due to extramedullary haemopoiesis, and there may be varices and
ascites. Secondary gout is a prominent feature,
and pneumonia is a major cause of death.

Urticaria pigmentosa (mastocytosis)

Large numbers of mast cells are present in the
skin and may produce skin nodules. In both
infants and adults, wheals are produced by
histamine release when the skin is traumatized.

In the bones, mast cell aggregates can cause
focal osteolysis, but usually new bone formation
results in thickened trabeculae with medullary
sclerosis (Figure 2.18a). Hepatosplenomegaly
and lymphadenopathy follow. In children, bone
changes in the long bones are said to predominate but, in adults, mainly the central skeleton is
affected, as active marrow is centrally confined.

In mastocytosis, splenomegaly is rarely as
marked as in myelosclerosis, where the spleen
often tips in the iliac fossa. Marrow and peripheral blood examination also distinguish the two
diseases. Lack of infarcts and bone modelling
deformities distinguish them both from haemolytic anaemias, Gaucher's disease and particularly
osteopetrosis. Generalized osteosclerosis is rare
in myeloma and the lymphomas (Figure 2.18b).

Leukaemia

Osteosclerosis is rare in leukaemic children,
nearly all of whom have changes of bone
destruction, which are also seen in adults.

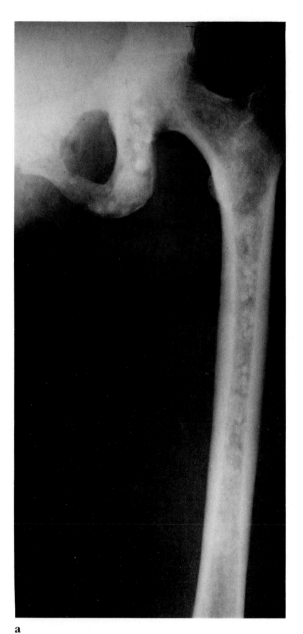

a

Figure 2.18

(**a**) Mastocytosis showing a
widespread diffuse increase in
medullary density.

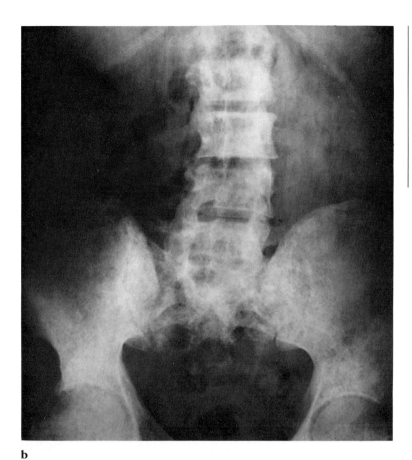

Figure 2.18 *continued*

(**b**) Sclerosing myeloma, with a widespread increase in trabecular density in the lumbar spine, sacrum and innominate bones as well as the proximal femora. This is a rare manifestation in untreated myeloma. Lytic lesions in myeloma may sclerose following chemotherapy or radiotherapy.

b

Lymphomas

Lesions originate in lymph nodes and there is probably no primary involvement of bone. Bone involvement is either direct, from adjacent nodes, or by haematogenous spread resulting from splenic involvement. Contiguous erosion of bone from diseased lymph nodes primarily affects the region of the sacroiliac and para-aortic nodes, therefore the spine and pelvis are most commonly involved in this form of the disease. Haematogenous metastases can occur anywhere in the axial skeleton. Two-thirds of the bony lesions are multiple and may be lytic, sclerotic or both. The incidence of sclerotic lesions varies greatly (between 20 and 45 per cent) because lytic lesions sclerose on therapy and sclerotic lesions may become lytic with progressive destruction. Widespread sclerosis is rare and generally only the pelvis and spine are affected. Anterior spinal erosions and fluffy periosteal reactions are seen (Figure 2.19). Erosions on the anterior aspects of contiguous vertebral bodies are seen in Hodgkin's disease due to pressure or

Figure 2.19

Lymphoma. Anterior erosion of a
thoracic vertebral body due to
disease in adjacent lymph nodes.

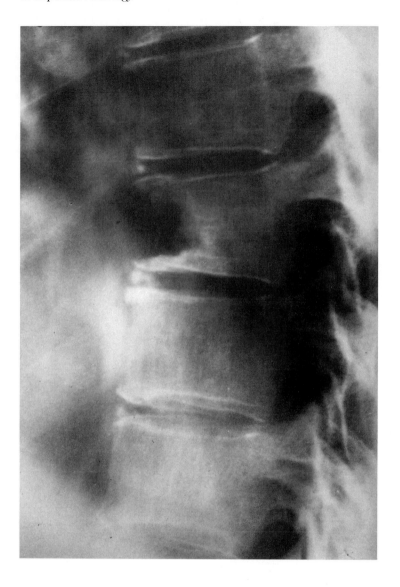

invasion by anteriorly situated abnormal lymph
nodes.

   A similar phenomenon may occur as a result
of pressure from an aortic aneurysm or invasion
from tuberculous lymph nodes (Figure 2.20).
Only in the latter condition will the adjacent disc
spaces usually be involved and narrowed. Destruction of vertebral bone is occasionally followed by radiological evidence of discal narrowing
in malignant disease as disc material herniates
into softened vertebral bone (Figure 2.21).
Assessment of the paraspinal pathology causing
spinal erosion is made by CT, ultrasound and
biopsy.

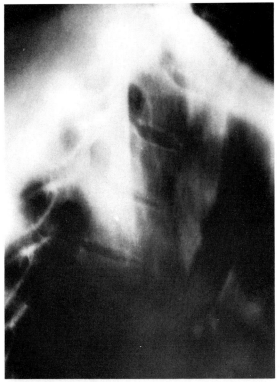

a

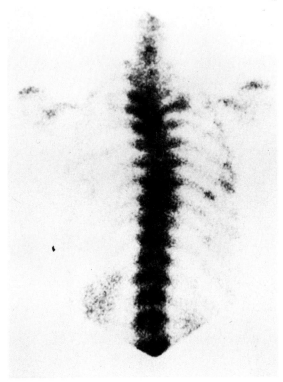

b

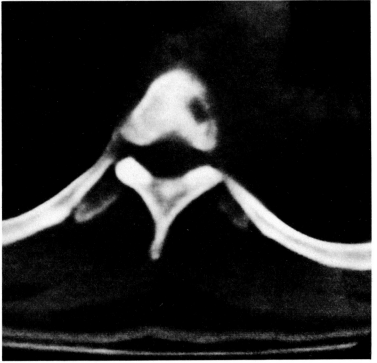

c

Figure 2.20

Tuberculosis. (**a**) The plain radiograph shows a soft tissue mass displacing the tracheal translucency anteriorly and eroding the anterior aspects of adjacent vertebral bodies. There is early discal narrowing. (**b**) In the radioisotope bone scan there is increased uptake in the upper thoracic spine and adjacent ribs in the region corresponding to the plain film change. (**c**) The CT scan shows a local erosion on the vertebral body with irregularity of the cortex and an overlying soft tissue mass.

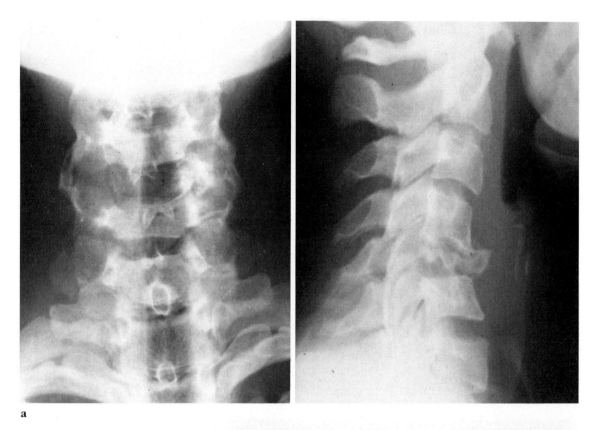

a

Figure 2.21

In this patient with osteogenic sarcoma, (**a**) the vertebral body of C5 is collapsed, and there is some anterior displacement of bony fragments. The adjacent discs vary in height and, anteriorly, they are narrowed due to herniation into the affected vertebral body. There is a local soft tissue mass. (**b**) The CT scan shows destruction of the vertebral body, encroachment upon the neural canal and some local expansion.

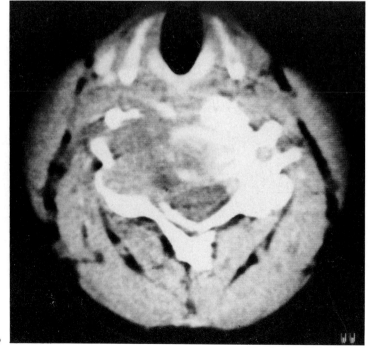

b

Focal areas of bone sclerosis (*Table 2.5*)

Osteopoikylosis

This is discovered as an incidental finding and is of no clinical significance. Genetically, the disease is caused by an autosomal dominant gene, and lesions may be present at birth and during infancy. The histology was first described by Schmorl. Small (2–5 mm), well-circumscribed, round or ovoid areas of uniform sclerosis are distributed in the bone around the major joints (Figure 2.22). The skull is not usually involved,

Table 2.5   Focal areas of bone sclerosis.

Bone islands Osteopathia striata Osteopoikylosis	Innocent conditions with no adverse features and normal bone modelling
Melorheostosis Tuberous sclerosis Multiple osteomas	Widespread osteosclerosis in symptomatic disorders with abnormal bone contours

Figure 2.22

Osteopoikylosis. Discrete islands of increased bone density are seen with a periarticular distribution around the sacroiliac and hip joints, and the symphysis pubis.

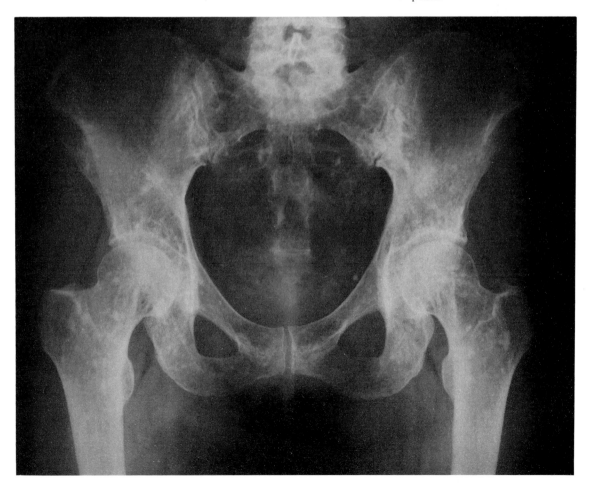

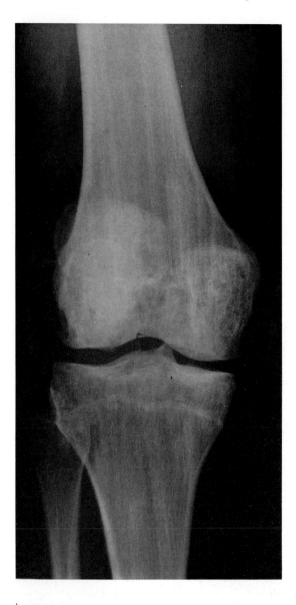

and bone remote from the articular regions is usually spared. The lesions are multiple at each site and only rarely change under observation during adult life and so are distinguishable from sclerotic metastases. Increased density is the result of bone trabeculae which are slightly thicker than normal, and regularly spaced in a parallel arrangement.

Osteopathia striata

This condition resembles osteopoikylosis and a mixture of the two types of lesion is found in some patients. Parallel, longitudinal rays of increased bony density stream backwards along the shafts of the long bones from the metaphyses in the immature skeleton, but appear to approach articular surfaces after fusion (Figure 2.23). Small bones are affected in their entirety. These asymptomatic lesions do not alter with time.

Streaks of abnormal bony density passing proximally from the growth plates are also seen in Ollier's disease. These are lucent rather than sclerotic and are usually associated with modelling abnormalities (Figure 2.24).

Bone islands

These may be solitary or multiple, are commonly situated in the femoral neck or acetabulum, and may be regarded as a forme fruste of osteopoikylosis, although the lesions are rather larger. They may occur anywhere and may increase in size under observation (Figure 2.25). They show some uptake on a bone scan and may cause slight confusion with focal metastases. Both lesions blend in with surrounding bone and may show peripheral infiltration into the adjacent medulla.

Widespread osteosclerosis in symptomatic disorders with abnormal bone contour

Melorheostosis

Clinically this condition is associated with pain in the limbs and skin contractures. Sclerotic bone

Figure 2.23

Osteopathia striata. Vertical parallel strands of increased bony density extend backwards from the articular surfaces in a mature skeleton.

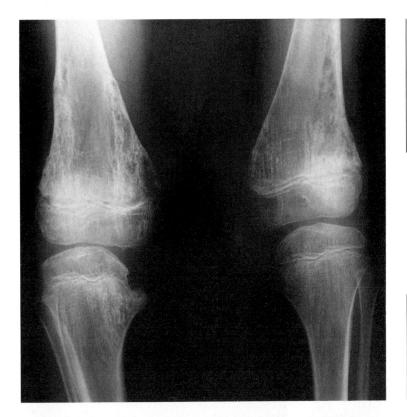

Figure 2.24

In Ollier's disease, abnormal bone texture is seen in the metaphyseal regions, consisting of strands of radiolucent cartilage streaming backwards from the epiphyseal plates. The changes are associated with abnormal modelling.

Figure 2.25

Growing bone island in the second metatarsal head in a patient with Sudeck's atrophy. With growth, the bone island in the second metatarsal head is seen to enlarge.

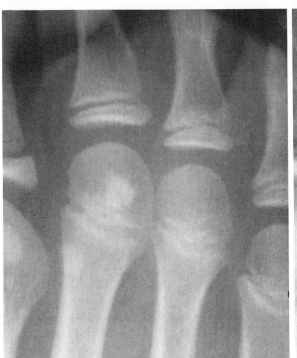

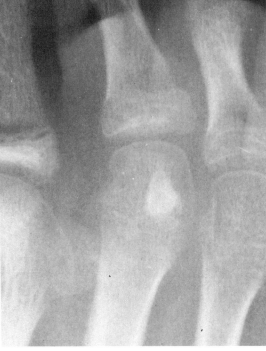

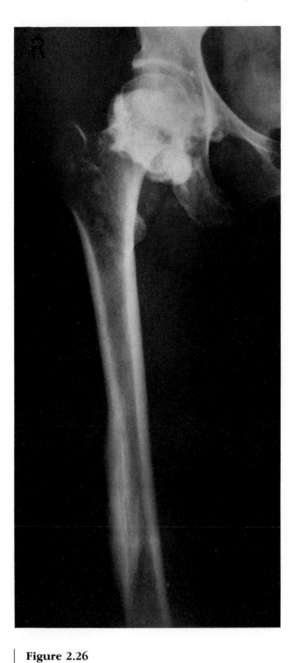

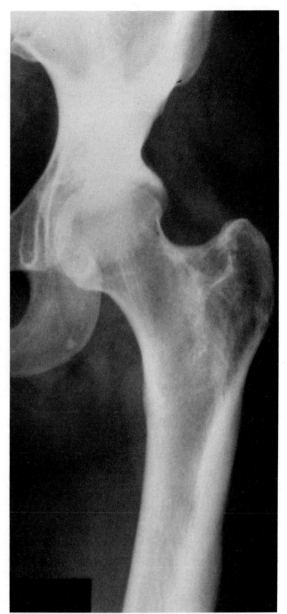

Figure 2.26

Melorheostosis. Marked new
bone formation is seen on the
lateral aspect of the midshaft
femoral cortex, and around the
femoral neck. The proximal
lesion resembles an osteoma.

Figure 2.27

Another patient with
melorheostosis showing
acetabular and femoral sclerosis.

is deposited on the internal and external aspects of the cortex of tubular bones, usually in the distribution of the sclerotomes, which are the sensory nerve supply to skeletal structures.

The external surfaces of the affected bones have a lobulated, undulant appearance similar to flowing candle-wax. The lesions cross joints, and ossification is seen in local soft tissues (Figures 2.26 and 2.27). Bones are both thickened and lengthened. (For other causes of bone lengthening, see Table 7.2., page 349.)

Often, only one half of a tubular bone is involved. It elongates along its long axis and a bowing deformity results. Large sclerotic lesions resemble osteomas and may cause gross expansion of bone. The ribs and vertebral bodies are rarely affected but no effects on the skull have been seen.

Tuberous sclerosis

This is one of the neurocutaneous syndromes or phakomatoses and has widespread manifestations, including facial adenoma sebaceum, mental defect and epilepsy. A fine honeycomb lung results in chronic pneumothorax and pulmonary arterial hypertension. Renal angiomyolipoma and lung, liver and adrenal hamartomas may also be present.

In the skull, the intracranial hamartomas or tubers may calcify and the vault itself undergoes a patchy increase in density (Figure 2.28). The long tubular bones show undulant cortical thickening, both endosteally and periosteally, and the metacarpals, metatarsals and phalanges show similar features with narrowing of the medulla (Figure 2.29). Cortico-medullary differentiation

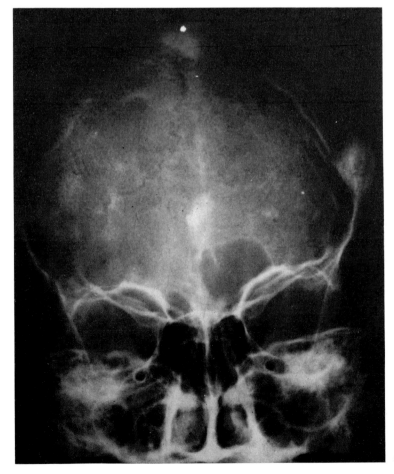

a

Figure 2.28

Plain radiographs (**a,b**) and CT (**c**) show periventricular tumours and areas of increased density in the skull vault of this patient with tuberous sclerosis.

Figure 2.28 *continued*

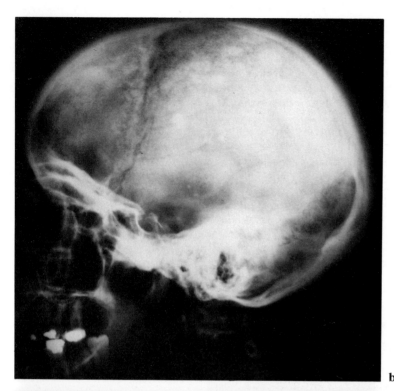

b

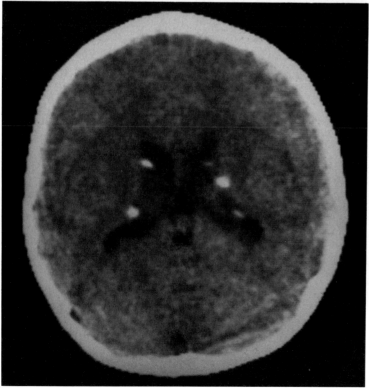

c

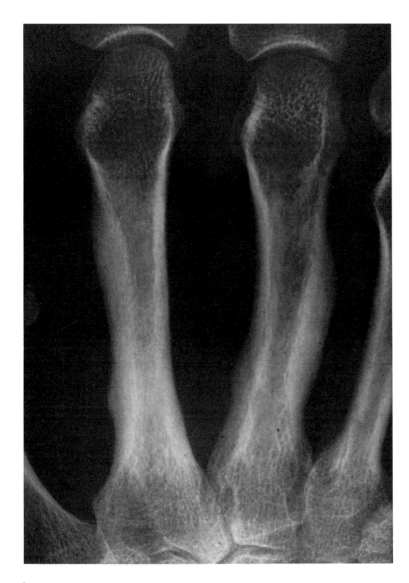

Figure 2.29

Tuberous sclerosis. Cortical thickening almost obliterates the medullary cavity. There is a smooth and undulant periosteal reaction.

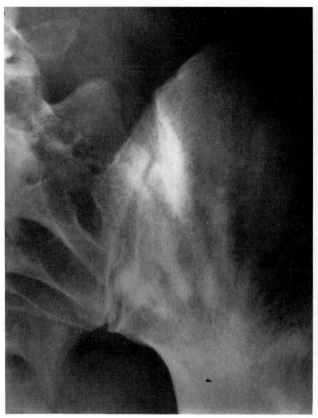

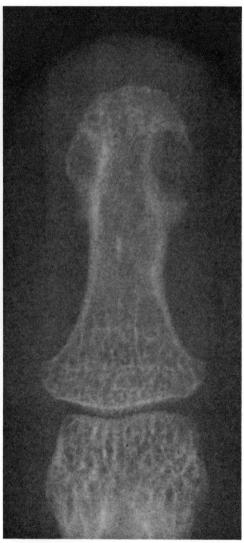

Figure 2.30

Large flame-shaped areas of
osteosclerosis are seen in the
iliac blade in this case of
tuberous sclerosis.

Figure 2.31

Tuberous sclerosis. Small, well-
corticated defects occur in the
distal phalanges, related to
subungual fibromas or
hamartomas within the bone.

is preserved. In the pelvis, large flame-shaped
areas of density occupy both iliac blades (Figure
2.30) and the vertebral bodies may show sclerosis affecting both bodies and appendages.

Hand changes are often associated with small
lytic defects, often at the distal phalanges, due to
local hamartomas or fibromas (Figure 2.31).
Skull sclerosis and hand lesions are found in 60–
65 per cent of cases and together are characteristic of the disease.

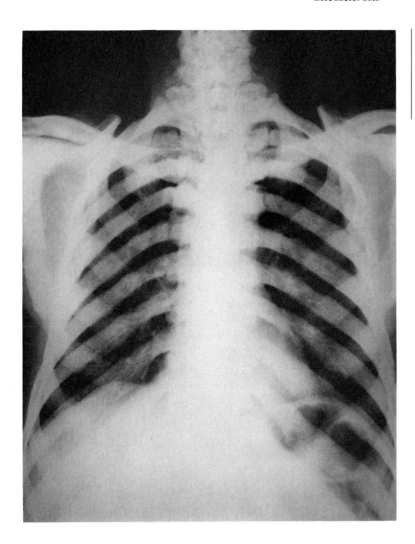

Figure 2.32

In this patient with fluorosis, there is an overall increase in bony density and the margins of the ribs are undulant due to ossification of muscle insertions.

Fluorosis

Ingestion of water containing 8 parts/million fluorine, or exposure to industrial waste, leads to fluorosis. Although low fluorine concentrations appear to protect teeth from caries, concentrations greater than 2 parts/million lead to dental enamel mottling and pitting.

Bone sections in fluorosis show cortical thickening and prominent medullary trabeculation. Radiologically, there is a pronounced, diffuse increase in bone density in the axial skeleton, with relative sparing of the cranium and peripheral bones. Cortico-medullary differentiation is lost and the bones become uniformly dense (Figure 2.32). There is marked 'fringing' or ossification of musculo-tendinous insertions into

Figure 2.33

A widespread diffuse increase in bone density with obliteration of cortico–medullary differentiation can be seen in this fluorotic patient. The ribs show osteosclerosis and are expanded with ossification of musculo-tendinous insertions.

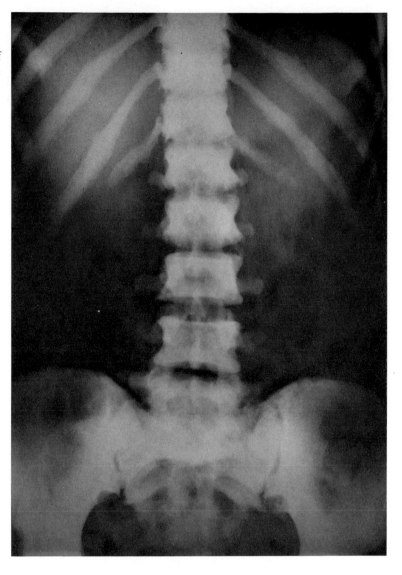

bone, resulting in lesions resembling the neostosis of ankylosing spondylitis and of diffuse idiopathic skeletal hyperostosis (ankylosing hyperostosis) (Figure 2.33) (see Chapter 6, page 339). Ligaments ossify, even in the spinal canal, and periostitis in the hands is always a feature of gross and widespread disease.

The combination of sclerosis and fringing also occurs in X-linked hypophosphataemic osteomalacia (Figure 2.34). Bowing, Looser's zones and sacroiliac joint fusion are seen in X-linked hypophosphataemic osteomalacia but not in fluorosis. The sclerosis in fluorosis does not seem to lead to bone weakening, softening or fracture, therefore fluorine therapy has been used in the treatment of osteoporosis.

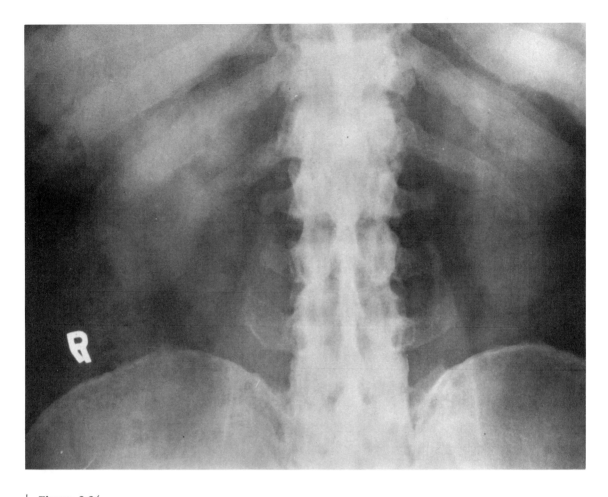

Figure 2.34

X-linked
hypophosphataemic
osteomalacia. Widespread
increase in bony density is
associated with increase in width
of the ribs and fringing.

Heavy metal poisoning

Apart from fluorine, other chemical elements cause changes in bone density and modelling. However these changes are generally epiphyseal and metaphyseal, and reflect ingestion during growth, so that isolated episodes limited in time cause local band-like metaphyseal and epiphyseal densities, more similar to osteopetrosis than fluorosis. An increase in metaphyseal density with undertubulation is best seen in children with lead poisoning (Figure 2.35) (see Chapters 5 and 7). Maternal ingestion of heavy elements, for example, matches, during pregnancy may give a similar change in the fetus due to

Figure 2.35

Metaphyseal bands of density are associated with local undertubulation in this patient with heavy metal poisoning.

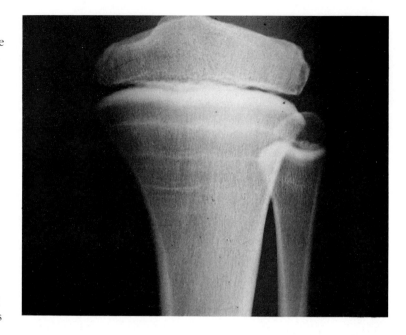

Figure 2.36

Phosphorus poisoning. Maternal ingestion of heavy metals results in the bone-within-a-bone appearance in the newborn infant.

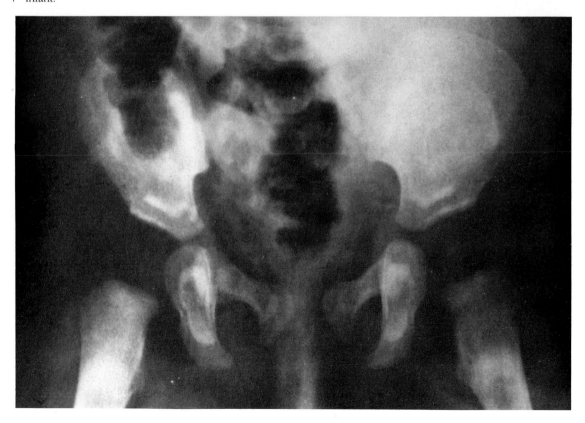

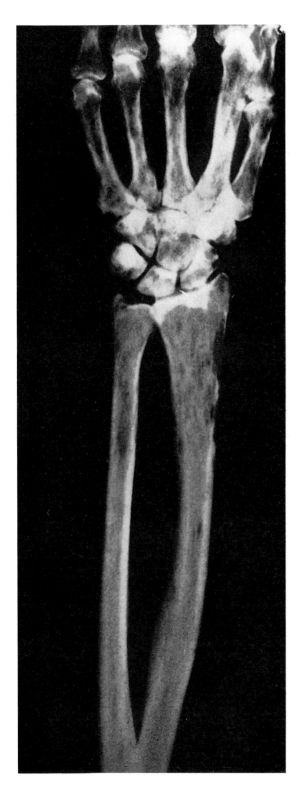

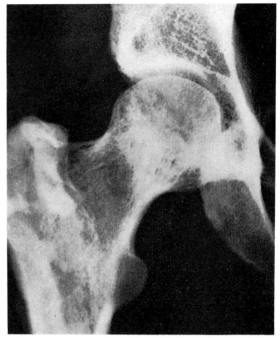

Figure 2.37

Ingestion of radium leads to areas of osteonecrosis, with resultant sclerosis and bone destruction.

phosphorus transmission across the placenta (Figure 2.36).

With radium poisoning, widespread areas of infarction and necrosis may produce areas of sclerosis and bone destruction (Figure 2.37).

Osteosclerosis, abnormal modelling, hepatospleno-megaly and pathological fractures

Osteopetrosis

This occurs in a severe recessive form known as congenita and a later, more benign form, tarda, which has a dominant inheritance.

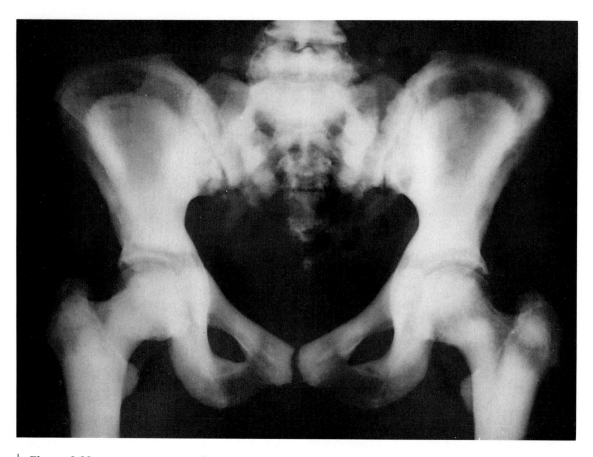

Figure 2.38

Osteopetrosis. A bone-within-a-
bone appearance is shown,
reflecting the intermittent nature
of the pathological process. This
is associated with
undertubulation, which is
particularly apparent in the
upper femora.

Bone changes occur due to failure of resorption of the primary spongiosa, which is normally
resorbed by vascular mesenchyme. Absence of
this process leads to preservation of fetal bone
with a high concentration of calcium and therefore increased bone density and metaphyseal
undertubulation. The increased density may be
uniform and all bones may be affected. In many
patients, however, the process is intermittent so
that normal bone is laid down between zones of
abnormal bone. The bands parallel the surfaces

Table 2.6 Causes of a bone-within-a-bone appearance.

Osteopetrosis

Paget's disease

Sickle-cell disease

Heavy metal poisoning

Stress lines

laying them down, so that arcuate dense curves are seen beneath the iliac crests, and cuboid densities are seen in vertebral bodies and tarsal and carpal bones—the bone-within-a-bone phenomenon (Figure 2.38) (Table 2.6).

In the congenita form, anaemia results in hepatosplenomegaly, retardation of growth and widening of bone, particularly in the diametaphyseal regions of long bones, which gives an Erlenmeyer flask appearance (see Table 5.4 in Chapter 5). Multiple fractures occur even in utero in this form and further contribute to small stature and deformity.

The tarda form is generally less severe and may not be noticed until two or three fractures are sustained in middle age due to inappropriate or minor trauma. Bone deformity due to softening occurs, and may be seen in the ribs, which can lose their normal upward convexity and slope downwards.

Pyknodysostosis

This rare form of increased bony density was distinguished from osteopetrosis by Maroteaux and Lamy in 1953. The patients are severely dwarfed, and the bones are intensely osteosclerotic, lack cortico-medullary differentiation and are susceptible to fracture.

The modelling abnormalities resemble those of cleidocranial dyostosis. Wormian bones, acroosteolysis and hypoplastic clavicles are seen, on a background of increased bony density (Figure 2.39). In addition, the angle of the mandible is

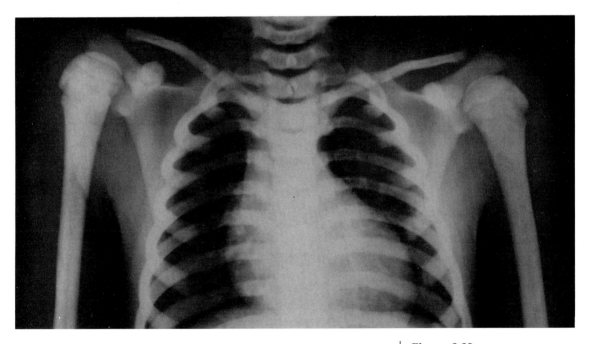

Figure 2.39

Hypoplastic clavicles can be seen in this patient with pyknodysostosis who has a uniform increase in bony density. There is undertubulation of the long bones, particularly in the metaphyses.

Figure 2.40

In pyknodysostosis, dwarfism is associated with an increase in bony density which is apparent in the parietal and occipital bones. The mandible does not have a normal angle.

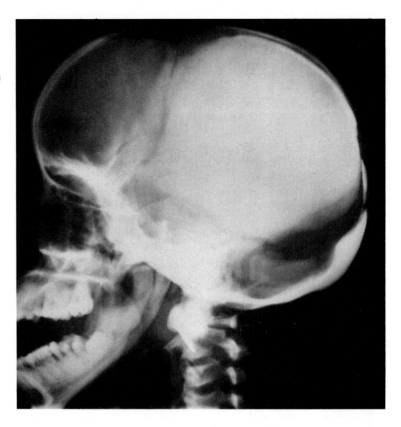

lost (Figure 2.40), the paranasal air sinuses do not develop and hepatosplenomegaly is prominent. The bones are abnormally modelled, not expanded, but rather gracile. In particular, the vertebral bodies have large anterior and posterior defects, and resemble cotton reels (Figure 2.41).

Renal osteodystrophy

In this condition, changes of secondary hyperparathyroidism are superimposed on those of osteomalacia.

An anabolic effect of parathormone on bone, tends to occur if levels are mildly elevated over a long period of time, in contrast to the bone destruction seen with higher levels of hormone in primary hyperparathyroidism (see Chapter 1). The anabolic effects include:

1 excessive maturation of osteoblasts leading to new bone formation;
2 increased laying down of osteoid, particularly in areas which have a relatively high blood supply. This osteoid calcifies under the influence of the secondarily elevated serum calcium levels.

Increased bone density in the axial skeleton and beneath the vertebral end-plates gives a 'rugger jersey' or 'sandwich spine' appearance (Figure 2.42). Trabeculae remain hazy and are not as

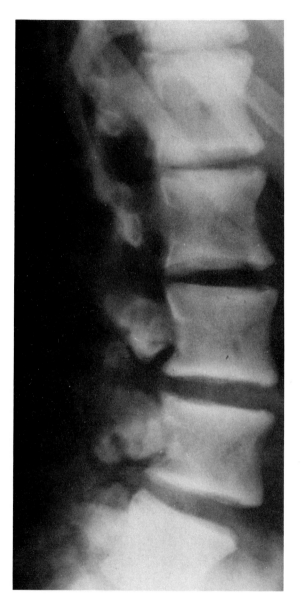

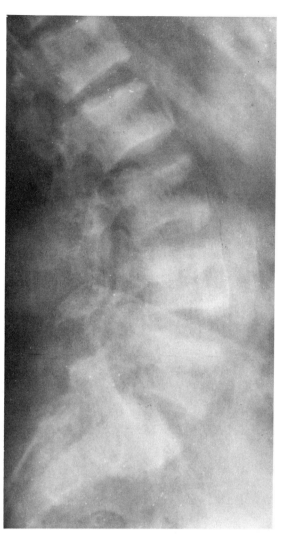

Figure 2.41

Pyknodysostosis. An increase in bony density is seen in the vertebral bodies of the lumbar spine. Anterior and posterior defects are also present, giving an appearance similar to a cotton reel. Pathological fractures have occurred in the pars interarticularis due to bone softness.

Figure 2.42

Renal osteodystrophy. There is generalized loss of bone density but sub-end-plate condensation of bone results in a rugger-jersey spine. The trabeculae are poorly defined.

well-defined or as dense as those seen in osteopetrosis, for instance (Tab.e 2.7). Diffuse sclerosis, with poor definition of affected trabeculae, is seen. Subperiosteal bone resorption also occurs at the usual sites, and cortico-medullary differentiation is poor. The major long bones may have cortical thickening, and Looser's zones may be visible. Soft tissue calcification may be seen in blood vessels, in and around joints, and occasionally in the lungs and other viscera.

Table 2.7 Causes of the rugger jersey appearance (sandwich spine or sub-end-plate condensation).

Osteopetrosis

Renal osteodystrophy

Heavy metal ingestion

Paget's disease

Growth arrest line

Figure 2.43

Avascular necrosis. Crescentic lucencies may be seen beneath the cortex of the humeral heads associated with subarticular density in this patient receiving steroids. A loose body is also present.

Avascular necrosis occurs at major articular surfaces and also at the condyles of the temporomandibular joints. This may be related to drug therapy rather than the disease and is particularly prominent at the humeral head (Figure 2.43), which is otherwise only rarely affected by avascular necrosis.

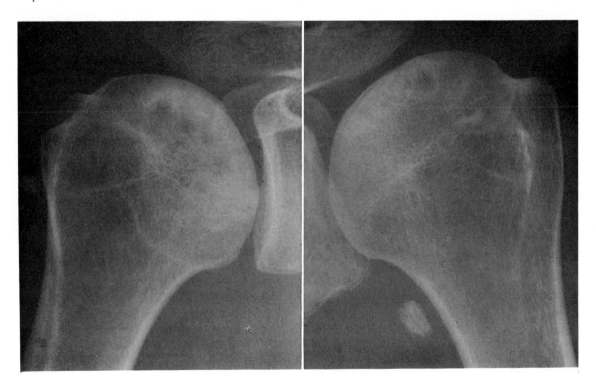

Osteosclerosis, abnormal modelling, hepatosplenomegaly and bone infarcts

Sickle-cell disease

Widespread osteosclerosis with coarsening of the trabecular pattern and loss of cortico-medullary differentiation is occasionally seen in sickle-cell disease (Figure 2.44). Radiologically, the changes predominantly involve the axial skeleton. Medullary infarction is followed by fibrosis with dystrophic calcification and the deposition of new trabecular bone upon the pre-existing trabecular framework during the healing process.

Although sickle-cell disease may be included in this diagnostic group, abnormal modelling due to medullary expansion is not usually seen in the disease in the USA or UK, although bone expansion does apparently occur in Africa, where the disease is more severe and the patients have other concurrent diseases. Marrow hyperplasia predominates in thalassaemia, as the anaemia is generally more severe, but marrow fibrosis with osteosclerosis is not seen in thalassaemia.

Splenomegaly occurs initially in sickle-cell disease, but progressive infarction causes subsequent hyposplenism. Infarcts occur at the cortices producing cortical splitting at the articular surfaces, causing avascular necrosis and articular collapse, and at vertebral end-plates resulting in

Figure 2.44

Sickle-cell disease. An increase in bone density is associated with cortical thickening and obliteration of the medullary cavity. This particularly affects the proximal femora.

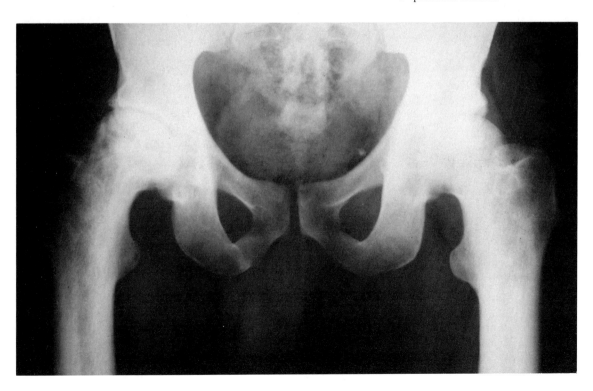

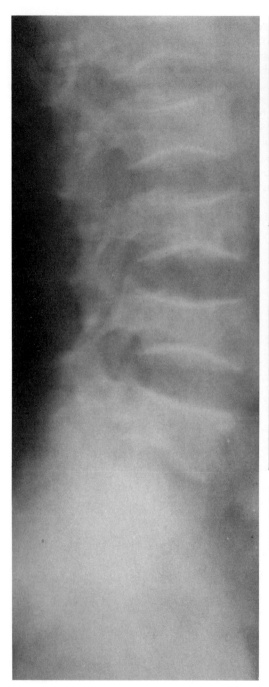

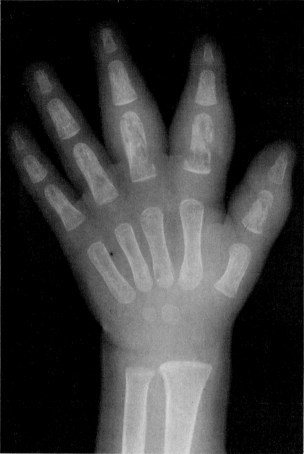

Figure 2.46

Sickle-cell disease, with soft tissue swelling associated with destruction of phalanges.

Figure 2.45

Sickle-cell disease with bone softening results in vertebral collapse and deformity of the codfish type.

a step deformity (Figure 1.66). These step-like end-plate depressions in this disease are caused by the occlusion of end-arteries, which also occurs in Gaucher's disease. Bone softening in sickle-cell disease also leads to vertebral collapse, of the codfish type (Figure 2.45). Infarcts of the hands, known as the 'hand–foot syndrome', may be aseptic or complicated by *Salmonella* or coliform osteomyelitis. Radiologically, it is often impossible to distinguish the two conditions which both have soft tissue swelling, periostitis, sequestration and pathological fractures (Figure 2.46). The lesions eventually heal with 'cone' epiphyses, premature epiphyseal fusion and phalangeal shortening.

Gaucher's disease

The acute form of this disease affects children and is fatal. Skeletal changes are rare. In the chronic form, which affects adolescents and adults, medullary infiltration results in expansion of bone with an Erlenmeyer flask appearance, as seen in thalassaemia. Focal osteolysis may be present but fibrosis and reactive sclerosis may occasionally occur as in sickle-cell disease (Figure 2.47). However, hepatosplenomegaly is much more prominent in Gaucher's disease (Figure 2.48a). Cortical, articular and end-plate infarcts are seen in both diseases. The abnormal bone fractures easily (Figure 2.48b).

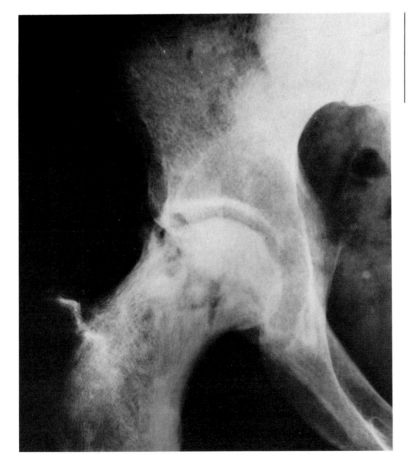

Figure 2.47

In this patient with Gaucher's disease there is widespread reactive sclerosis in the proximal femur and avascular necrosis of the femoral head.

Orthopaedic radiology

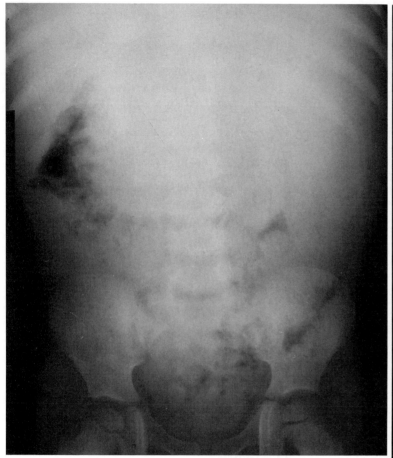

a

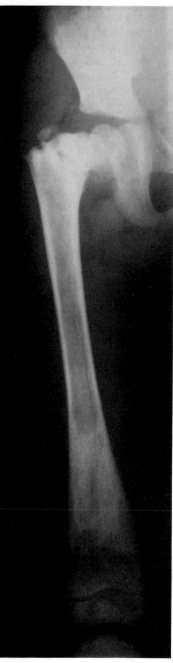

b

Figure 2.48

Gaucher's disease. (**a**) Splenomegaly. (**b**) An Erlenmeyer flask appearance of the distal femur is visible, and there is an area of medullary sclerosis proximal to it caused by infarction. Infarction at the femoral neck has resulted in sclerosis and a pathological fracture with varus deformity.

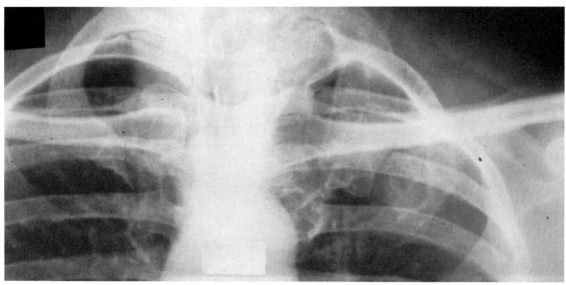

a

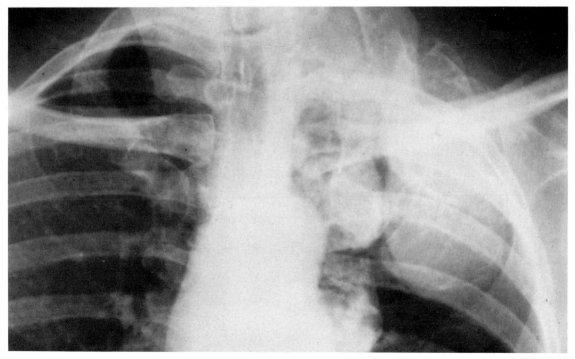

b

Figure 2.49

Fibrous dysplasia. Progressive
expansion of the ribs is shown in
this patient with polyostotic
disease.

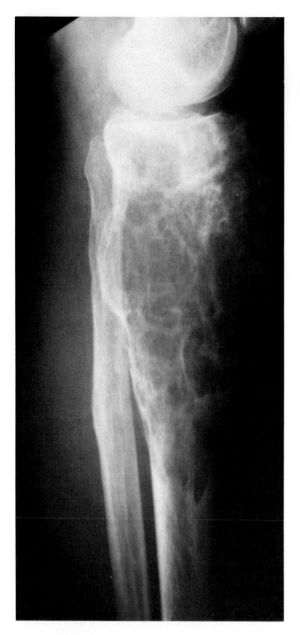

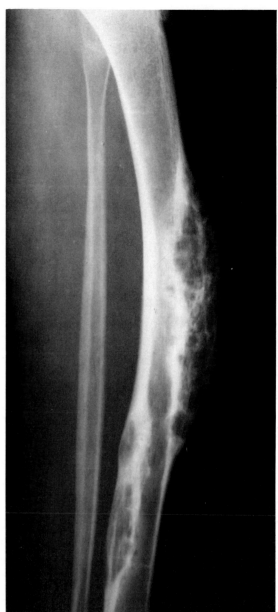

Figure 2.50

Fibrous dysplasia in the tibia
extends to the proximal articular
surface after epiphyseal fusion.

Figure 2.51

Fibrous dysplasia of the tibia. A
number of well-defined
lucencies related to the anterior
cortex are present and bowing is
also seen. This appearance is
similar to adamantinoma, but the
latter often looks much more
aggressive.

Fibrous dysplasia

This occurs in the more common monostotic form and a polyostotic form. The lesions start in infancy and childhood, but patients with monostotic disease are often older. Pathologically, normal bone is very sharply demarcated from areas of fibrous tissue which may be multilocular and also contain cysts. The fibrous tissue undergoes ossification with horseshoe-shaped whorls of woven bone. The changes are usually diametaphyseal. Their growth often, but not inevitably, ceases with skeletal maturity. Occasionally they may progress in size even in the sixth and seventh decades (Figure 2.49). After epiphyseal fusion, the tumours approach the articular surfaces and often expand bone (Figure 2.50).

Lesions are common in the femoral neck, the anterior midshaft of the tibia (Figure 2.51), the ribs (Figure 2.52) and the face (Figure 2.53). The skull is often affected, especially in polyostotic disease, and a characteristic 'blister' lesion results.

In polyostotic disease, lesions, although widespread, have a predominance for one side of the

Figure 2.52

Fibrous dysplasia. There is a cigar-shaped expansion of a rib which is typical of a benign lesion of bone. The cortex is thinned but preserved, and the lesion has a ground-glass texture.

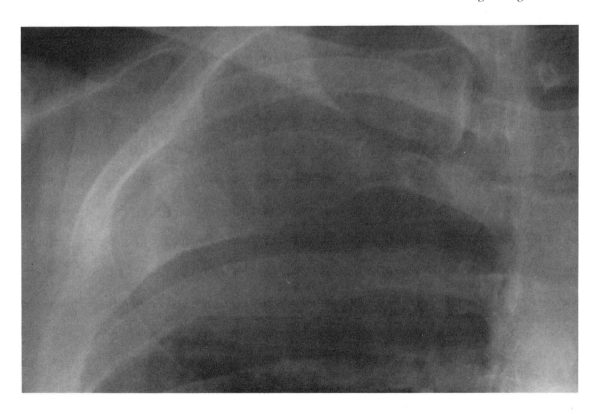

Figure 2.53

Fibrous dysplasia of the maxilla. The left maxillary antrum is expanded and sclerotic. Facial deformity is often considerable, and characteristic of this disease.

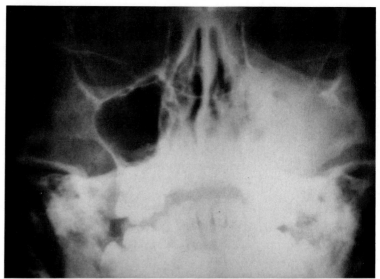

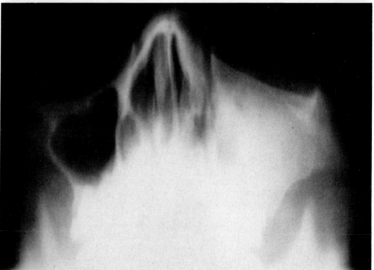

body. However, there is a more random distribution to brown tumours in hyperparathyroidism and secondary deposits, where the lesions may have a similar appearance.

Although initially radiolucent, the increasing ossification of the lesions in fibrous dysplasia gives them a mixed density, often with a very sclerotic margin or 'rind' (Figure 2.54). A ground-glass density may result (Figure 2.53). Expansion of bone occurs if the lesions reach cortices, which may be scalloped. Since the lesions are soft, bowing and pathological fractures occur.

In the femoral neck the lesions may resemble bone islands (Figure 2.55). In the ribs, a cigar- or sausage-shaped lesion is common (Figure 2.52).

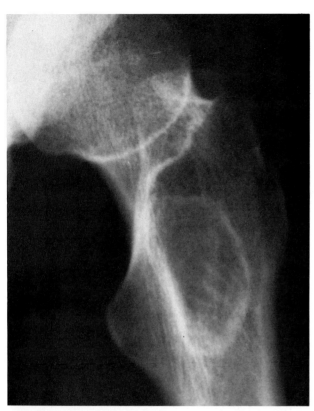

Figure 2.54

Fibrous dysplasia. A typical appearance in the proximal femur with a well-demarcated rind.

Figure 2.55

In this patient with fibrous dysplasia, the lesion is intensely sclerotic but the site and size are characteristic.

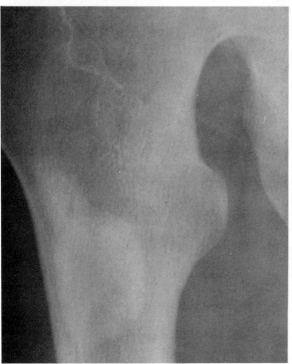

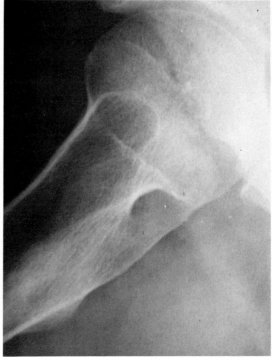

Figure 2.56

Fibrous dysplasia. A localized expansion and sclerosis of the skull vault results in a blister lesion.

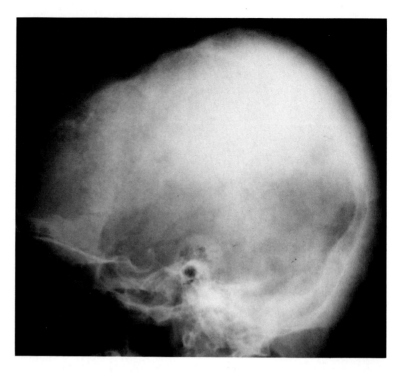

Figure 2.57

Cherubism. Numerous cysts are present in the mandible of this 14-year-old child, producing marked interruption of dentition. Some of these lesions will be truly cystic but others have radiolucent fibrous tissue within them.

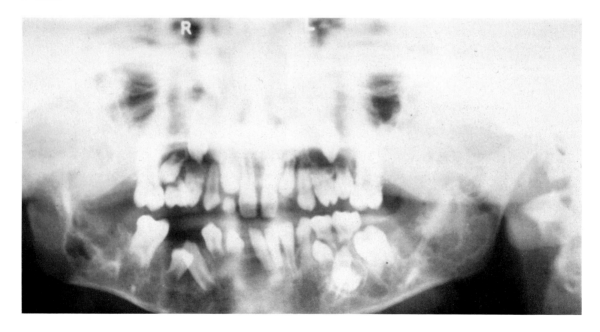

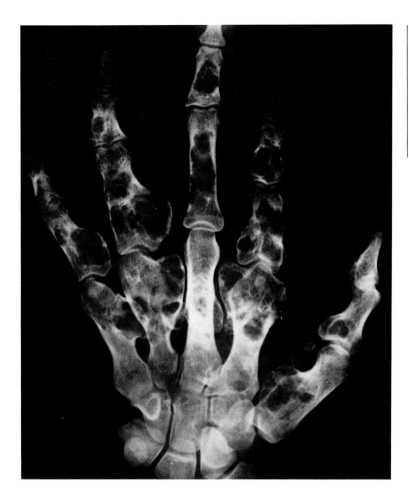

Figure 2.58

Abnormalities of growth are seen in this patient with multiple enchondromas. There is quite marked metacarpal shortening. The lesions have caused gross deformity. They are well corticated, expansile and some contain punctate calcification.

Generally, benign tumours enlarge along the long axis of a bone rather than centrifugally as in malignant lesions. In the skull, a classic lesion of the vault is the blister, a lenticular local expansion of bone of mixed or sclerotic density (Figure 2.56). Paget's disease of the vault tends to be more widespread, crosses sutures and is less locally expansile, but the texture may be similar in both diseases. The maxilla and the mandible of affected patients, usually children, show expansion, sclerosis and loss of normal bony markings, with obliteration of facial sinuses (Figure 2.53).

A familial form, called cherubism, is localized to the maxilla and mandible and is unrelated to disease elsewhere (Figure 2.57).

Punctate ossification within fibrous lesions, with bone expansion, may cause the lesions to resemble enchondromas. However these lesions may be more peripheral, commonly affecting the hands, feet, vertebral appendages and ribs. In enchondroma, a ground-glass texture is less usual than in fibrous dysplasia and the zone of reactive sclerosis around the lesions tends to be thinner and sharper (Figure 2.58).

The spine is rarely involved in this disease (Figure 2.59).

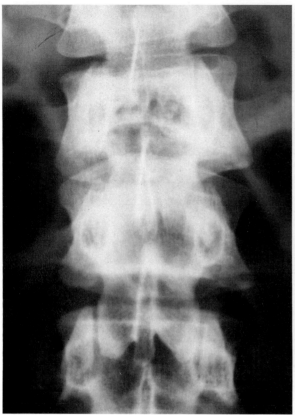 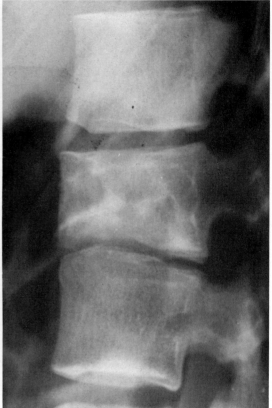

Figure 2.59

The spine is a very unusual site for fibrous dysplasia, which has caused collapse, and shows a fairly well-demarcated area of rather indolent sclerosis within which a ground-glass appearance may be seen.

Avascular necrosis and infarction of bone

Cell death in the epiphysis following local cessation of blood flow is known as avascular necrosis. Infarction is the term used when the bone shafts are affected by medullary or cortical/periosteal changes.

Cellular elements within bone die 36–48 hours after loss of blood supply, but initially the basic trabecular framework remains unaltered. Therefore, radiological change is *not* to be expected in the acute stage of ischaemia although later, reactive hyperaemia in surrounding vital bone causes the vital bone to become osteoporotic. This process does not involve avascular bone which, therefore, appears relatively sclerotic (Figure 2.60). Its density is initially unaltered. Subsequent healing takes place from the periphery of the infarcted area,

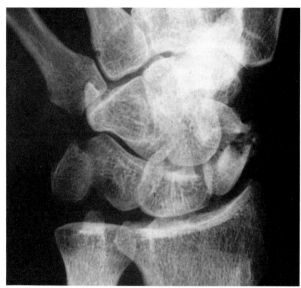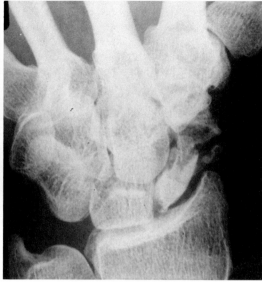

Figure 2.60

Avascular necrosis of the scaphoid follows a waist of scaphoid fracture. The proximal pole shows an increase in density. The radiographs are taken four years apart.

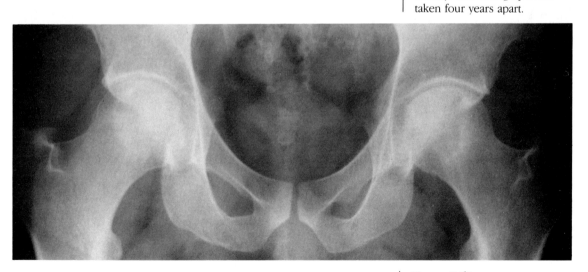

Figure 2.61

Avascular necrosis of the femoral head. Relative radiolucency in both femoral heads is surrounded by a serpiginous zone of density, the zone of creeping substitution.

with neo-vascularity, fibroblast proliferation and laying down of new bone on the framework of the old. The infarcted area of the medulla becomes surrounded by a serpiginous or ring-like zone of reactive sclerosis, termed the 'zone of creeping substitution', which represents the advancing front of neo-ossification. It may also show a central sclerosis (Figure 2.61). These changes are classically seen in the diametaphyseal regions of long bones.

Causes of diametaphyseal infarction

Infarction causing diametaphyseal sclerosis is commonly seen in the humeral and femoral necks of elderly patients. Fine, localized, medullary stippling is usually seen at multiple sites, and the surrounding medulla is normal in density with the cortex intact and the bone normally modelled (Figure 2.62).

Figure 2.62

In this example of a distal femoral infarct, there is spotty calcification of the distal femur; however, the surrounding bone shows normal density and the cortex is preserved. Note the defect on the distal femur caused by the patellar osteophyte.

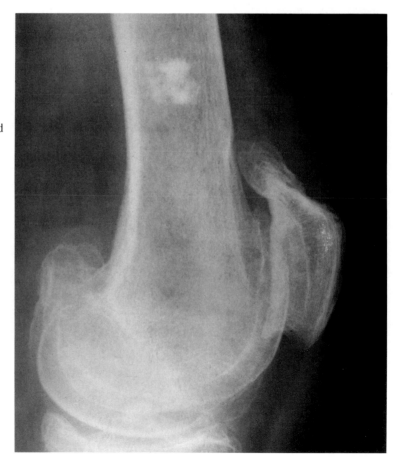

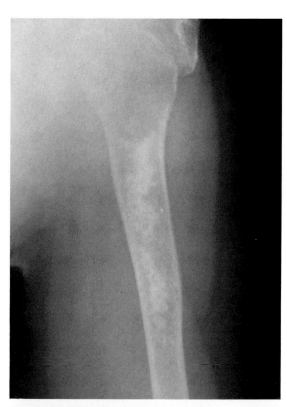

Figure 2.63

This large medullary infarct could be confused with an enchondroma or chondrosarcoma. However, the overlying cortex is preserved and the surrounding bone shows no radiolucency to suggest the presence of non-mineralized osteoid.

Figure 2.64

In this patient with caisson disease, avascular necrosis of the humeral heads has resulted in collapse with secondary degeneration. Well-demarcated medullary infarcts are visible and split cortices are also shown.

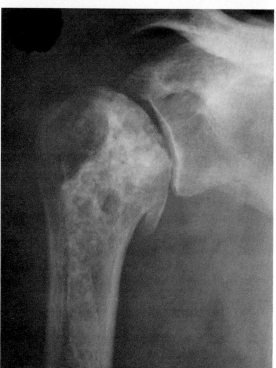

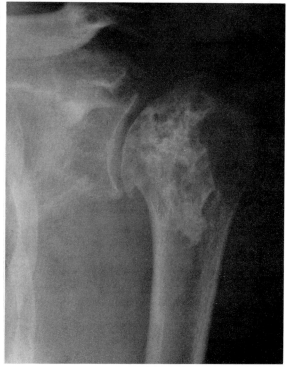

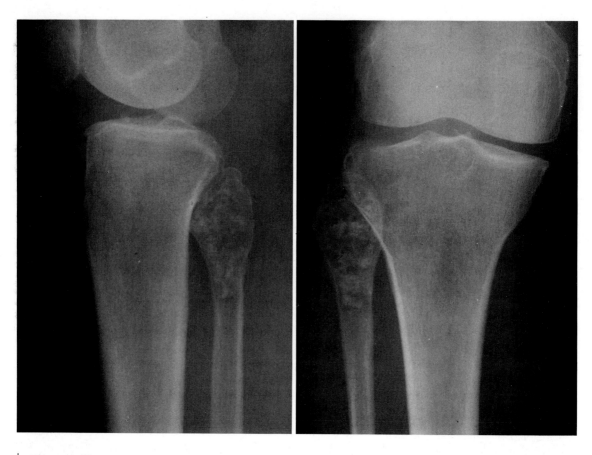

Figure 2.65

This example of enchondroma shows expansion of the proximal fibula with thinning of the cortex which is not breached. The abnormal matrix shows the speckled calcification which is characteristic of benign cartilaginous tumours.

More prominent infarctive changes are seen in sickle-cell disease, dysbaric osteonecrosis and Gaucher's disease, when larger serpiginous densities are prominent and associated with cortical and epiphyseal infarctive changes (Figures 2.63 and 2.64).

Enchondromas and chondrosarcomas may occasionally be seen in the areas typical for infarction, particularly the femoral and humeral necks. The basic chondral matrix is radiolucent and calcification or ossification may make the lesion indistinguishable from an infarct. However, these lesions are unlikely to be distributed at the multiple and symmetrical diametaphyseal sites of infarction. More importantly, the bone is likely to be expanded locally, the cortex scalloped endosteally and possibly thickened periosteally (Figure 2.65). Expansion does not occur with medullary infarcts, which will also tend not to change on serial films. Chondrosarcomas may be expected to show features of

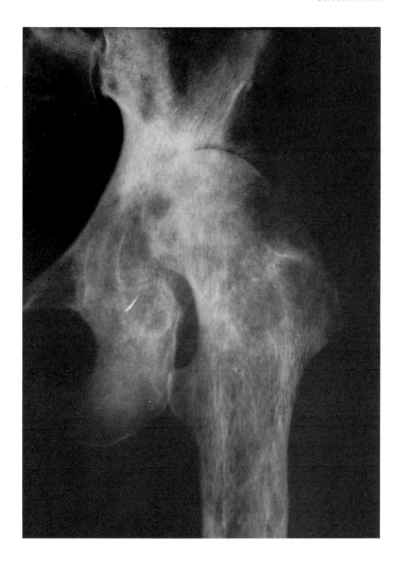

Figure 2.66

Sickle-cell disease. Widespread infarction of bone has resulted in the generalized increase in bone density. In the upper femur, linear densities representing old infarcted cortex are present.

malignant change, even if this is slow. Sarcomatous change does occur in infarcts but it is extremely rare. Cortical infarcts result in a 'bone-within-a-bone' appearance or split cortex.

Causes of cortical splitting

The dead cortex remains within the medulla due to apposition of bone beneath the elevated periosteum, and is separate from the new vital cortex (Figure 2.66). It appears dense and cannot be resorbed or become osteoporotic because of local avascularity. This density represents the tombstone of the old cortex. A split cortex may be the result of septic as well as aseptic necrosis and may also be seen with rapidly growing tumours, but still represents devascularized bone. Cortical splitting is a prominent feature of infection, sickle-cell and Gaucher's diseases.

3 | Localized lesions in bone

Localized lesions in bone may be solitary or multiple, and their distribution may be assessed by radiological skeletal survey or isotope bone scans. Multiple lesions are often due to the spread of malignant disease, especially if the patient is over 45 years of age. Therefore, the assumption is that multiple lesions are malignant until proven otherwise. Even if a lesion is seen to be solitary and has the radiological features of malignancy, it is still more likely to be a secondary deposit than a primary malignant tumour of bone as these are rare. It is most important to distinguish between benign and malignant lesions. Most bone lesions are distinctive in appearance but some cannot easily be diagnosed radiologically or even histologically (Table 3.1).

Differentiation between benign and malignant lesions of bone

Zone of transition

This defines the nature of the interface between normal and abnormal bone. In general, malignant lesions are characterized by rapid growth which may be assessed on serial radiographs. Tumour permeation results in a wide and poorly-defined

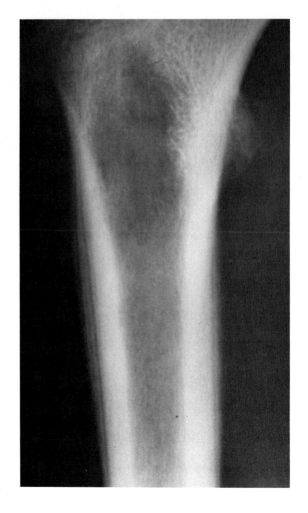

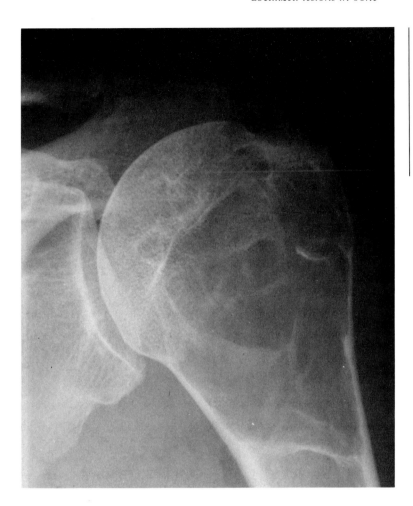

Figure 3.1

In this patient with Ewing's sarcoma, the zone of transition between normal and abnormal bone is wide, particularly inferiorly. Permeation extends beyond the main mass of the lesion, as shown by the presence of a lamellar periostitis extending to the midshaft.

Figure 3.2

This simple bone cyst is at a characteristic site, the proximal humerus, and shows endosteal scalloping. There is a narrow zone of transition between normal and abnormal bone with a thin zone of reactive sclerosis. The cyst shows slight trabeculation.

zone of transition between normal and abnormal bone (Figure 3.1). Infection may give a similar appearance.

Benign lesions grow slowly and often do not alter on serial radiographs. Their lack of local permeation results in a narrow zone of transition, so that the lesion is surrounded by normal bone (Figure 3.2). This may be altered by infection, fracture, surgery or healing. Malignant transformation of benign lesions occasionally occurs, for example, from chondroma to chondrosarcoma,

Table 3.1   Classification of primary bone tumours and tumour-like lesions.

	Benign	Malignant
A Presumed to arise from skeletal connective tissue		

Tumours forming bone	Osteoma
	  Exostosis
	Osteoid osteoma
	Benign osteoblastoma
	  (Giant osteoid osteoma)
		*Osteosarcoma
		Parosteal osteosarcoma
		Periosteal osteosarcoma

Tumours forming cartilage	Enchondroma
	  Solitary or multiple
	Benign chondroblastoma
	Chondromyxoid fibroma
	Cartilage-capped exostosis
	  (Osteochondroma)
	  Solitary or multiple
		Chondrosarcoma

Tumours forming fibrous tissue	Non-ossifying fibroma
	  Fibrous cortical defect
	  Metaphyseal fibrous defect
	Fibrous dysplasia
	  Probably not neoplastic
		Fibrosarcoma
		Malignant fibrous
		  histiocytoma

Tumours forming osteoclastic tissue		Giant-cell tumour Locally malignant
B Tumours of unknown histogenesis		
	Simple bone cyst	Ewing's tumour Undifferentiated sarcomas Ameloblastoma of long bones

	Benign	Malignant
C Presumed to arise from other skeletal components		

Blood and lymph vessels	Haemangioma
	    Solitary or multiple
	Haemangiomatosis
	    Massive osteolysis
	    Vanishing bone disease
	Lymphangiomatosis
	Aneurysmal bone cyst
	Glomus tumour
	    Haemangiopericytoma
		Angiosarcoma

Nerves	Neurofibroma Neurilemmoma	Neurosarcoma
Fat	Lipoma	Liposarcoma
Notochord		Chordoma Locally malignant
Epithelium	Implantation dermoid cyst	
Dental epithelium	Ameloblastoma of jaw	
Lymphoid and haemopoietic tissues		Leukaemia Lymphadenoma Hodgkin's disease Lymphosarcoma Plasmacytoma Myelomatosis Reticulum cell sarcoma

*Paget's sarcoma is usually osteosarcomatous but may be a fibrosarcoma, a reticulum cell sarcoma or, rarely, a chondrosarcoma.
Adapted from Sutton D (ed.), *Textbook of radiology* 1st edn., (E & S Livingstone: Edinburgh 1969), with permission.

Figure 3.3

Fibrosarcoma in fibrous
dysplasia. There is a pathological
fracture of the upper femur with
resultant deformity and soft
tissue ossification. Expansion is
longstanding, as shown at the
greater trochanter. The abnormal
bone extends down the shaft of
the femur, which is expanded,
curved and, in places, a ground-
glass appearance may be seen.

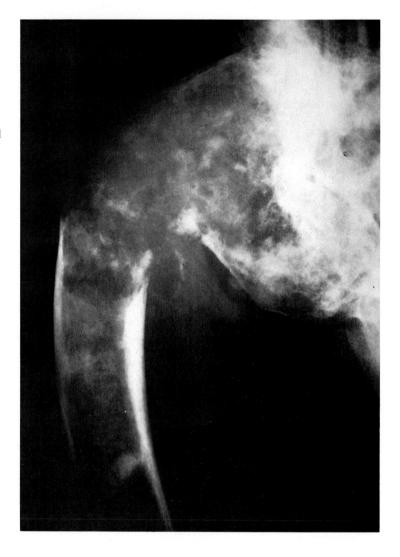

or fibrosarcoma in fibrous dysplasia (Figure 3.3).
This is associated with a change in the nature of
the lesion, rapid growth and loss of definition,
resulting in a wide zone of transition, and often
pain.

Zone of reactive sclerosis

The slow growth of benign lesions enables the
surrounding bone to form a shell of reactive new
bone. In some conditions, such as fibrous cortical
defect, this is thin and well defined (Figure 3.4).
Fibrous dysplasia tends to have a fairly well-
defined zone of reactive sclerosis, 2–4 mm wide,
whose appearance is similar to that of the rind of
an orange, giving the so-called 'rind sign' (Figure
3.5). Osteoblastomas tend to be surrounded by
gross reactive sclerosis (Figure 3.6), which is
often poorly defined. Osteoclastomas, although
usually benign, are often surprisingly poorly
defined (Figure 3.7).

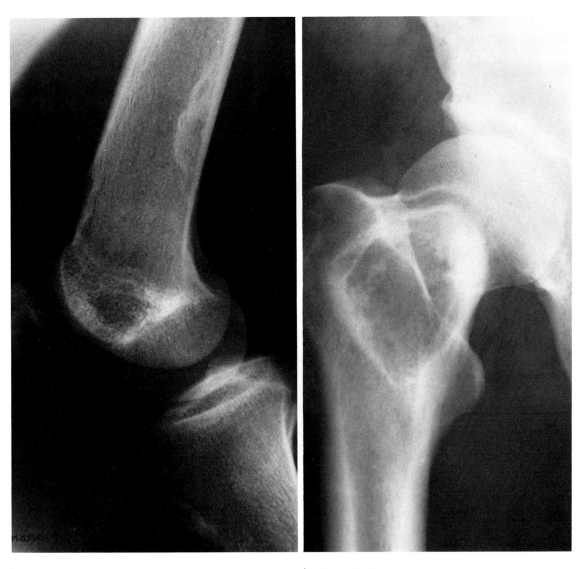

Figure 3.4

Fibrous cortical defect. These lesions characteristically occur at the metaphyses around the knee, often posteriorly. They are characterized by their subcortical location and a narrow zone of reactive sclerosis.

Figure 3.5

In this patient with fibrous dysplasia, the lytic lesion in the pertrochanteric region of the upper femur is surrounded by a thick rind of reactive sclerosis. There is some matrix calcification within it. The femoral neck is slightly expanded.

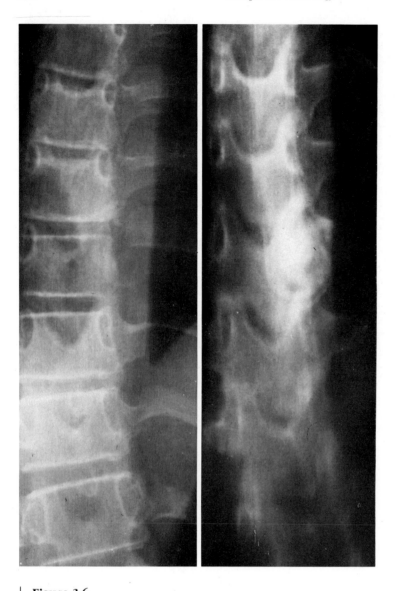

Figure 3.6

Osteoblastoma. A scoliosis is
associated with expansion of the
left pedicle of the ninth thoracic
vertebra at the apex of the curve.
On the concavity, an expansile
lesion, shown on tomography, is
seen as a very dense nidus of
bone surrounded by a thin
radiolucent rim. These
appearances are characteristic of
osteoid osteoma and
osteoblastoma in the spine.

Malignant tumours are permeative and usually
have little surrounding reactive sclerosis. An
exception is the chondrosarcoma, perhaps
because its growth is often slow (Figure 3.8).

The nature and shape of the bone lesion

Benign lesions arising in the medulla are often
round or ovoid until they reach the cortex where

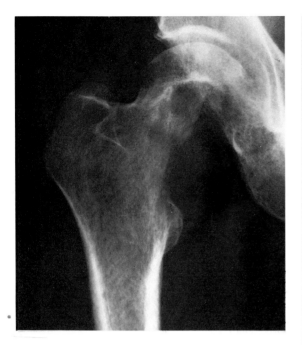

Figure 3.7

Giant-cell tumour. Superiorly, the lesion has a fairly well-demarcated rim of reactive sclerosis but inferiorly and medially, where the calcar has been destroyed, the tumour is poorly defined. It may be diagnosed as a giant-cell tumour because it reaches the articular surface of the femoral head, although only marginally.

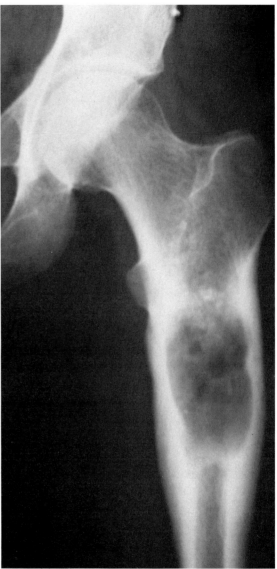

Figure 3.8

Chondrosarcoma. Despite the medullary bone destruction and endosteal cortical scalloping, smooth periosteal new bone is laid down on the outside of the cortex. The centre of the lesion shows punctate calcification. The zone of transition inferiorly is narrow with a well-demarcated zone of sclerosis but superiorly the lesion is permeative.

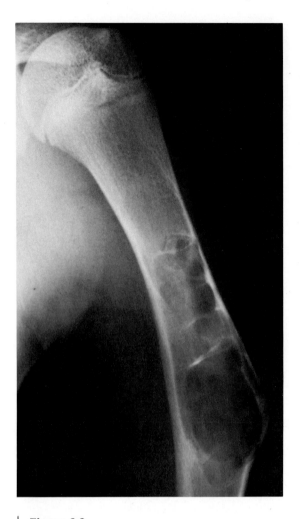

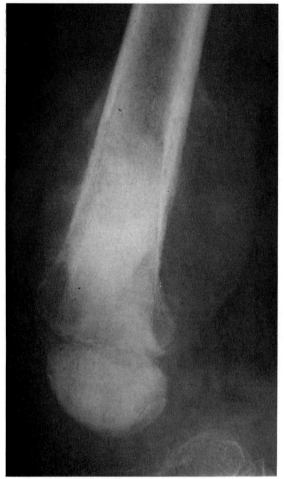

Figure 3.9

Simple bone cyst. The
multilocular expansile lesion lies
at the midshaft, having been left
behind by bone growth at the
epiphyseal plate. There is a
narrow zone of transition with a
thin rim of reactive sclerosis. The
cortex shows endosteal
scalloping but is not breached.

Figure 3.10

Osteogenic sarcoma. There is a
well defined soft tissue mass
around the distal femur. The
periphery of the tumour is
marked by a Codman's triangle
and the tumour extends to the
distal epiphyseal plate. The
epiphysis is also dense, possibly
because of invasion by tumour or
avascular necrosis. There is
perpendicular sunray
spiculation.

their shape is modified. Endosteal scalloping may occur (Figure 3.9), and the resorption of cortex is smooth. Some malignant lesions, such as osteogenic sarcoma, expand centrifugally, breaking through the cortex into soft tissues to form well-defined masses (Figure 3.10), whereas other malignant lesions, such as Ewing's tumour and fibrosarcoma, tend to infiltrate along the shaft of the bone, irregularly permeating cortices before invading soft tissues.

In general, bone replacement in benign lesions is total, within the confines of the circumscribed tumour. Malignant lesions tend to be permeative, patchy and infiltrative so that destruction and replacement is not always uniform. Tumours are not uniformly radiolucent; their appearance depends upon their nature and subsequent behaviour.

Cortical and periosteal changes

Benign lesions can cause such endosteal cortical scalloping, thinning and displacement that the displaced cortex is no longer radiologically visible. This unusual sequence occurs, for example, with aneurysmal bone cysts (Figure 3.11).

Generally, malignant lesions rapidly breach the cortex, elevating the periosteum, beneath which new bone is laid down. Primary malignant tumours of bone often result in large well-defined soft tissue masses which are visualized because of the displacement of overlying and intact fat planes (Figure 3.10). This is also seen in some secondary malignant tumours originating in renal and thyroid primary lesions, but most secondary deposits are not associated with significant soft tissue masses. Following the collapse of thoracic vertebral bodies, displacement of the paraspinal lines is seen against radiolucent lung. Infective soft tissue masses are poorly defined because oedema infiltrates local fat planes which are therefore no longer visible.

Where a tumour mass breaks centrally through the elevated layers of periosteal new bone, a Codman's triangle is formed at the margins of the extracortical lesion. This can also be seen in infections. A similar appearance occurs with marginal buttressing with rapidly growing benign lesions, such as aneurysmal bone cysts and giant-cell tumours.

Matrix and soft tissue calcification

Table 3.1 classifies tumours according to their cell of origin and benignity or malignancy. Usually, tumours are of osteoid, chondroid, fibrous, lipoid or angiomatous origin and may be benign or malignant. Each of these basic matrices may calcify or ossify in bone and soft tissue, usually in a fairly typical, diagnostic manner, for example, progressive ossification occurs centrally in osteoid osteomas, and punctate calcification in chondral tumours. Classically, fibrous dysplasia ossifies producing a speckled or ground-glass appearance. Fibrosarcomas ossify in a rather cloudy and irregular way, while the osteoid matrix in osteosarcoma is heavily and irregularly ossified, both in bone and soft tissues (Figure 3.12).

Age of incidence of benign and malignant lesions

The patient's age is invaluable for the correct diagnosis of bone tumours. Osteogenic sarcoma should not be diagnosed below the age of five years, and giant-cell tumours below the age of local epiphyseal fusion. Simple bone cysts and non-ossifying fibromas are not generally seen after skeletal fusion, although exceptions occasionally occur. Giant-cell tumours can arise in children and also in the seventh decade, but these lesions are rare exceptions to the rule. Most primary tumours of bone present before skeletal maturity (Tables 3.2, 3.3 and 3.4).

Sites

The site of a tumour before skeletal fusion may be epiphyseal, metaphyseal or diaphyseal (Tables 3.5–3.8), and is often specific. Thus, chondroblastoma occurs before fusion in the epiphysis, simple bone cyst in the metaphysis and fibrous dysplasia in the diametaphysis. After fusion, giant-cell tumours occur in subarticular sites and should not be diagnosed elsewhere. Ewing's

Figure 3.11

Aneurysmal bone cyst. (**a**) These
lesions can grow faster than any
other tumour. They
characteristically enlarge the
bone, giving a balloon-like
appearance. The cortex may
become so thin that it is invisible,
but will re-appear after
radiotherapy. (**b**) The
arteriogram shows the highly
vascular nature of the lesion and
its extent.

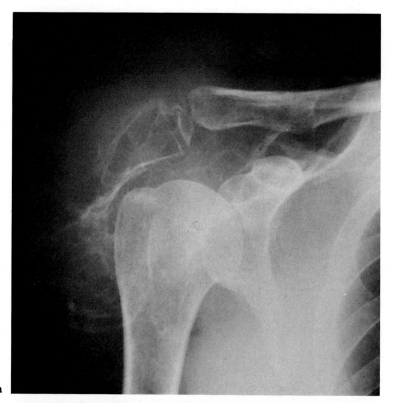

a

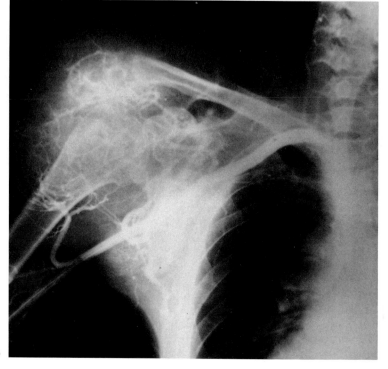

b

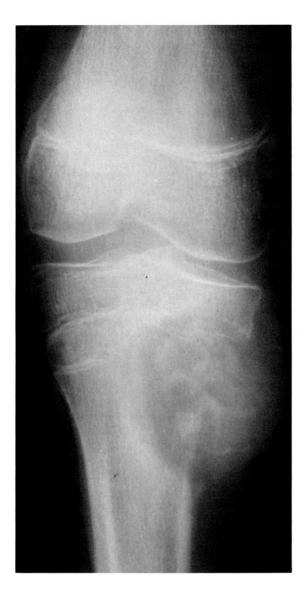

Figure 3.12

Osteosarcoma. There is a fairly well defined metaphyseal area of bone destruction which has breached the cortex. A large soft tissue mass contains amorphous calcification and there is a minor Codman's triangle. Elsewhere, quite marked osteoporosis is shown by loss of medullary trabeculation and thinning of the cortices, which are now prominent.

Table 3.2   Age of incidence of benign lesions.

Lesion type	Age (years)
Eosinophilic granuloma	2–30
Simple bone cyst	5–20
Non-ossifying fibroma	5–20
Osteoid osteoma	5–30
Osteoblastoma	5–30
Aneurysmal bone cyst	10–30
Chondroblastoma	10–20
Chondromyxoid fibroma	10–20
Giant-cell tumour	20–45

Table 3.3   Age of incidence of malignant lesions.

Lesion type	Age (years)
Leukaemia	0–5
Neuroblastoma	0–5
Ewing's sarcoma	5–25
Osteogenic sarcoma	10–25; 60–80
Periosteal osteosarcoma	20–30
Reticulum cell sarcoma	25–40
Parosteal osteosarcoma	25–35
Fibrosarcoma	30–45
Chondrosarcoma	35–55
Malignant fibrous histiocytoma	40 +
Secondary lesions and myeloma	45–80

Table 3.4   Solitary cyst-like lesions of bone.

	Calcifies	Expands	Before skeletal fusion
Echondroma	C	E	B
Nonossifying fibroma	—	—	B
Fibrous dysplasia	C	E	B
Aneurysmal bone cyst	—	E	B
Hyperparathyroidism	—	E	—
Chondroblastoma	C	—	B
Chondromyxoid fibroma	C	—	—
Cystic infection, particularly tuberculosis	C	—	—
Eosinophilic granuloma	—	—	B
Giant-cell tumour	—	E	—
Hydatid	—	E	—
Haemophilic pseudotumour	—	E	B
Metastasis from carcinoma of kidney and thyroid	—	E	—
Plasmacytoma	—	E	—
Simple bone cyst	—	—	B
Osteoid osteoma	C	—	B
Osteoblastoma	C	E	B
Vascular lesions	C	E	—
Malignant fibrous histiocytoma	—	E	—

Table 3.5   Tumours and tumour-like lesions appearing in epiphyses or apophyses.

Chondroblastoma (in the immature skeleton)

Fibrous dysplasia ⎫ After skeletal
Giant-cell tumour ⎭ maturity

Malignant fibrous histiocytoma (late adult life)

Cysts or geodes associated with arthritides ⎫
Synovial tumours ⎬ Usually on both sides of a joint
Osteomyelitis, especially cystic tuberculosis ⎭

Secondary deposits after 45–50 years of age

Table 3.6   Tumours and tumour-like lesions of the metaphysis.

Simple bone cyst

Non-ossifying fibroma, fibrous cortical defects

Malignant fibrous histiocytoma

Fibrous dysplasia

Enchondroma, chondromyxoid fibroma

Eosinophilic granuloma

Simple and tuberculous infections

Osteogenic sarcoma

Parosteal osteosarcoma

Chondrosarcoma

Leukaemia

Neuroblastoma

Table 3.7 Tumours and tumour-like lesions occurring in the diaphysis.

Ewing's tumour, reticulum cell sarcoma

Less commonly, osteogenic sarcoma

Metastases and myeloma

Simple bone cyst (late)

Enchondroma

Fibrous dysplasia

Brown tumour in hyperparathyroidism

Eosinophilic granuloma

Adamantinoma (of the tibia)

Table 3.8 Focal lesions occurring in specific sites.

Site	Lesion
Ribs	Metastases
	Myeloma
	Brown tumours in hyperparathyroidism
	Fibrous dysplasia
	Hydatid disease
	Angioma
	Paget's disease
Fingers	Enchondroma
	Cysts or geodes associated with arthritides
	Sarcoidosis ⎫
	Leprosy ⎬ Granulomas
	Tuberculosis ⎫
	Syphilis ⎬ Spina ventosa
	Enlarged nutrient foramina in Sarcoidosis
	Leprosy
	Haemolytic anaemia
	Implantation dermoid ⎫
	Subungual fibroma ⎬ Distal phalanx
	Tuberous sclerosis ⎭
	Glomus tumour
	Brown tumour in hyperparathyroidism
	Secondary deposit, usually pulmonary in origin
Sacrum	Anterior sacral meningocoele
	Myeloma
	Chordoma
	Neurofibroma
	Ependymoma
	Dermoid
	Invasion from rectal or ovarian cancer
Skull	Fibrous dysplasia
	Osteoporosis circumscripta (Paget's disease)
	Neurofibromatosis
	Eosinophilic granuloma
	Sarcoidosis
	Osteomyelitis, including tuberculosis
	Fungal infections (Madura skull)
	Developmental defects
	Hydatid
	Erosion from skull tumours
	Leptomeningeal cyst
	Brown tumour of hyperparathyroidism
	Arteriovenous malformation, haemangioma
	Metastasis, myeloma, occasionally tumours, eg osteoblastoma
	Meningioma
	Cholesteatoma
	Burr hole

Table 3.9 Focal lucent area containing calcification surrounded by sclerosis.

Osteoid osteoma	(<1.5 cm)	⎫
Osteoblastoma	(>1.5 cm)	⎬ Generally solitary and painful
Brodie's abscess		
Chondrosarcoma		⎭
Lipoma of bone		⎫ Generally painless,
Enchondroma		⎬ solitary or
Fibrous dysplasia		⎭ multiple
Infarcts		Often painful, generally multiple

tumours are classically diaphyseal and osteogenic sarcomas metaphyseal.

Calcification or ossification occurs in tumours originating in osteoid, chondroid and fibrous tissue, as well as in lipomatous or vascular tumours. Usually the appearance of the lesion is characteristic, enabling the diagnosis to be made (Table 3.9).

Specific lesions

Osteoid osteoma

This is a small (<1.5 cm) lesion found in children and young adults, which is more common in males and may present in any bone producing pain characteristically at night. It is usually seen in the major long bones and vertebral appendages (Figure 3.13). Radiologically the lesion has a lucent central nidus consisting of vascular osteoid which undergoes progressive ossification, starting with a small central fleck of density (Figure 3.14). The surrounding reactive sclerosis may be so marked

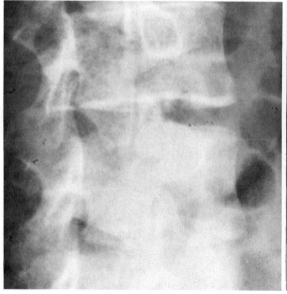
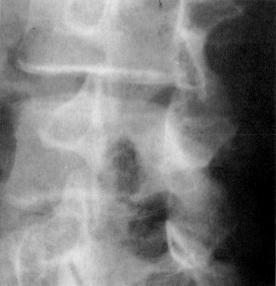

Figure 3.13

Oblique views show unilateral sclerosis and expansion of vertebral appendages. This appearance is typical of osteoid osteoma.

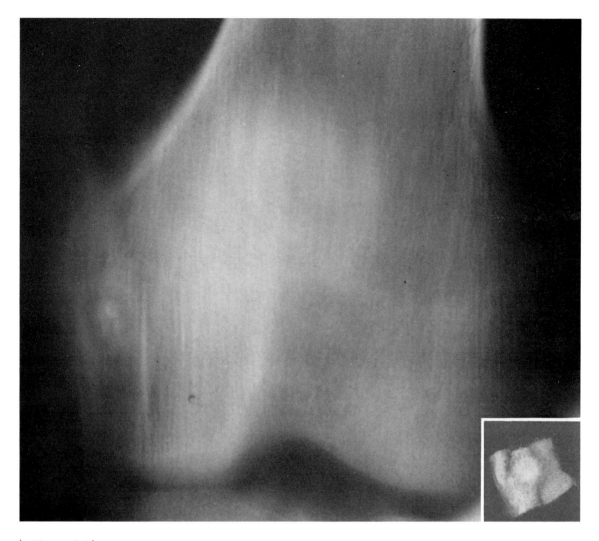

Figure 3.14

Ossification of an osteoid
osteoma in the femoral condyle.
Insert: Surgical specimen.

that it obscures the tumour, particularly if the lesion is related to the cortex (Figure 3.15). This classically occurs in the region of the lesser trochanter of the femur (Figure 3.16), when tomography may be helpful. Alternatively, if the lesion is in a bone which has little or no periosteum, such as the talus, it may not be visualized because of a lack of surrounding sclerosis, although it may be seen on tomography (Figure 3.17). The entire tumour is often extruded from the neck of the talus into the local soft tissues, resembling an osteochondroma (Figure 3.18). An osteoid osteoma is characteristically well visualized on isotope bone scans, both in the immediate vascular phase and on the delayed images (Figure 3.19). The lesion often cannot be

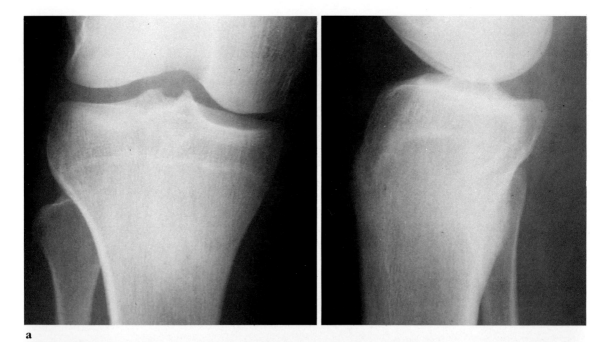

a

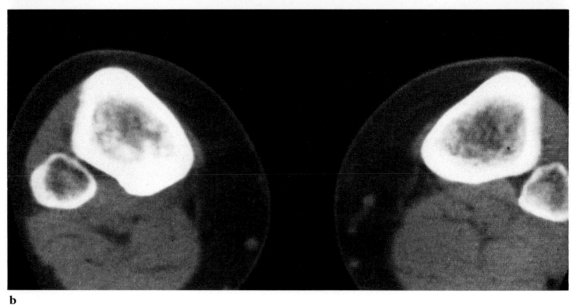

b

Figure 3.15

Osteoid osteoma. (**a**) There is diffuse osteosclerosis of the proximal tibia on the anteroposterior view, while the lateral view shows the change to lie posteriorly. There is cortical thickening, but no central lucency is seen. (**b**) In the CT scan the right tibia shows posterior cortical thickening with local encroachment upon the medulla by dense new bone, but a central lucency cannot be identified.

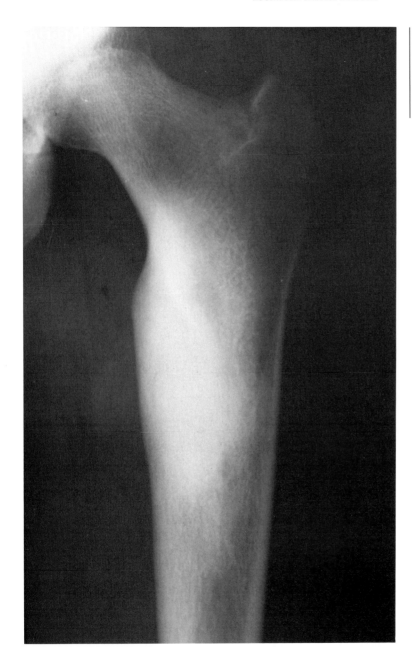

Figure 3.16

An osteoid osteoma in the region of the lesser trochanter presents as a sclerotic mound of cortical bone, often without visualization of the causative lesion.

Figure 3.17

Osteoid osteoma. (**a**) The
radiograph shows osteoporosis
but, at the medial aspect of the
femoral head, there is patchy
sclerosis with buttressing
periostitis on the calcar. (**b**) The
tomogram clearly reveals the
radiolucent osteoid osteoma with
a central fleck of density. Osteoid
osteomas excite little reactive
sclerosis at joints in the absence
of local periosteum.

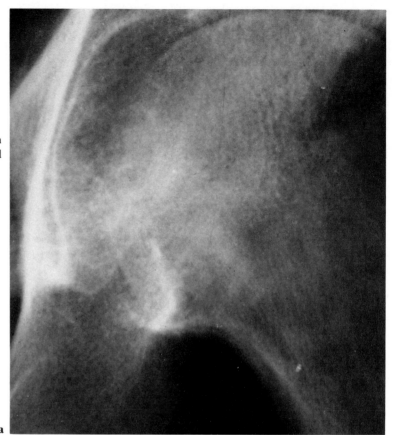

a

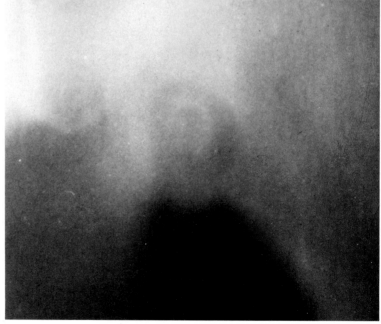

b

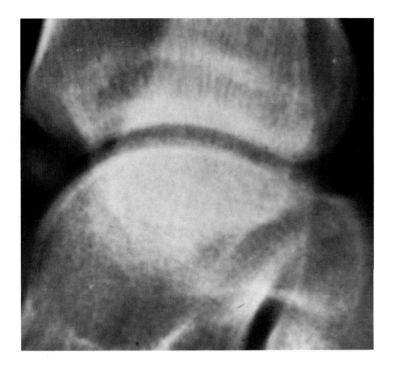

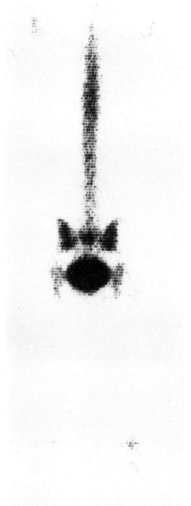

Figure 3.18

This osteoid osteoma of the talus resembles a small extruded fleck of bone, or an osteochondroma, and may be confused with local degeneration or trauma.

Figure 3.19

A radioisotope bone scan of an osteoid osteoma shows an increase in uptake in the left heel due to an osteoid osteoma of the calcaneum which was not obvious on the plain radiograph. This is not uncommon at this site and leads to a delayed diagnosis. Constant or long-term pain in a child with an apparently normal radiograph should always be followed by radioisotope bone scanning to exclude this lesion.

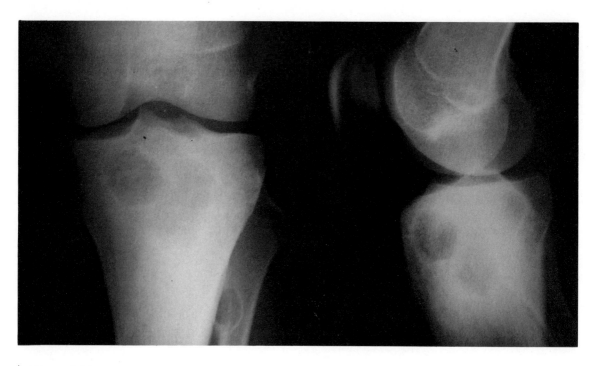

Figure 3.20

Brodie's abscess. Well-defined
radiolucent areas of bone
destruction are seen in the
proximal tibia surrounded by
quite gross local reactive
sclerosis. The lesion of the
proximal fibula is a non-ossifying
fibroma. It has a thinner margin
and the surrounding bone is
normal.

distinguished from a Brodie's abscess in chronic
osteomyelitis, which may be seen in areas atypical for osteoid osteoma, for example, the skull,
and is often metaphyseal since, in childhood, the
metaphysis is commonly the site of an infection.
Dystrophic calcification which occurs in the
centre of the destructive lesion is surrounded by
reactive sclerosis (Figure 3.20) and there may be
an overlying periositis as occurs with osteoid
osteoma. The osteoid osteoma is more vascular
and so shows up strongly on the blood pool

isotope image, while the centre of the Brodie's
abscess is avascular.

Osteoblastoma

This is larger than the osteoid osteoma, has
surrounding reactive sclerosis and may be painful during the day as well as at night. The lesion
commonly occurs in the spinal appendages,
which are enlarged and sclerosed (Figure 3.21).

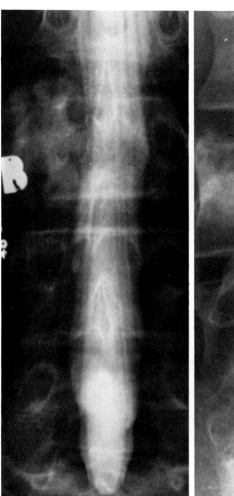
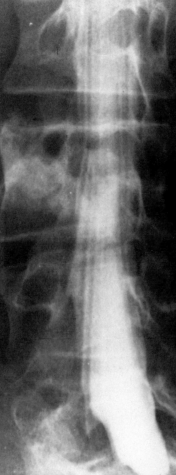

a

Figure 3.21

Osteoblastoma in the right pedicle of the third lumbar vertebra. (**a**) This 17-year-old male patient was referred for chronic back pain. A previous radiculogram had been negative. The plain film shows the expanded, sclerotic vertebral appendage, which obliterates the local nerve root seen at radiculography. (**b**) The CT scan demonstrates marked sclerosis of the pedicle and transverse process, which is expanded and contains a lytic lesion with a central nidus of density. The adjacent part of the vertebral body also shows reactive sclerosis and enlargement.

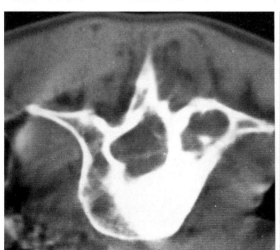
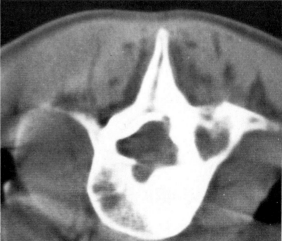

b

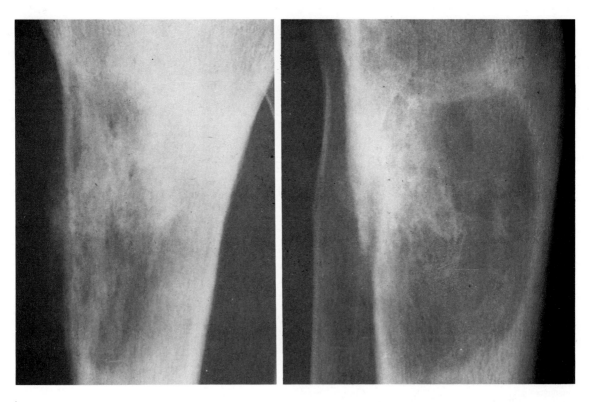

Figure 3.22

Malignant osteoblastoma. A lytic
lesion of the proximal tibia is
well demarcated in parts but has
broken through the cortex
posteromedially and looks
aggressive. There is ossification
of soft tissues and within the
large lesion, which is
indistinguishable in many ways
from an osteosarcoma.

Malignant degeneration and metastasis have been
described in this lesion (Figure 3.22).

Lipoma of bone

Matrix calcification is also seen in this rather rare
condition. In this lesion, which is slightly expansile and often seen in the calcaneum, the central
calcification is extremely dense, and the zone of
reactive sclerosis narrow (Figure 3.23).

Enchondroma

This is the commonest benign tumour of bone,
and occurs most frequently in the hand. Statisti-
cally, therefore, a lucent phalangeal tumour is
likely to be chondral in origin. It may be
discovered incidentally, and pain is usually the
result of fracture or malignant degeneration.

A solitary enchondroma is often metaphyseal
in a small bone but extends to the bone end after
skeletal fusion. With growth of the lesion, or in
a small bone, the cortex is scalloped and thinned,
and the bone expanded. The zone of reactive
sclerosis is always narrow, and calcific densities
within the tumour may be multiple. The lesions
can vary greatly in size so that soft tissue
deformities result (Figure 3.24).

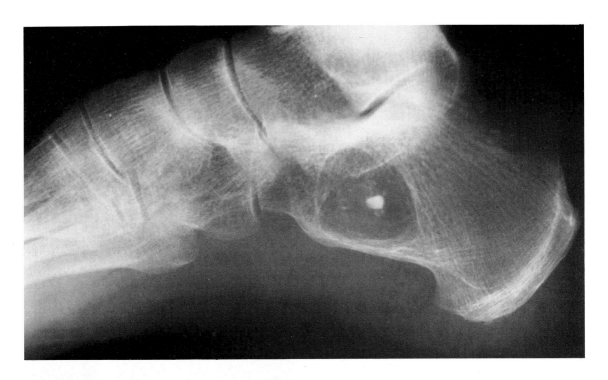

Figure 3.23

Intraosseous lipoma. A characteristic site for this lesion, which is generally well defined with a thin zone of reactive sclerosis and contains a central fleck of calcium.

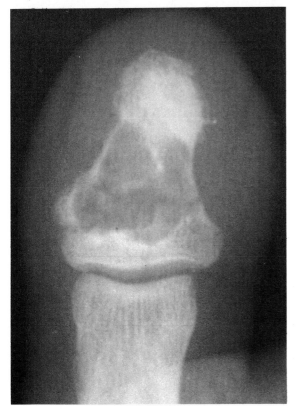

Figure 3.24

Enchondroma. A pathological fracture has occurred, associated with soft tissue swelling. The lesion expands bone, thins the cortex endosteally and contains a few specks of calcification.

Malignant transformation is less common in single enchondromas than in patients with enchondromas in Ollier's disease or the Maffucci syndrome. Rapid growth and loss of margination accompanied by pain are associated with this change.

Fibrous lesions

Fibrous dysplasia

This usually ossifies so that the initially spherical, lucent lesion later shows a mixture of patchy

Figure 3.25

Fibrous dysplasia. Various appearances of this lesion are shown at the proximal femur. These may be associated with bowing (*bottom left*) and expansion (*top left* and *bottom left*). The lesions may be totally sclerotic or mixed with sclerosis and lysis. They are usually well defined and may be monostotic or polyostotic.

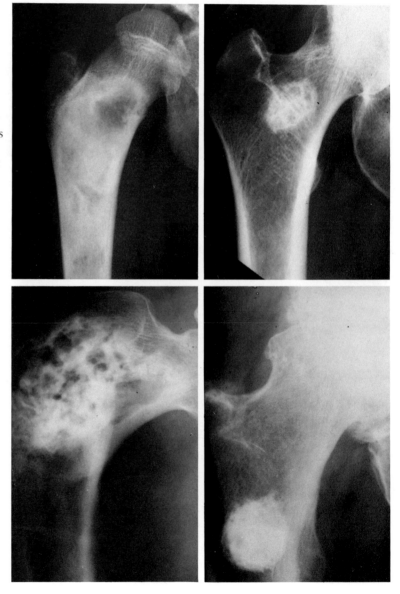

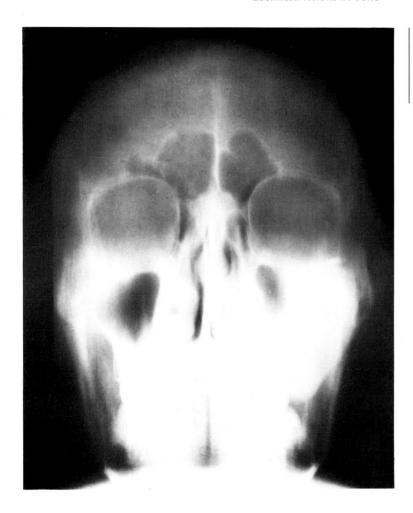

Figure 3.26

Facial fibrous dysplasia.
Expansion and obliteration of the
left antrum by a homogeneous,
dense bony mass.

central sclerosis, a ground-glass texture and
cystic lucency (Figure 1.56). The surrounding
zone of sclerosis is thicker than the zone around
enchondromas, and has the appearance of an
orange rind, being well defined and 2–4 mm
thick. The lesions vary in size and may cause
marked expansion of bone, but their softness
leads to deformity (Figure 3.3). Solitary lesions
are common, and often occur around the hips, in
the upper femur (Figure 3.25), around the knee
and in the ribs. Facial lesions are usually sclerotic
(Figure 3.26). The vertebral column is not often
involved in fibrous dysplasia.

Infarcts

These result from deprivation of the blood
supply to bone leading to death of its cellular
elements with the trabecular framework remaining intact initially. The surrounding vital bone
often loses density so that the infarcted area
appears relatively sclerotic. Subsequent healing
of the infarct involves peripheral revascularization, followed by laying down of a peripheral
serpiginous zone of sclerosis of new bone at the
margins of the infarct, which is referred to as the
zone of creeping substitution. Centrally, fibrous

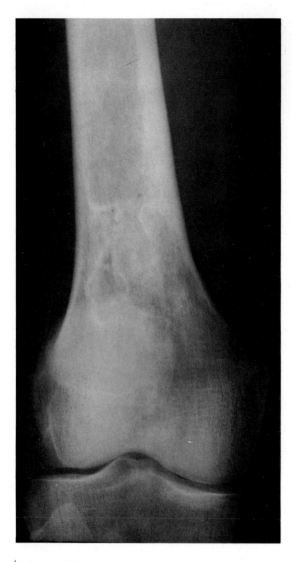

Figure 3.27

Infarction in caisson disease.
There is widespread abnormality
in the texture of the distal
femoral metaphysis. Serpiginous
and amorphous densities are
superimposed upon areas of
relative radiolucency. The cortex
is intact. The bone is not
enlarged, and there is no
periosteal reaction.

tissue undergoes dystrophic calcification, resulting in an ovoid or circular sclerotic rim surrounding a central area of relative lucency which
contains speckled densities (Figure 3.27).

These lesions are usually at epiphyseal and
metaphyseal sites, are often multiple and symmetrical (Figure 3.28), but occasionally are
solitary. Collapse results in epiphyses such as the
hip. The local bone is never enlarged.

The lesions most closely resemble fibrous
dysplasia, enchondroma, and chondrosarcoma
(Figure 3.29); however, expansion or bowing are
not present. The zone of peripheral sclerosis is
serpiginous, poorly defined and possibly 2–3 mm
thick. A detailed patient history often elicits the
cause of infarction (Table 3.10).

Fibrous dysplasia may be 'warm' (Figure 3.30)
or 'hot' (Figure 3.31) on an isotope bone scan.
Initially the infarcted area is 'cold' on the scan,
may be hot during the phase of active repair, but
is subsequently quiescent.

**Table 3.10   Causes of medullary
infarction.**

Old age, presumably due to atheroma

Sickle-cell anaemia

Gaucher's disease

Caisson disease

Infection

Radiation

Pancreatitis

Vasculitis

Chemotherapy

Lytic lesions

Geodes—cysts in the arthritides

These usually present as cysts of varying size in
the subarticular regions, in weight-bearing areas,
such as hips, knees, and ankles, but are also seen
in the wrists and elbows. Rheumatoid and

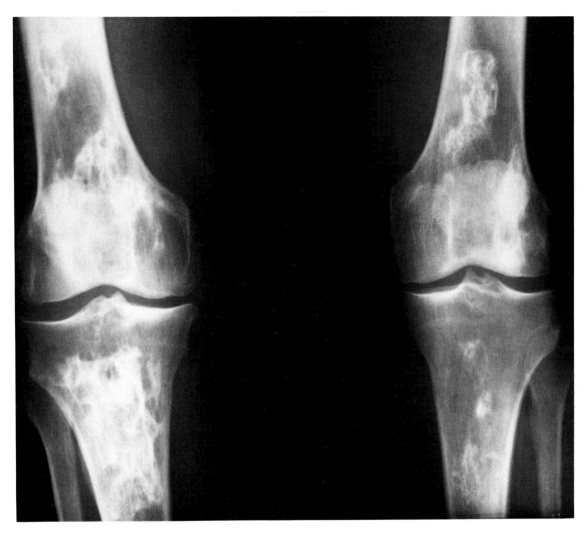

Figure 3.28

Infarction in caisson disease. Metaphyseal areas of increased density are shown in all the bones around the knee joints. The densities are well defined, particularly peripherally, and although the increase in density is not uniform, there is no overt bone destruction surrounding them. The bones are not expanded, there is no endosteal scalloping and no periosteal reaction.

osteoarthritis are the usual causes of these lesions, and therefore they are usually associated with evidence of major joint disease, such as joint narrowing, deformity, erosions or osteophytosis.

These well-defined cystic lesions usually reach the articular surface and are totally lucent (Figure 3.32). They vary in size, may be 5 or 6 cm in diameter, and multiple. The cyst may fill with

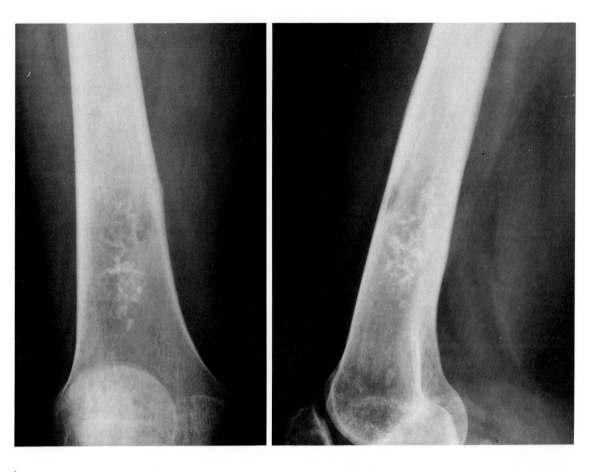

Figure 3.29

Many of the features of early
chondrosarcoma are similar to
those seen in the infarct due to
caisson disease (Figure 3.27).
There is distal femoral medullary
stippling associated with
proximal areas of radiolucency.
In this patient, however, there is
an early periosteal reaction with
slight expansion of the bone
which is maximal in the region of
the bony lucency.

Figure 3.30

Fibrous dysplasia. The
radioisotope scan of Figure 2.51
shows minimal increase in
uptake in the region of the
abnormal femoral neck.

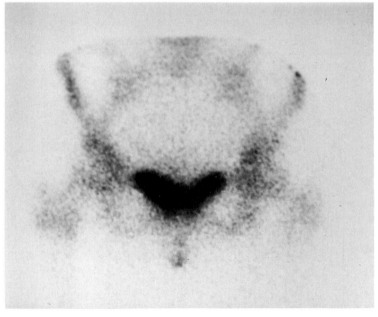

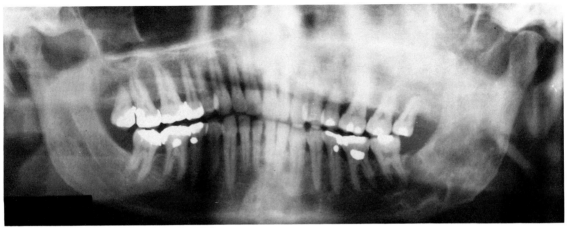

a

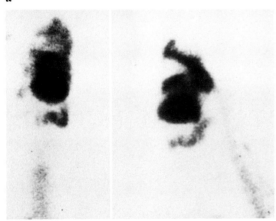

b

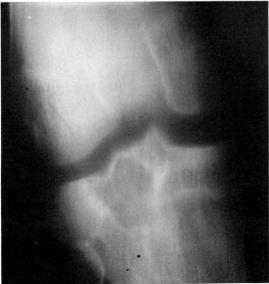

Figure 3.31

In this patient (**a**) The left antrum shows increased density and the left maxillary alveolus is enlarged by a sclerotic area of fibrous dysplasia. In the left side of the mandible, the lesion is more radiolucent. (**b**) On the radioisotope bone scan, the anterior and lateral scans show a gross increase in uptake in the left maxillary antral region. Expansion is also confirmed. The abnormality extends to the base of the skull at the anterior cranial fossa. The lytic mandibular lesion seen on the plain radiograph is also seen as an area of increased uptake but, as expected, is not as prominent.

Figure 3.32

This subarticular cyst was associated with local collapse of the weight-bearing surface of the joint.

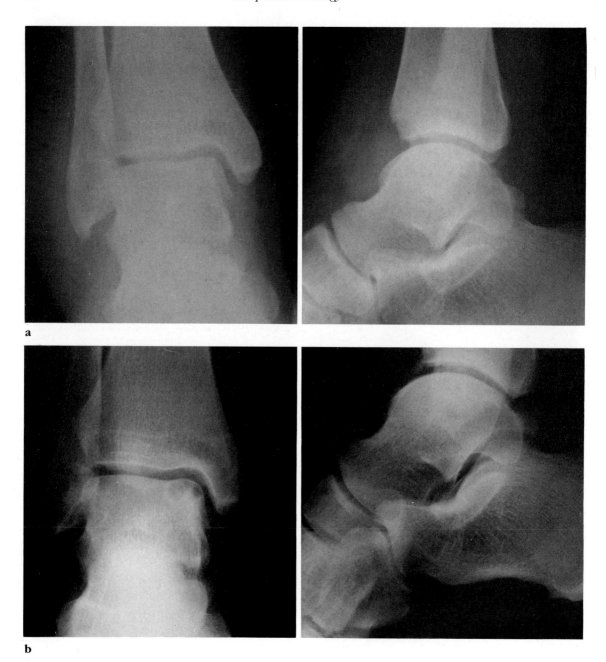

a

b

Figure 3.33

Post-traumatic subchondral cyst.
(**a**) The initial radiograph shows
soft tissue swelling around the
ankle but no other abnormality.
(**b**) Six months after trauma, a
cyst is seen in the talus, but the
joint is not narrowed.

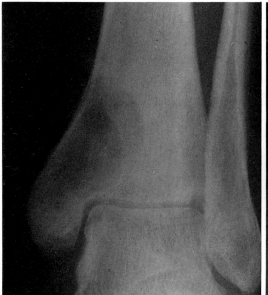
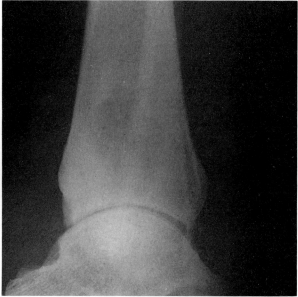

Figure 3.34

Chronic osteomyelitis. In this patient with an immune defect, expansion of the medial malleolus associated with a large cystic lesion can be seen, due to chronic infection.

contrast at arthrography. The thinned, overlying articular cortex is weakened and may collapse producing structural failure. The aetiology of the cyst is usually seen on inspection of the local joint and any other joints involved in rheumatoid disease, for example.

Patients may be middle-aged or elderly, but an identical lesion is found in young, often athletic, patients. The solitary traumatic subchondral cyst is probably the result of microfracture with synovial intravasation, so that the surrounding joint will be normal (Figure 3.33).

Chronic osteomyelitis

This is occasionally the cause of a lytic lesion at the end of a long bone in the metaphysis before skeletal fusion, but reaching the joint line in the mature skeleton. One or many bones may be affected. If cystic lesions are multiple, the cause may be tuberculosis or chronic granulomatous disease. The surrounding bone may be expanded, there may be a periostitis, and the adjacent joint narrowed because of cartilage destruction by the inflammatory process (Figure 3.34). Cystic

Figure 3.35

Rheumatoid arthritis. A lytic
lesion is present in the greater
tuberosity on the anteroposterior
view. This change may be found
with rheumatoid arthritis,
tuberculosis or may even follow
repeated anterior dislocation
(hatchet defect). In this patient
there is also upward subluxation
of the humeral head with para-
articular erosions and eburnation
of the articular surface. The joint
space is narrow.

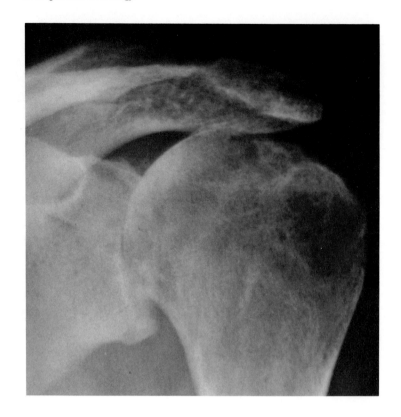

change at the greater tuberosity of the humerus
may be due to rheumatoid arthritis or tuberculosis (Figure 3.35). A similar appearance may
follow recurrent dislocation and formation of a
Hill–Sachs hatchet defect.

Chondroblastoma

This is a rare, benign tumour of cartilaginous
origin, which occurs before epiphyseal fusion
and is a cause of local pain. It is usually seen in
the epiphyses around the knee, the upper
humerus and greater tuberosity, the greater

trochanter, ankle and patella. Therefore, the
lesion is usually subarticular, but in the unfused
skeleton (Figure 3.36). Giant-cell tumours occur
at the same sites after skeletal fusion; however,
the chondroblastoma is usually smaller. It is
typically surrounded by a well-demarcated zone
of reactive sclerosis and, therefore, is better
defined than a typical giant-cell tumour. Approximately 50 per cent of these lesions show central
calcification. In the immature skeleton, both
enchondroma and fibrous dysplasia are initially
metaphyseal and, although both lesions usually
show matrix calcification, they reach the bone
end only after fusion. The chondroblastoma can
straddle the growth plate and extend into the
metaphysis before fusion (Figure 3.37).

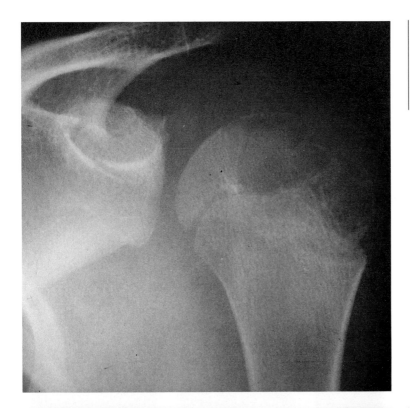

Figure 3.36

Chondroblastoma. A lytic lesion of the epiphysis before skeletal maturity is not due to a giant-cell tumour but is much more likely to be due to a chondroblastoma.

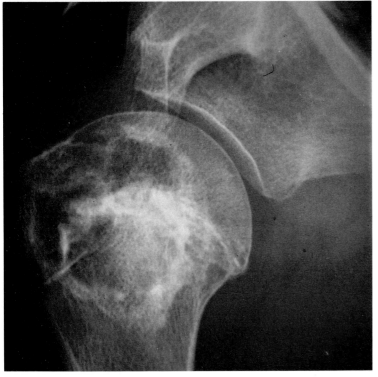

Figure 3.37

Chondroblastoma. The growth plate is on the point of fusing and a lytic lesion containing calcification straddles it.

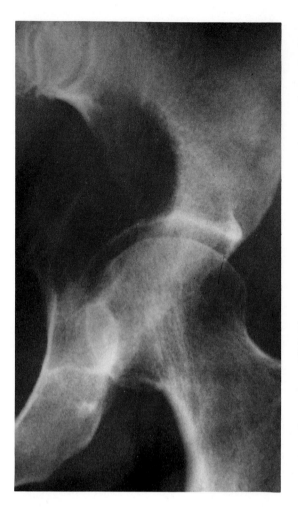

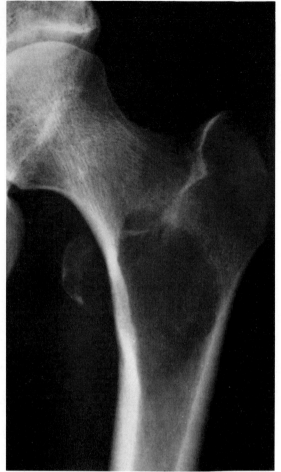

Figure 3.38

Giant-cell tumour. Although
apparently atypical, a poorly
defined lytic lesion extends to
the articular surface at the hip
joint, and is characteristic for a
giant-cell tumour.

Figure 3.39

Giant-cell tumour. A lytic lesion
erodes the lesser trochanter
which has been expanded and
avulsed. This sequence is also
seen with metastatic deposits in
this region, but these usually
occur over the age of 45 years.
Between 20 and 40 years of age,
a giant-cell tumour is perhaps
more likely at this previous
apophysis.

Giant-cell tumour

This is a relatively common, often highly expansile lesion lying at the joint surface of a mature bone (Figure 3.38). Both previous epiphyses and apophyses are affected (Figure 3.39). The most common sites are around the knee, the distal radius and shoulder, but any bone may be affected (Figure 3.40). It is occasionally described in the metaphysis of an immature skeleton, but should not be diagnosed before epiphyseal fusion. Inevitably, the lesion extends to an articular surface at a joint, although this may not always be obvious. Therefore, on the anteroposterior view of the knee, the tumour may not appear to extend to the distal femoral articular surface, but the lateral view shows that it extends to the femoral condyles at the patello-femoral articulation (Figure 3.41).

The lesion is generally lucent and may contain a few strands of residual trabecular bone. It is unusual to see the speckled, punctate calcification seen in fibrous and cartilaginous lesions. Fibrous lesions, such as fibrous dysplasia and

Figure 3.40

Giant-cell tumour. (**a**) A poorly-defined lytic lesion extends to the distal tibial articular surface. There is slight expansion of bone and residual septation.

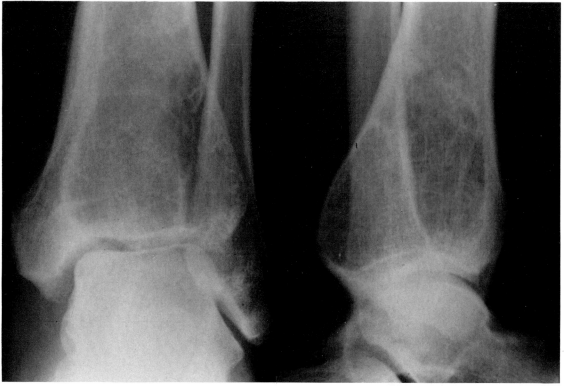

a

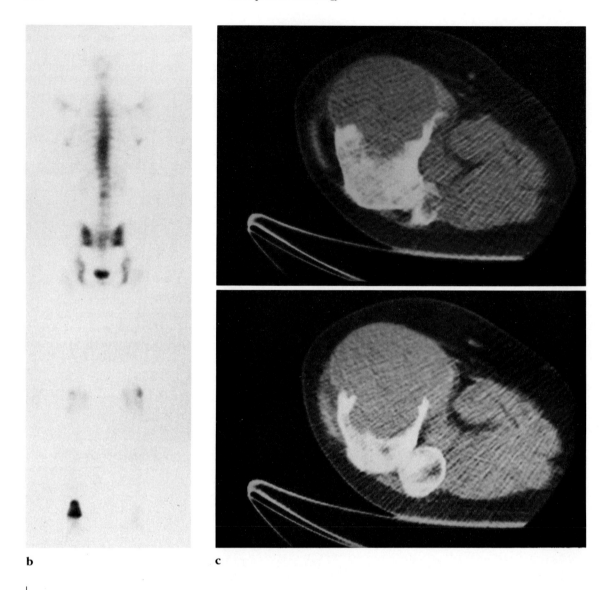

b   c

Figure 3.40 *continued*

(**b**) The radioisotope
bone scan shows
this to be a solitary lesion. (**c**)
The CT scan shows the expansile
and destructive nature of the
lesion, but a thin rim of bone
remains at its periphery.

Figure 3.41

Giant-cell tumour. (**a**) On the
anteroposterior view the lesion
does not seem to extend to an
articular surface, but, on the
lateral view, the patello-femoral
joint is affected by a well-defined
lytic lesion in a mature skeleton.
(**b**) The isotope scan confirms
the highly vascular nature and
cellularity of the tumour.

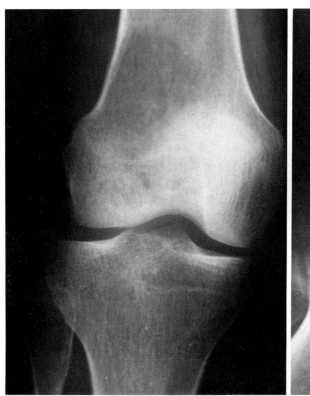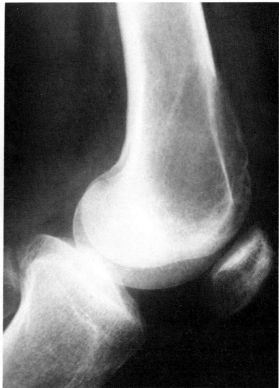

a

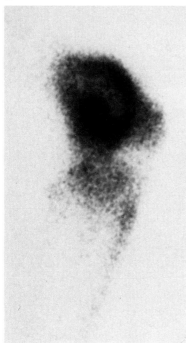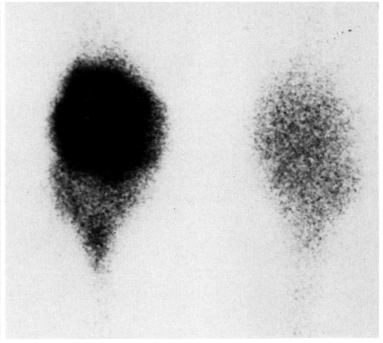

b

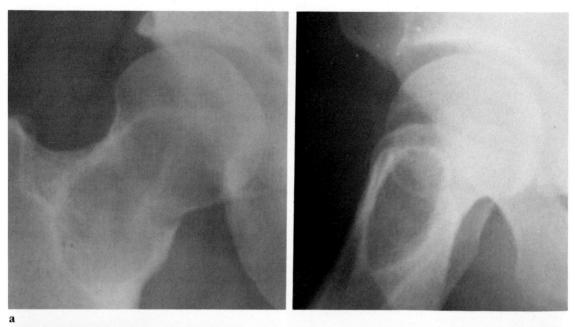

a

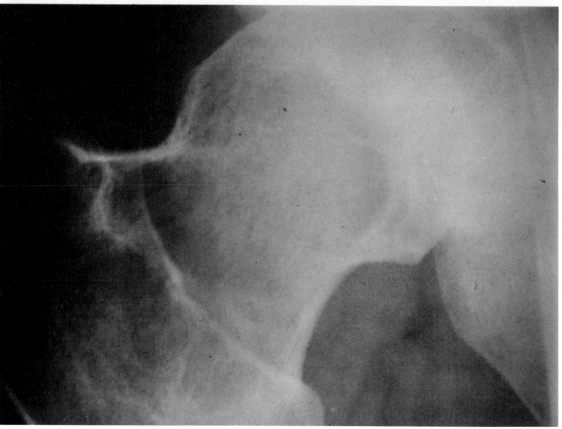

b

malignant fibrous histiocytoma, may be subarticular and have little or no matrix calcification; therefore occasionally they cannot be differentiated from giant-cell tumours (Figure 3.42).

The margin of a giant-cell tumour is never very sclerotic and is often blurred. In places, there may be quite a wide zone of transition, suggesting local bone infiltration, which is also a feature of malignant fibrous histiocytoma.

A giant-cell tumour may be eccentric, extending to the corner of the articular surface but, with growth, may occupy the entire subarticular zone. This is seen at the distal radius, proximal humerus and fibula. The cortex of the articular surface is often markedly thinned but remains faintly visible and the adjacent shaft often bulges aneurysmally (Figure 3.43). The junction between the bulging tumour and the normal adjacent shaft may be quite angular and buttressed with periosteal new bone, resembling a Codman's triangle. This is a feature of large, rapidly growing lesions such as the giant-cell tumour and aneurysmal bone cyst. It is not seen with a simple bone cyst. A renal or thyroid metastasis may also resemble a giant-cell tumour but the latter is solitary and usually seen between 18 and 45 years of age.

Malignant transformation and metastases do occur. Local recurrence may follow curettage, and is often from the periphery of the lesion, with resorption of packed bone chips (Figure 3.44). Very aggressive-looking margins may indicate malignant potential but generally there is no correlation between the radiological appearance and the behaviour of the tumour.

The spine is rarely involved. The vertebral body is usually affected rather than the appendages, normal bone is completely replaced by the lucent tumour, and early expansion causes cord compression.

Figure 3.42

(**a**) Fibrous dysplasia. A typical appearance in the upper femur is of an area of ground-glass bone texture surrounded by a thick rind of reactive sclerosis. The bone is expanded, and the appearance resembles that of a giant-cell tumour reaching the margins of the articular surface but, in this case, the lesion is much better defined. (**b**) Giant-cell tumour. A lytic expansile lesion is shown in the neck of the femur which extends to the articular surface of the head. There is a fairly narrow zone of transition with a little reactive sclerosis.

Malignant fibrous histiocytoma

Most patients with this lesion are middle-aged or elderly, but occasionally adolescent. The lesions are commonest at the ends of the long bones, as are giant-cell tumours. Radiologically, an expansile lytic lesion is visualized, often with cortical breakthrough, associated with a soft tissue mass (Figure 3.45). These appearances are also very similar to those seen with a giant-cell tumour. However, the soft tissue mass occasionally ossifies and the lesion then resembles a fibrosarcoma rather than a giant-cell tumour.

The malignant fibrous histiocytoma is an aggressive tumour which recurs and metastasizes. Therefore, in behaviour, it is usually more like a fibrosarcoma than a giant-cell tumour.

Figure 3.43

Subarticular giant-cell tumour of the balloon type. (**a**) The tumour extends to the articular surface of the femoral head but there is no opportunity for expansion adjacent to the acetabulum. It also extends into the greater trochanter. It may have arisen here because this was an apophysis. Here, there is no obstruction to expansion, and the greater trochanter is hugely enlarged. (**b**) The subsequent film shows further expansion of the lesion. There is a well-defined soft tissue mass, hugely expanding the greater trochanter. A few strands of cortex remain around the lesion. Aneurysmal bone cysts also cause balloon-like lesions, but these occur in younger patients. Large lesions of this type are rarely seen in the UK.

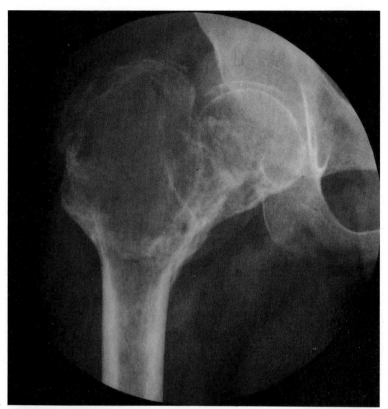

a

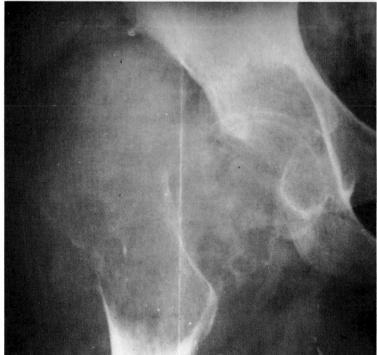

b

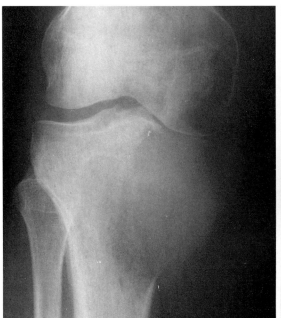
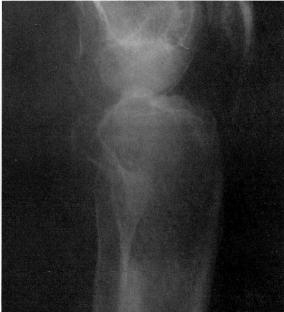

a

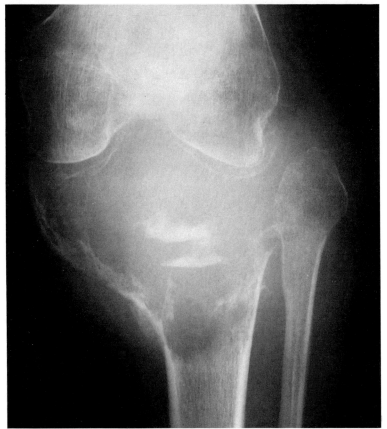

b

Figure 3.44

(**a**) Another patient with giant-cell tumour has a typical lesion at the proximal tibia. (**b**) The lesion has been curetted and packed with bone chips but has recurred. Further expansion results in a 'balloon' tumour.

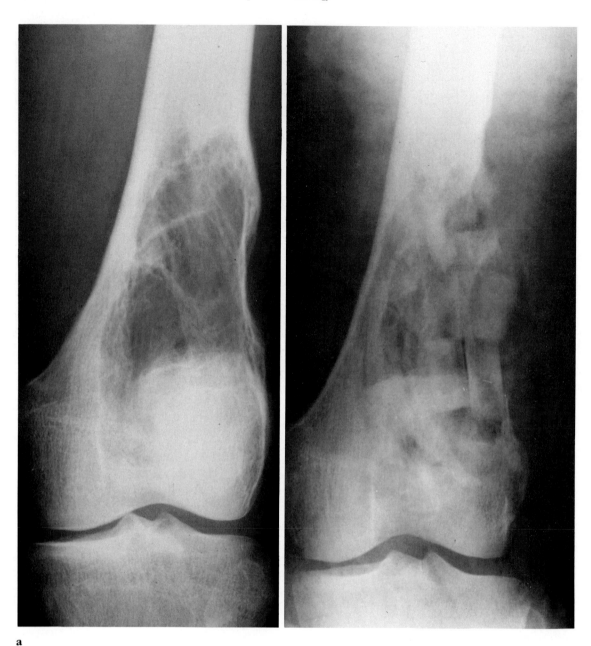

a

Figure 3.45

Malignant fibrous histiocytoma. (a) The lesion is similar to, but perhaps more extensive proximally than a giant-cell tumour. The cortex is scalloped endosteally and the bone marginally expanded by this eccentric lesion. Residual trabeculation remains. (b) In the same patient following surgery, the lesion has been curetted and packed with bone chips. (b) The bone chips have resorbed and the lesion has expanded. There is now quite obvious cortical breakthrough with the formation of a partially ossifying soft tissue mass, revealing the aggressive nature of this lesion.

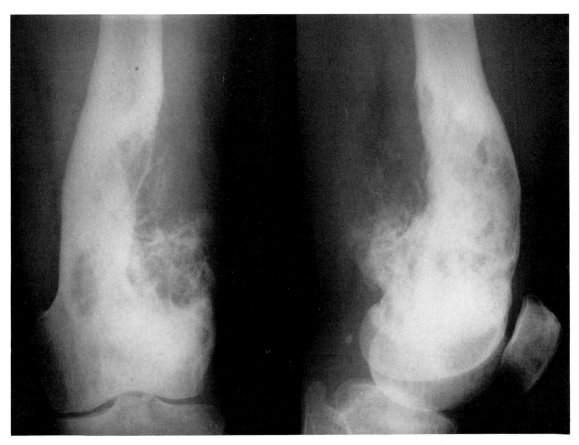

b

Aneurysmal bone cyst

This originates in the metaphysis of a long bone before skeletal fusion and, therefore, is totally unlike a giant-cell tumour. After fusion, the lesion can extend to the articular surface, and may be so expansile that occasionally the thinned and elevated cortex is not radiologically visible, and may often only reappear after radiotherapy (Figure 3.46). The angle between the cyst and the cortex is often filled with lamellar buttressing periostitis (Figure 3.47) as seen with giant-cell tumours. Its zone of transition may be sharp or poorly defined.

A feature of this lesion (Figure 3.48) is rapid growth under observation which often is faster than in malignant lesions such as renal or thyroid metastases. These usually occur after the age at which the aneurysmal bone cyst or giant-cell tumour are seen. The lesions are lightly trabeculated and commonly occur in the femur and humerus. In the spinal appendages, they show expansion and lucency (Figure 3.46), unlike the similarly situated osteoblastomas and enchondromas which show density (Figure 3.6). In the spine, an aneurysmal bone cyst can occasionally cross posteriorly from one set of vertebral appendages to the next.

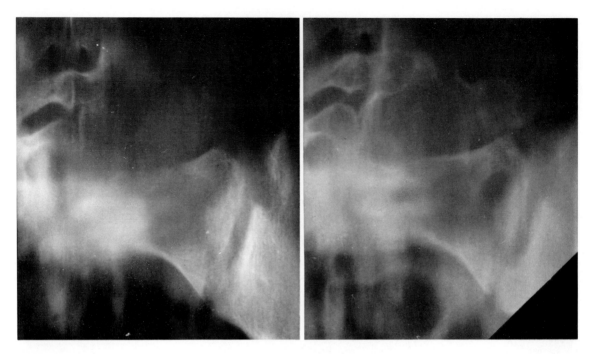

Figure 3.46

The initial radiograph of an aneurysmal bone cyst shows expansion and lysis of the vertebral appendages on the left with a large soft tissue mass. After radiotherapy the cortex is visualized and the expansile nature of the lesion can be seen.

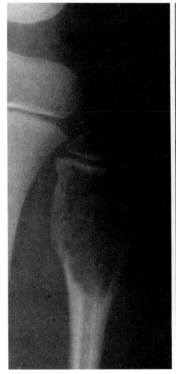
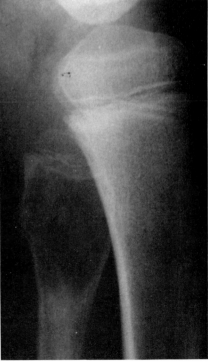

Figure 3.47

An aneurysmal bone cyst showing an expansile lesion of the fibular metaphysis in an immature skeleton. The cortex is thinned but not broken through and the zone of transition is narrow. There is cortical buttressing at the angle between normal and abnormal bone.

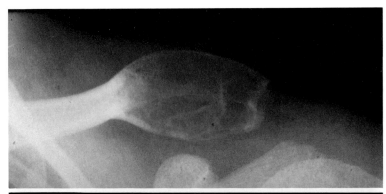

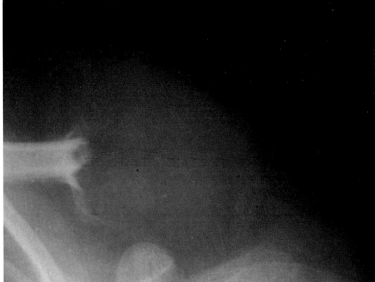

Figure 3.48

The initial radiograph of an aneurysmal bone cyst of the clavicle, shows a highly expansile lytic lesion resembling a giant-cell tumour of the distal end of the clavicle (*top*). Rapid growth produces a balloon tumour (*bottom*). Aneurysmal bone cysts tend to occur in a slightly younger age group but, occasionally, the lesions cannot be distinguished.

Simple bone cysts

These occur in children before epiphyseal fusion, and usually before aneurysmal bone cysts. They occur in the proximal humeral and proximal femoral metaphyses, as well as in the calcaneum (Figure 3.49). The lesions are well demarcated, only minimally expansile (Figure 3.50), and contain little or no residual trabeculation with no marginal periosteal buttressing. With time, they are left behind by growth at the epiphyseal plate so that they appear to migrate to the midshaft of the bone (Figure 3.51). They are not usually seen in the mature skeleton. Presentation usually occurs because of a pathological fracture. Occasionally, there may be a 'falling leaf' sign of cortical fragments moving in the serous contents of the cyst (Figure 3.52).

Figure 3.49

(**a**) There is a well-demarcated lucency representing a simple bone cyst in the anterior aspect of the calcaneum. This has no central calcification as seen with a lipoma (Figure 3.23). It should also not be confused with a normal variant, the pseudocyst, which lies between the major groups of trabeculae. (**b**) Pseudocyst. Bilateral, rather poorly defined defects are seen as a normal variant. Note also the sclerosis and irregularity of the calcaneal apophyses and thickening of the overlying soft tissues. If pain is present, a diagnosis of Sever's disease can be made.

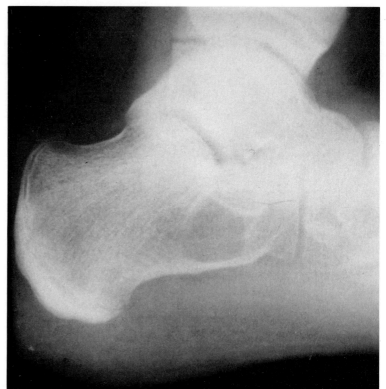

a

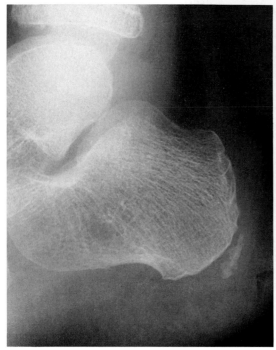
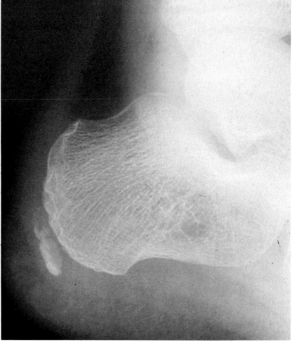

b

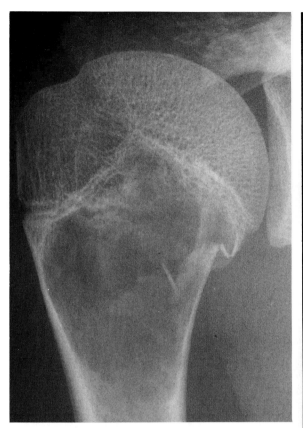

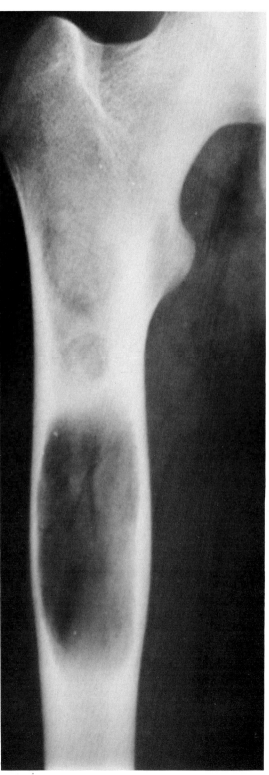

Figure 3.50

Simple bone cyst. There is no expansion of the proximal humeral metaphysis. The lesion scallops the cortex endosteally, but the absence of aneurysmal dilatation and the site of the lesion indicates that this is not an aneurysmal bone cyst. A pathological fracture has occurred and a free-floating fragment of cortex is seen centrally within the lesion.

Figure 3.51

This simple bone cyst, in a mature skeleton, appears as a slightly expansile, monolocular lytic lesion situated in the midshaft of the femur and has sustained a pathological fracture.

Figure 3.52

Simple bone cyst with fracture. In the immature skeleton, this is a typical, slightly expansile lesion reaching up to the metaphysis. It appears multilocular, but this is probably because of endosteal scalloping. The expansion is not accompanied by a buttressing periostitis at the junction between normal and abnormal bone, as is the case with aneurysmal bone cyst and giant-cell tumour. A fracture has occurred and fragments of bone may be observed to float if the arm is subsequently radiographed in an erect position.

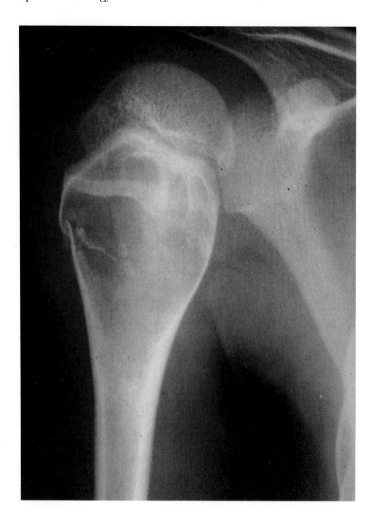

Fibrous cortical defect and non-ossifying fibroma

The fibrous cortical defect is a small (<3 cm), lucent, fibrous lesion seen as an incidental finding in children. The lesion is metaphyseal in a long bone, usually the distal femur, oval in shape, thinning the cortex with a very thin endosteal zone of reactive sclerosis. There may be slight cortical expansion (Figure 3.53) and,

occasionally, the lesion fractures. The majority ossify with age, leaving either normal or sclerotic bone. Occasionally they enlarge and migrate to the centre of the bone, giving a multilocular, spherical or cigar-shaped lucency, called the non-ossifying fibroma, which causes expansion and cortical thinning (Figure 3.54). These are diametaphyseal, well demarcated and multilocular, but are not as expansile as an aneurysmal bone cyst. They may be confused with simple bone cysts of the femur. These lesions also present because of pathological fracture.

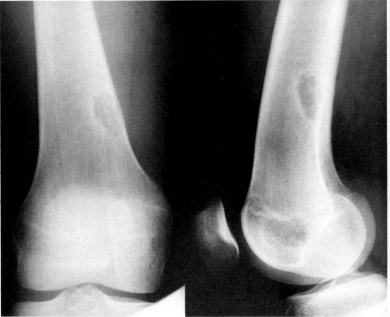

Figure 3.53

Fibrous cortical defect. This
lesion is seen in young patients.
There is slight expansion of the
bone locally with thinning of the
cortex. The lesion is multilocular
and has a very narrow zone of
transition with a thin rim of
reactive sclerosis. Fibrous
cortical defects usually fill up
with normal bone and vanish.
They are normally asymptomatic
but may fracture occasionally.

Eosinophilic granuloma

This is a disease of children and occasionally of
young adults. Solitary or multiple lytic lesions
preferentially occur in the axial skeleton and
skull, and resemble those seen with chronic
cystic infections such as tuberculosis and occasionally chronic granulomatous disease. The
areas of lysis are initially well defined and lucent
(Figure 3.55), but in their healing phase the
sharp margin is lost and they ossify from within
(Figure 3.56). In a narrow bone, a periostitis may

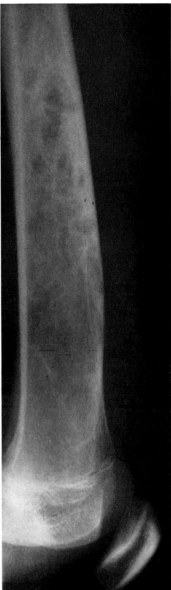

Figure 3.54

Non-ossifying fibroma. This
resembles the fibrous cortical
defect but is obviously larger and
occupies the medulla of the
bone. Otherwise, it has the same
thin zone of transition and rim of
reactive sclerosis, and causes
slight expansion of bone with
endosteal cortical scalloping.

Figure 3.55

Eosinophilic granuloma. A
solitary well-defined lytic lesion
with a bevelled edge in the
posterior parietal region.

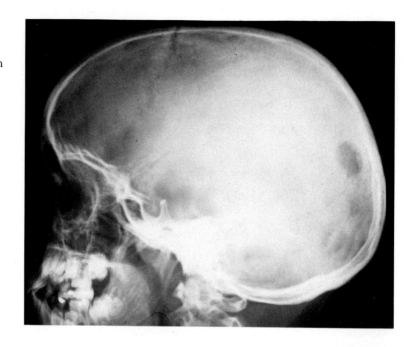

Figure 3.56

Eosinophilic granuloma. The
well-defined margins seen on the
previous radiograph have
disappeared as the lesion is
slowly healing with central
ossification.

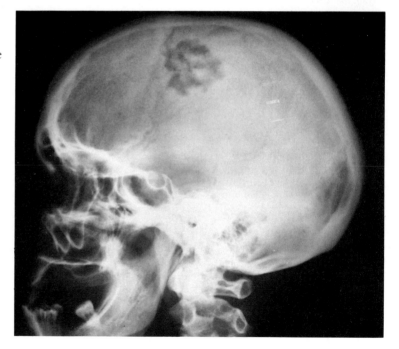

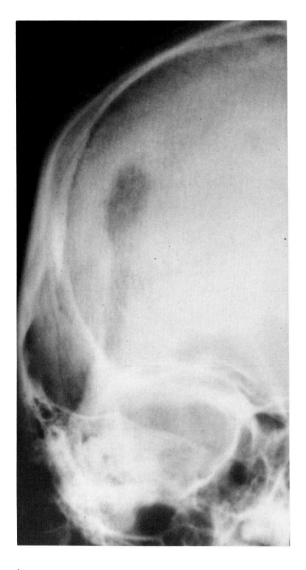

Figure 3.57

In this patient with tuberculosis of the skull, the solitary osteolytic lesion is poorly defined, but this can be seen in a healing eosinophilic granuloma. However, the long finger-like process or tunnel leading from the lesion is a feature of infection.

be seen and, in the skull, a 'bevelled edge' effect occurs (Figure 3.55). Unfortunately, bevelled edges are also seen in tuberculosis, while the margin of an eosinophilic granuloma can be irregular. 'Tunnelling', however, is not a feature of eosinophilic granuloma but of infection (Figure 3.57).

Multiple lesions of six or more may cause great alarm, and may even mimic leukaemia in children (Figure 3.58); however, they undergo spontaneous remission, only for further lesions to reappear. Eosinophilic granuloma and fibrous dysplasia should always be considered when solitary or multiple lytic lesions are seen in children (Figure 3.59).

Cystic lesions in haemophilia

This disease is rare and will be diagnosed before presentation to the radiologist. Large cysts due to subperiosteal or intraosseous bleeding are found in the iliac blades or long bones (Figure 3.60), through which pathological fractures can occur. The patients have other bone changes; the epiphyses are overgrown due to hyperaemia and the joint spaces are narrow and irregular (see Chapter 4, page 231) due to synovial proliferation (Figure 3.61).

Hydatid disease

This is common in sheep-farming regions, but bone lesions account for only 2 per cent of total lesions. The cysts are occasionally single (Figure 3.62) but usually multiple (Figure 3.63) and are well defined, varying in size from small (1–2 mm) to very large. The cortices may be scalloped endosteally and the bone may be expanded with large cysts. Lesions occur around joints, and affect both sides similarly to other infections (Figure 3.64). In a long bone, the lesions can resemble fibrous dysplasia and brown tumours in hyperparathyroidism (Figure 3.65). They are obviously uncommon outside endemic areas but may be seen elsewhere because of population migration.

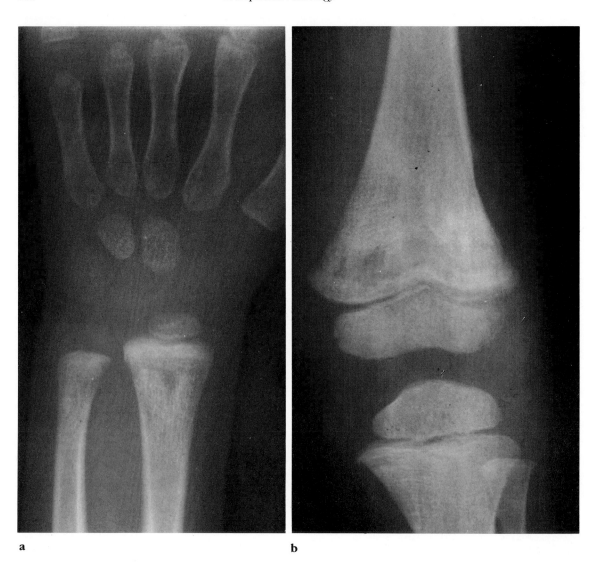

a   b

Figure 3.58

Multicentric eosinophilic
granuloma. Irregular medullary
bands of bone destruction are
seen at the distal radius (**a**) and
distal femur (**b**), closely
mimicking leukaemia in
appearance.

Figure 3.59

Eosinophilic granuloma. (**a**) In
this immature skeleton, the
acetabulum is thickened and
shows a generalized increase in
density. (**b**) The radioisotope
scan shows this region to be the
site of increase in uptake. (**c**) The
CT scan confirms the expansion
of the acetabulum and shows an
osteolytic lesion within it.

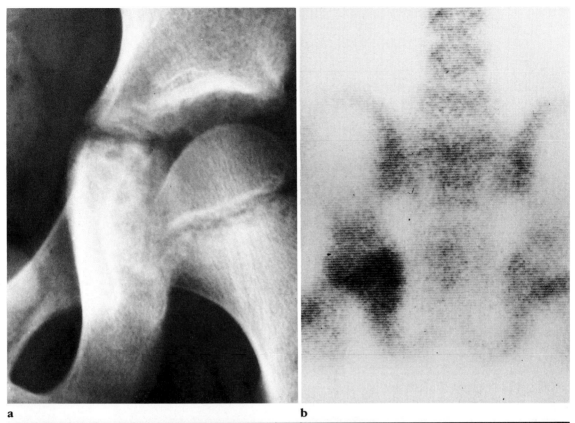

a

b

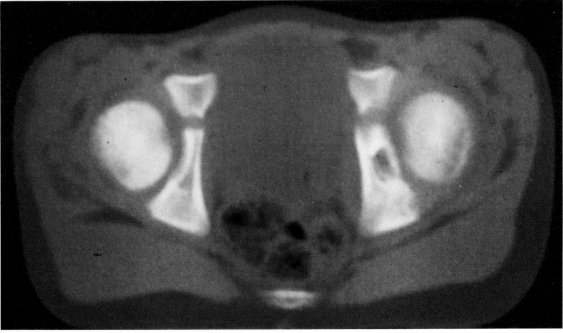

c

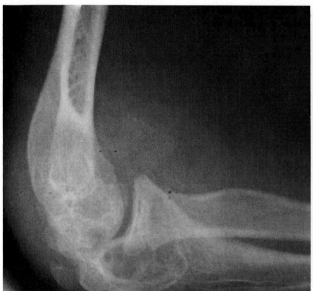
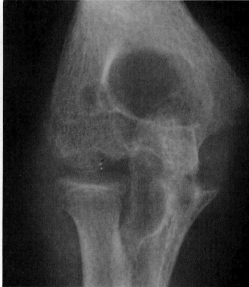

Figure 3.60

Haemophilia. The lateral view
shows soft tissue swelling around
the elbow joint associated with
cysts in the proximal ulna and
distal humerus. The appearances
are compatible with synovial
proliferation and erosion of
bone. Similar appearances may
be seen in juvenile chronic
arthritis and tuberculosis.
Osteolytic defects in haemophilia
may also be produced by
intraosseous bleeding.

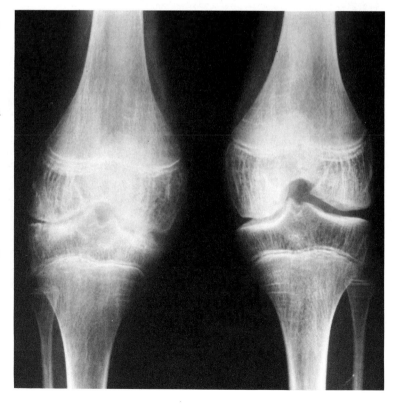

Figure 3.61

Haemophilia. There is soft tissue
wasting and osteopenia. Growth
arrest lines are seen, and the
epiphyses are expanded and
bulbous with angular margins.
The intercondylar notches are
deepened and the joint spaces
narrowed. Intercondylar notch
deepening is a characteristic
feature of haemophilia.

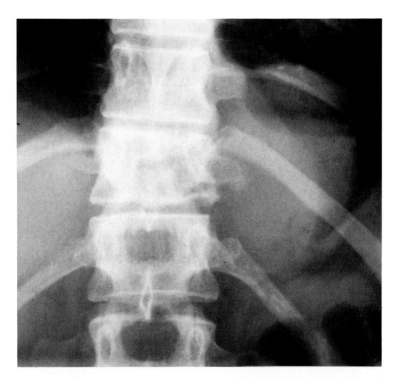

Figure 3.62

In this patient with hydatid disease, an osteolytic lesion is present in the body of the eleventh thoracic vertebra, which is associated with a large paraspinal swelling and early collapse.

Figure 3.63

Hydatid disease. Multiple cysts in the distal femur expand the bone and break through the cortex with the formation of soft tissue masses. The cysts within the bone are fairly well marginated and may occasionally resemble those seen in fibrous dysplasia, in which cortical breakthrough does not occur.

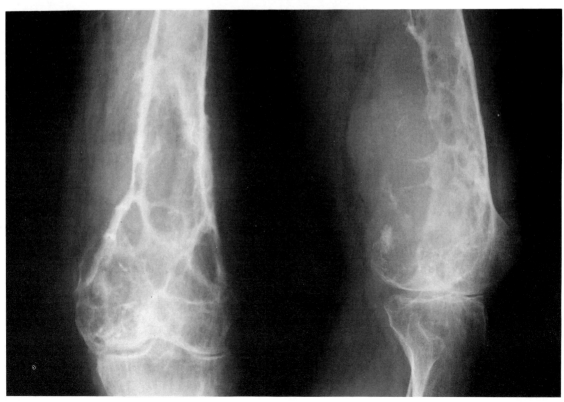

Figure 3.64

Hydatid disease commonly
involves the hip, affecting both
sides of the joint. There is quite
widespread destruction of bone
which is neuropathic in type, but
cystic change is seen in the
surrounding bone in this patient.

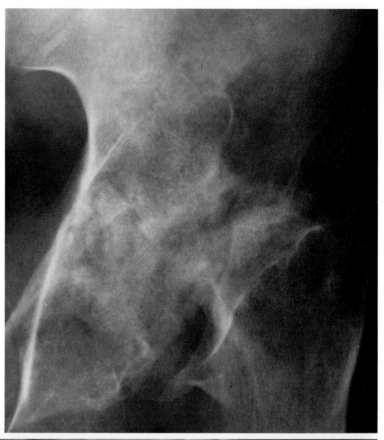

Figure 3.65

Hydatid disease. A large,
expansile, multicystic lesion
associated with cortical thinning
is seen affecting the pubic bones.
The lesions have well-defined
margins with a narrow zone of
transition and a thin rim of
reactive sclerosis. The lesions
mimic those seen in
hyperparathyroidism and fibrous
dysplasia.

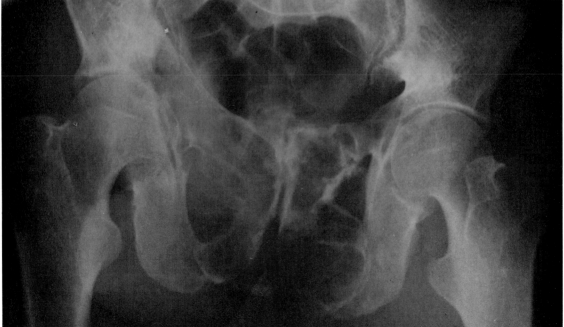

Malignant lesions of bone

Solitary malignant lesions of bone have characteristics which usually enable them to be distinguished from benign lesions. These are:

- Rapid growth
- Wide zone of transition
- Ill-defined or absent zone of reactive sclerosis
- Cortical breach
- Periostitis and possibly a Codman triangle
- Soft tissue mass
- Matrix calcification (see page 139)

Age incidence is often highly specific (Table 3.3), but the sex of the patient is less useful for diagnosis. The site is often characteristic, both generally, for example, Ewing's tumours are diaphyseal, and specifically, that is, they often occur in ribs.

An important decision is made when malignancy is diagnosed, as it is sometimes more difficult to make a distinction between malignancy and infection than between benign and malignant lesions. The common malignant tumours are listed in Table 3.1 and their sites in the skeleton and within a bone are shown in Tables 3.5–3.8. The nature of malignant periostitis is described in Chapter 6, page 315).

Osteogenic sarcoma

This occurs as a primary lesion between 5 and 25 years of age, and is more common in males. In elderly patients, secondary lesions are often superimposed on Paget's disease and irradiated bone, and occur very rarely as a complication of fibrous dysplasia.

Lesions commonly arise around the knee and shoulder, and in the pelvis, but any bone may be involved. The mandible is often involved in the third and fourth decades (Figure 3.66). The lesions are typically metaphyseal. The resultant malignant osteoid destroys bone and undergoes irregular ossification.

A radiological spectrum exists. The commonest appearance is of gross central medullary destruction of bone in the metaphysis, with a broad zone of transition. Cortical breakthrough and a well-defined soft tissue mass with a Codman's triangle are seen. Matrix ossification in bone and soft tissue is irregular and dense. The periostitis is coarse and may be lamellar or perpendicular (Figure 3.67). Occasionally, purely lytic and sclerotic metaphyseal tumours are encountered (Figures 3.68, 3.69 and 3.70).

Osteogenic sarcoma metastasizes to other bones and to the lungs. These secondary deposits are often osteoblastic and can be detected on isotope bone scans (Figure 3.71). CT scans are sensitive in the detection of pulmonary metastases.

Ewing's sarcoma

This is the other significant primary malignant tumour of bone which occurs between 5 and 25 years of age. Multiple malignant round cells infiltrate the shaft of a long bone, or a flat bone in the axial skeleton. This produces a widespread 'moth-eaten' permeative and destructive lesion, aligned along the shaft of a bone, unlike the focal expansile lesion seen in osteogenic sarcoma. The central lesion is destructive and not osteogenic (Figure 3.72).

The periosteal reaction is often finer and more delicate than in osteogenic sarcoma, but is also associated with cortical breakthrough and a soft tissue mass (Figure 3.73).

In children, the ribs are frequently involved and extrapleural masses and effusions are formed (Figure 3.74). In flat bones, such as the pelvis and scapula, reactive sclerosis and lamellar periostitis cause bone expansion (Figure 3.75), which often obscures permeative destruction.

Reticulum cell sarcoma

This occurs between 25 and 40 years of age and causes diffuse malignant infiltration with cortical breakthrough, lamellar periostitis and a Codman's triangle. This tumour resembles Ewing's sarcoma both microscopically and radiologically (Figure 3.76).

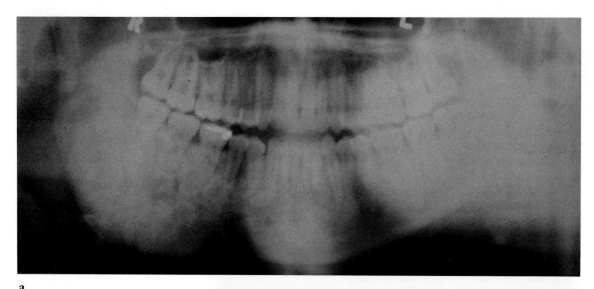

a

Figure 3.66

Osteogenic sarcoma of the
mandible. (**a**) The right side of
the mandible shows expansion
by a tumour which causes fairly
well-defined new bone
formation. (**b**) The CT scan of the
same patient shows extensive
bone destruction with an
ossifying soft tissue mass.

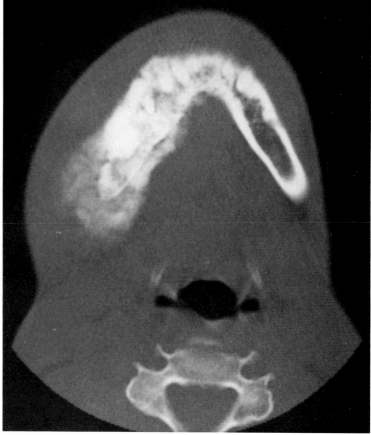

b

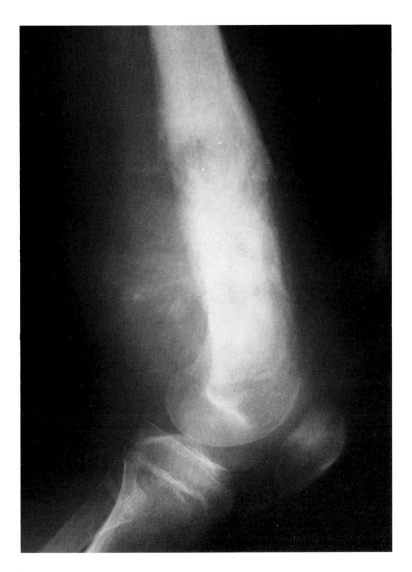

Figure 3.67

Osteogenic sarcoma. A large soft tissue mass is associated with a metaphyseal destructive lesion. There is much new bone proliferation, both within the shaft of the femur and in the soft tissues. There is a 'sunray' or hair-on-end spiculation which is coarse, as well as periosteal elevation at the margin of the lesion with the formation of a Codman's triangle.

Figure 3.68

Osteogenic sarcoma. (**a**) There is
a large soft tissue mass at the
distal femur. Remnants of dead
cortex may be seen anteriorly,
and the lesion is predominantly
lytic posteriorly. There is some
poorly defined tumour new bone
and posterior 'saucerisation' or
erosion of the cortex,
characteristic of malignant re-
entry. (**b**) On the CT scan, the
tumour permeates and
eventually breaks through the
medulla of the femur, with the
formation of a large anterior soft
tissue mass containing a few
areas of ossification. The bulk of
the tumour new bone lies
postero-laterally and is associated
with another large soft tissue
mass. (**c**) Following radiotherapy
further ossification takes place
within the tumour. This is coarse
and shaggy, and is both
amorphous and sunray in type.

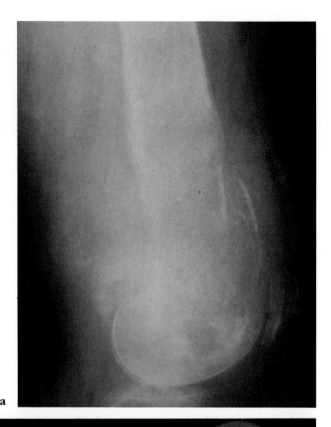

a

b

Figure 3.68 *continued*

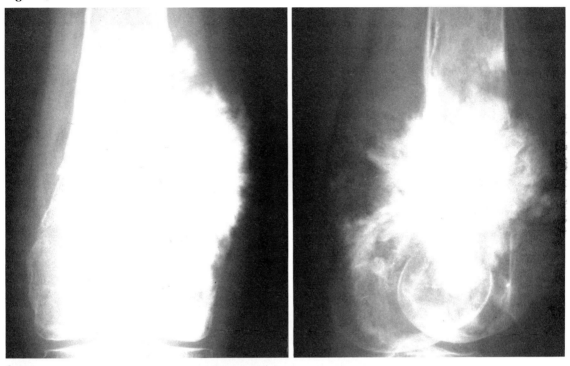

c

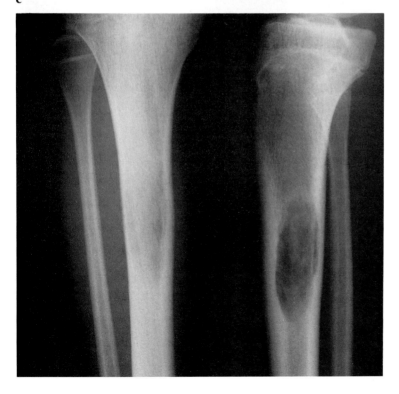

Figure 3.69

Lytic osteogenic sarcoma. This lesion resembles a simple bone cyst, although the site might be unusual. It is poorly defined and causing endosteal scalloping, but as yet there is no significant expansion of the bone or obvious periostitis. The clinical findings might be helpful in such a patient.

Figure 3.70

Osteogenic sarcoma of the
calcaneum. There is sclerosis of
the entire calcaneum which is
only slightly expanded. There is
also some cortical irregularity
and soft tissue ossification. The
appearances may resemble
Paget's disease but, in the latter,
soft tissue swelling will not be
evident, and there is usually no
visible soft tissue ossification.
The age of the patient is an
important diagnostic tool.

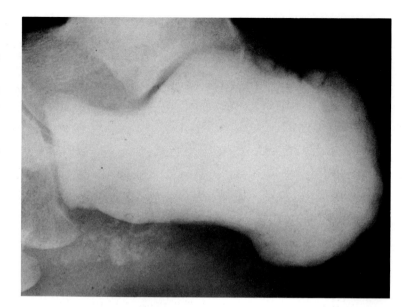

Figure 3.71

In this patient with
osteogenic sarcoma (**a**) a
large ossifying tumour arises
on the proximal fibula. (**b**)
The lesion is seen on the
radioisotope bone scan and
there is quite marked
increase in uptake
throughout both lung fields
and, particularly, at the hilum
of the left lung. (**c**) The chest
radiograph shows multiple
pulmonary metastases
which have added areas of
density due to ossification.
(**d**) A further radioisotope
bone scan shows increase of
uptake in both lungs and in
the lymph nodes of the
groin on the affected side.

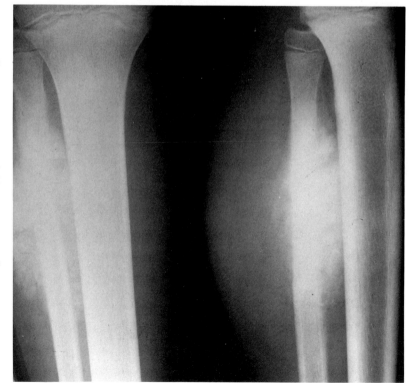

a

Figure 3.71 *continued*

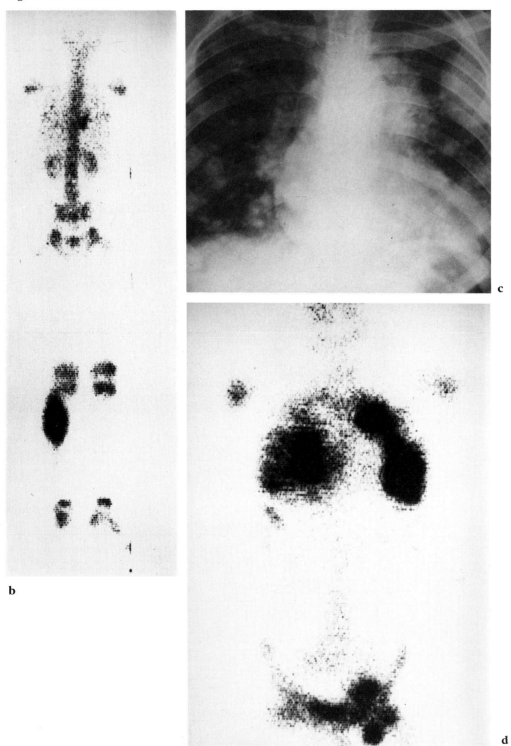

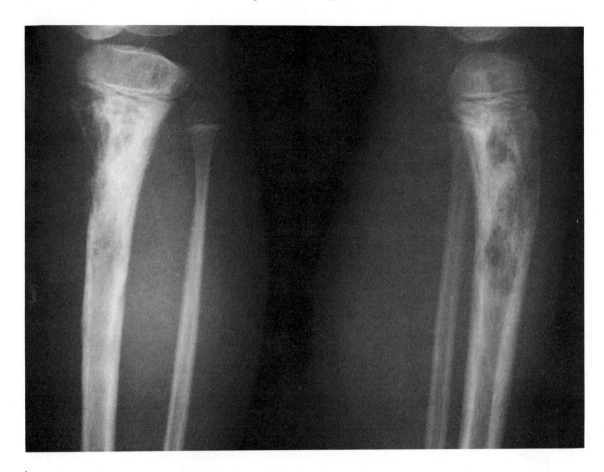

Figure 3.72

Ewing's sarcoma. A permeative
and destructive lytic lesion of the
proximal tibia is associated with
disuse osteoporosis. There is
sclerotic reaction locally but no
new bone formation in the soft
tissues.

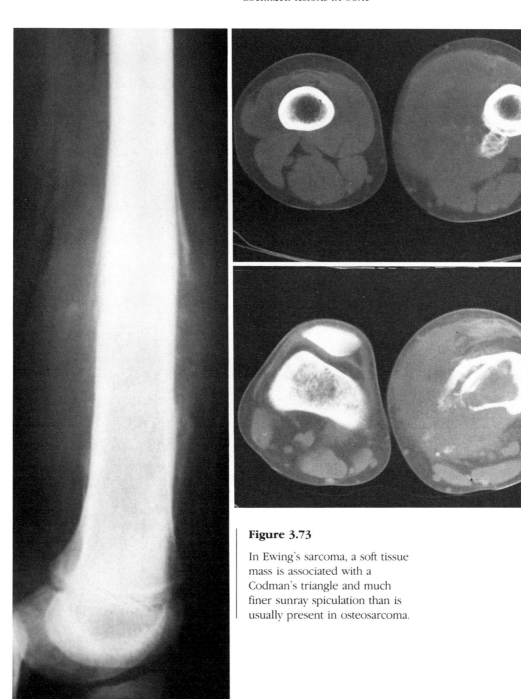

Figure 3.73

In Ewing's sarcoma, a soft tissue mass is associated with a Codman's triangle and much finer sunray spiculation than is usually present in osteosarcoma.

Figure 3.74

The left fourth rib is irregular
and increased in density. There is
a large associated soft tissue
swelling. This lesion in a child is
strongly suggestive of Ewing's
sarcoma.

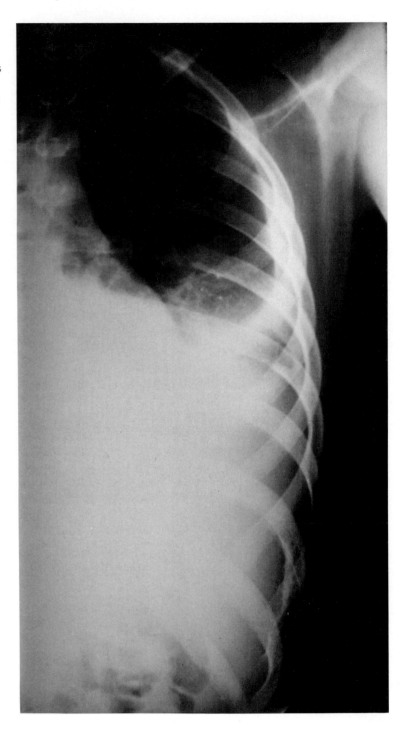

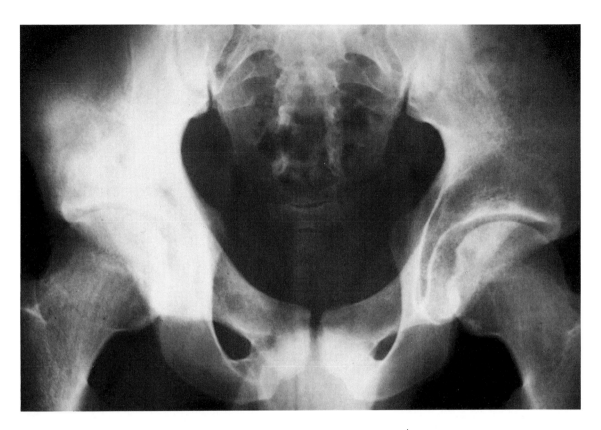

Leukaemia

Below five years of age, any malignant lesion which has the infiltrative features of a Ewing's sarcoma is likely to be due to leukaemia or neuroblastoma. These lesions are usually multiple and associated with metaphyseal bands of lucency and sutural widening in the skull. Lucent bands are also present beneath vertebral endplates, rib cortices and iliac crests (Figure 3.77).

Fibrosarcoma

This is a rare primary malignant tumour of bone which also occasionally arises on pre-existing fibrous dysplasia, Paget's disease and bone infarcts. The lesion has a maximal incidence in the fourth decade and is probably more common

Figure 3.75

Ewing's sarcoma in the pelvis. In common with other malignant tumours at this site, the appearance is of slight expansion with a soft tissue mass and reactive sclerosis. These changes should be assessed with a CT scan which confirms the soft tissue swelling and often shows new bone formation (Figure 3.82b).

Figure 3.76

Reticulum cell sarcoma. Diffuse
infiltration along the shaft of the
humerus causes lysis, although
there is some reactive sclerosis.
There is no new bone formation
and very little evidence of a soft
tissue mass, but cortical
sequestration is present.

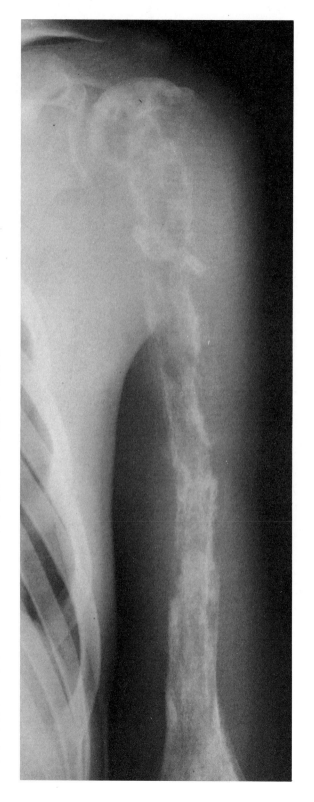

in males. Although most commonly seen in the
metaphyses around the knee, ribs and flat bones
are also involved (Figures 3.78 and 3.79). The
tumour is highly destructive, breaking through
the cortex, invading soft tissues, forming a mass,
and causing diffuse and ill-defined destruction of
the medulla within which residual bony sequestra may be seen. The lesion may extend to an
articular surface and the poorly-marginated area
of destruction may then resemble a giant-cell
tumour (Figure 3.80); however, these patients
are usually older than those with giant-cell
tumour. Destruction is probably more localized,
less permeative and moth-eaten than with reticulum cell sarcoma.

Chondrosarcoma

Malignant tumours of cartilage can arise *ab initio*
or, rarely, secondary to a single enchondroma, to
an enchondroma in multiple enchondromatosis
(Figure 3.81), on a cartilage-capped exostosis or
in diaphyseal aclasia.

Loss of marginal definition, rapid growth and
pain in a pre-existing lesion may all suggest
malignant change. Primary lesions occur in the
pelvis and major long bones, most commonly in
males in their fifth and sixth decades (Figure
3.82).

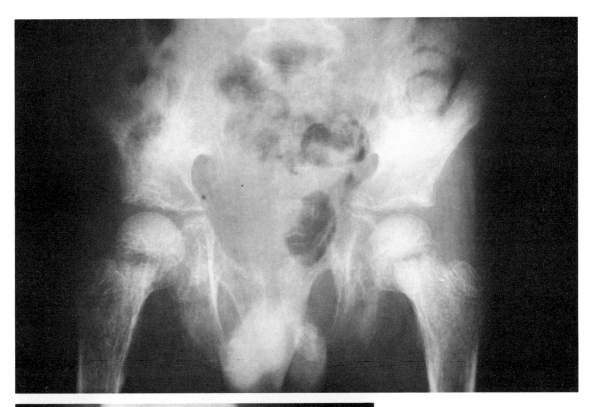

Figure 3.77

In this patient with leukaemia, there is widespread demineralization of bone which is accentuated in subcortical regions. The cortices are thinned.

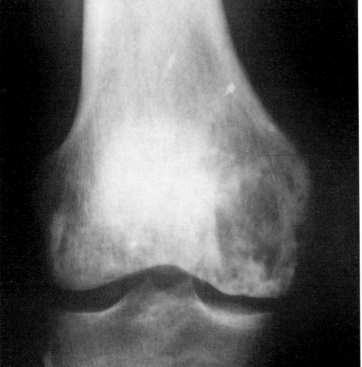

Figure 3.78

Fibrosarcoma. The distal femur has a moth-eaten appearance due to a mixture of areas of osteolysis and osteosclerosis. There is very little evidence of a soft tissue mass, cortical breakthrough or periostitis.

Figure 3.79

In this patient with fibrosarcoma, quite marked destruction of bone on the medial aspect of the acetabulum extends to the symphysis pubis. This is associated with a soft tissue mass, but there is no new bone formation.

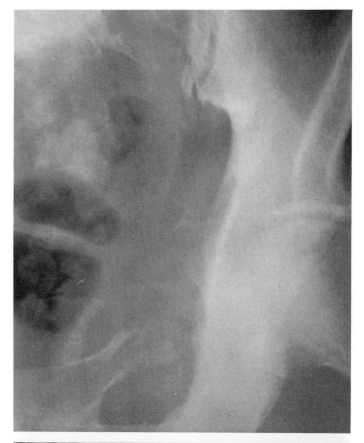

Figure 3.80

Fibrosarcoma. A diffuse, permeative, destructive lesion of the distal radius causes some local reactive sclerosis but minimal periostitis and no soft tissue mass.

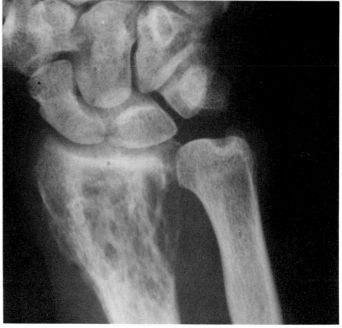

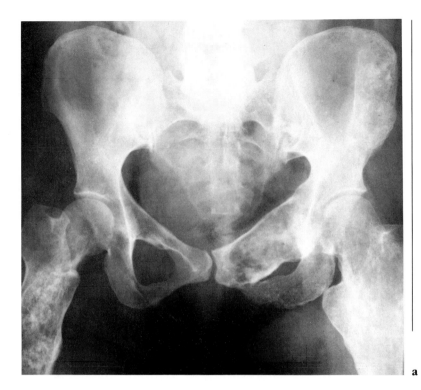

a

Figure 3.81

(**a**) Chondrosarcoma in multiple enchondromatosis. Expansile lesions are present in the left iliac blade, left ischium and pubis and right proximal femur. They are well defined and have thin sclerotic margins. (Compare these appearances with those seen in hyperparathyroidism, fibrous dysplasia and even hydatid disease.) This lesion shows spotty matrix calcification. (**b**) The same patient showing transformation of the lesion in the left pubis into chondrosarcoma. The lesion has expanded, become poorly defined and is associated with a soft tissue mass. A pathological fracture has occurred.

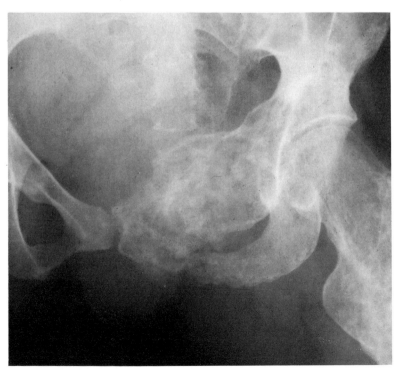

b

Figure 3.82

Chondrosarcoma. (**a**) There is
destruction of the left iliac blade
associated with marked tumour
new bone formation. (**b**) On the
CT scan, soft tissue masses are
seen anterior and posterior to
the left iliac blade which is
expanded, irregular and
sclerotic. The soft tissue masses
show new bone formation.
Therefore, the appearances are
those of a highly aggressive
malignant tumour of bone.
Similar appearances may be seen
with an osteogenic sarcoma at
the same site.

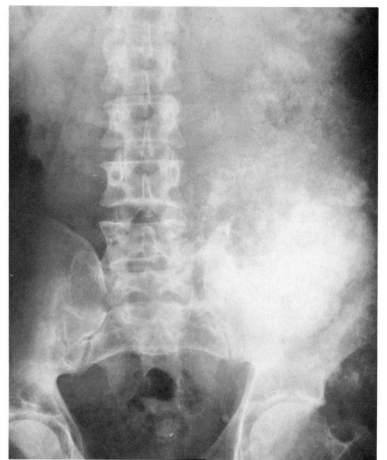

a

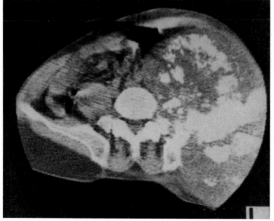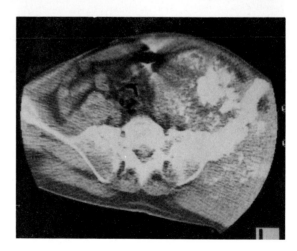

b

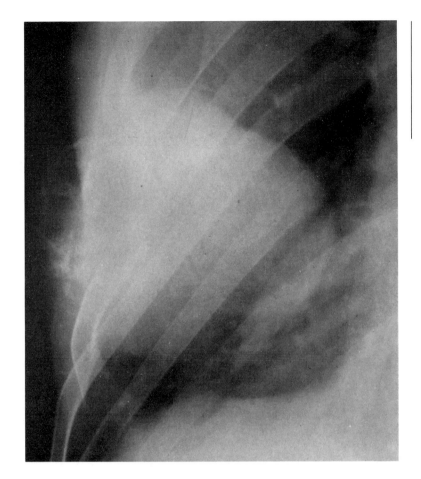

Figure 3.83

Chondrosarcoma of rib. Destruction of a rib is associated with a large soft tissue mass, part of which shows patchy ossification characteristic of a malignant tumour of cartilaginous origin.

The typical appearance is of an osteolytic lesion with a wide zone of transition, whose cartilaginous matrix undergoes patchy amorphous ossification. The cortex may be eroded and broken through, with the formation of a soft tissue mass (Figure 3.83), but often a typical tumour grows so slowly that it stimulates the overlying periosteum. The bone expanded by the tumour shows endosteal cortical scalloping, but external cortical thickening (Figure 3.84). Matrix ossification occurs centrally within the lesion rather than at its margin. Radiologically, a chondrosarcoma can resemble an infarct, but infarcts do not expand bone and often show marginal sclerosis, the zone of creeping substitution.

Differentiation between infection and malignancy

Chronic osteomyelitis (Brodie's abscess) and osteoid osteoma (or osteoblastoma)

Both of these lesions occur in children and young adults and are associated with pain, but night pain is a characteristic of osteoid osteoma. In both conditions, a central lucency surrounded by reactive sclerosis may contain foci of density, which are due to sequestra in granulation tissue

Figure 3.84

Chondrosarcoma. A permeative destruction of the medulla is associated with patchy tumoural calcification. The medullary lesion is poorly defined and infiltrative with a wide zone of transition but no surrounding reactive sclerosis. The cortex over the lesion however is thickened externally, even though in places it is scalloped endosteally.

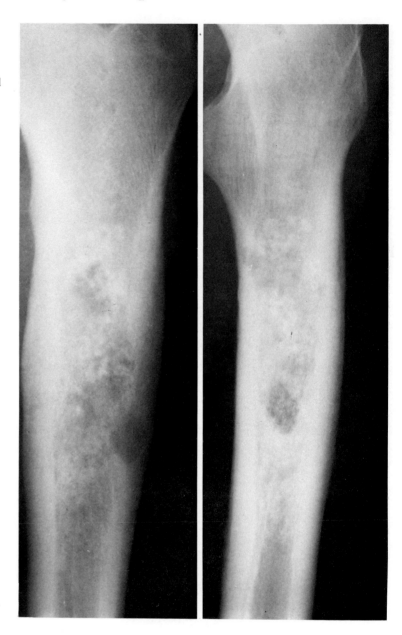

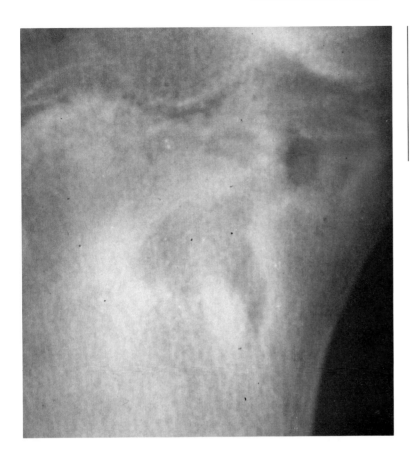

Figure 3.85

Osteomyelitis. This metaphyseal lesion in a child is associated with a well-defined zone of transition and a rather thick zone of reactive sclerosis but, most importantly, there is tunnelling, indicating the infective nature of the lesion.

in a Brodie's abscess or matrix ossification in the tumour (see page 150). Finger-like extensions of the destructive process called tunnelling only occur in infections (Figure 3.85). The osteoid osteoma is a highly vascular tumour and therefore is well displayed at angiography and isotope scanning, whereas the central lucent area in the Brodie's abscess is avascular.

Acute infection and malignant round cell tumours—leukaemia, neuroblastoma and Ewing's sarcoma

Both types of lesion may have similar clinical and laboratory features of pain, fever, local swelling and a raised erythrocyte sedimentation rate (ESR). Aggressive infiltration of bone causes a permeative lesion which destroys the cortex and elevates the periosteum, causing a periostitis with a soft tissue mass. Infections progress more rapidly than tumours and, although the initial radiological examination of the acutely painful limb may be normal, rapid progress usually confirms infection. Sequestra are the hallmark of infection, but are not usually seen in tumours with the exception of fibrosarcoma which usually occurs in an older age group. Linear sequestration in infections is often very dense and should not be confused with matrix ossification in malignant tumours of bone such as osteogenic sarcoma. This tumour occurs in the same age group as infection and often at the same metaphyseal site. Sequestra are often very dense. Soft tissue masses in infection are generally poorly defined because of oedema of displaced fat planes, whereas malignancy displaces, but does not invade, the fat planes.

4 | Lesions affecting the epiphyses

John Poland, FRCS, Consultant Surgeon to the City Orthopaedic Hospital, London, the forerunner of the Royal National Orthopaedic Hospital, published his *Atlas of skiagraphic development of the hand and wrist* in 1898 (Figure 4.1). Standards for skeletal development have subsequently been established by Greulich and Pyle, and Tanner and Whitehouse (see Appendix). In particular, Pyle and co-workers have produced atlases of skeletal development for the hand and wrist, knee and foot.

Causes of delay in skeletal maturity (Table 4.1)

Hypothyroidism

There is a delay in skeletal and dental maturation, accompanied by short stature (Figure 4.2). Epiphyses appear and fuse late, and are often abnormal in appearance, with increased density and fragmentation particularly at the femoral and humeral heads (Figure 4.3). The changes are symmetrical, unlike in Perthes' disease, when the fragmentation of the ossific nucleus of the upper femoral epiphysis is almost inevitably asymmetrical, even if bilateral (Figure 4.4). In dysplasia epiphysealis multiplex, the femoral heads are also occasionally symmetrically flattened or fragmented, but there is no delay in fusion of the epiphyses (Figure 4.5).

Table 4.1 Causes of delay in skeletal maturity.

Congenital heart disease

Hypothyroidism

Hypogonadism

Hypopituitarism

Diabetes

Severe generalized disease—renal failure, coeliac disease

Haemolytic anaemia

Malnutrition

Steroid therapy

Rickets

Skeletal dysplasias, eg the mucopolysaccharidoses

206

SKIAGRAPHIC ATLAS

SHOWING

THE DEVELOPMENT

OF THE

BONES OF THE WRIST AND HAND

FOR THE USE OF STUDENTS AND OTHERS

BY

JOHN POLAND, F.R.C.S.

LONDON
SMITH. ELDER, & CO., 15 WATERLOO PLACE
1898

a

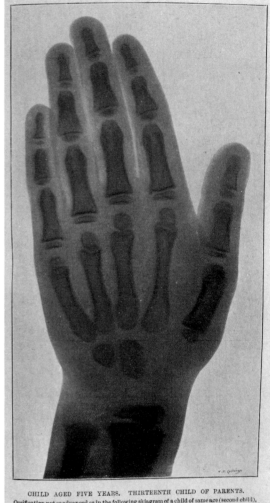

CHILD AGED FIVE YEARS. THIRTEENTH CHILD OF PARENTS.
Ossification not so advanced as in the following skiagram of a child of same age (second child), and in some respects no further advanced than in skiagram of child of three years.
Taken by Mr WM. WEBSTER.

b

In hypothyroidism, a flattened or fragmented epiphysis may persist into adult life (Figure 4.6). In the shoulder, there may be humerus varus which has a 'telephone receiver' appearance (Figure 4.7). Other radiological changes include Wormian bones and vertebral body hypoplasia, particularly at the thoracolumbar junction. Bone density may be increased generally.

In the other diseases with Wormian bones, osseous density is *reduced* in osteogenesis imperfecta and hypophosphatasia, while pathological fractures and bony bowing are not a feature of cretinism. However, bone density is *normal* in

Figure 4.1

(**a**) The title page of *Atlas of skiagraphic development of the hand and wrist*, published in 1898, by John Poland, FRCS. (**b**) A specimen from the book assessing skeletal development.

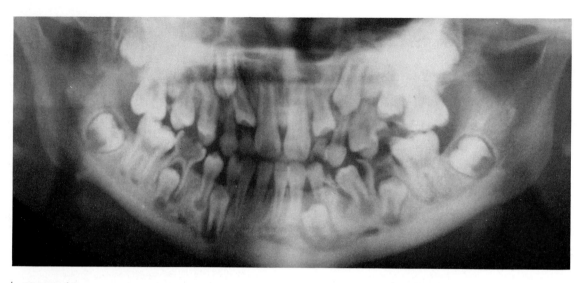

Figure 4.2

This patient has hypothyroidism. The secondary dentition has failed to develop, and much of the primary dentition remains. Therefore, there is gross retardation of dental age.

Figure 4.3

Cretinism. Symmetrical fragmentation of the femoral heads resembles Perthes' disease; however, in the latter condition the changes are rarely symmetrical. There is associated broadening of the irregular femoral necks. The synchondrosis at the ischio-pubic ramus is still open. This is another feature of retarded skeletal maturity and is not to be confused with a Looser's zone.

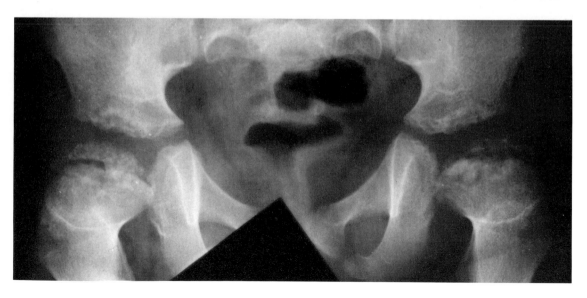

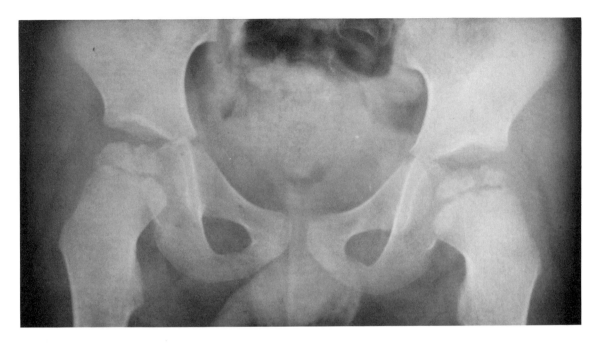

Figure 4.4

Perthes' disease. In this patient the changes are seen at both femoral heads but there is asymmetry. Acetabular and supra-acetabular modelling are more normal.

Figure 4.5

Dysplasia epiphysealis multiplex. Both femoral heads are irregular and flattened, but not fragmented. Changes at the acetabular roof reflect this change. In this patient abnormalities were also present at other large joints.

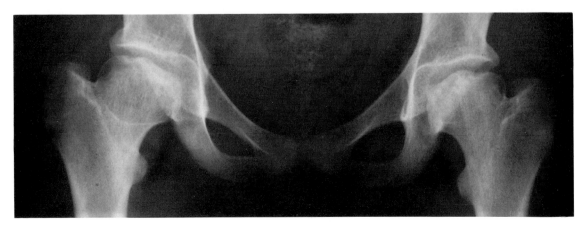

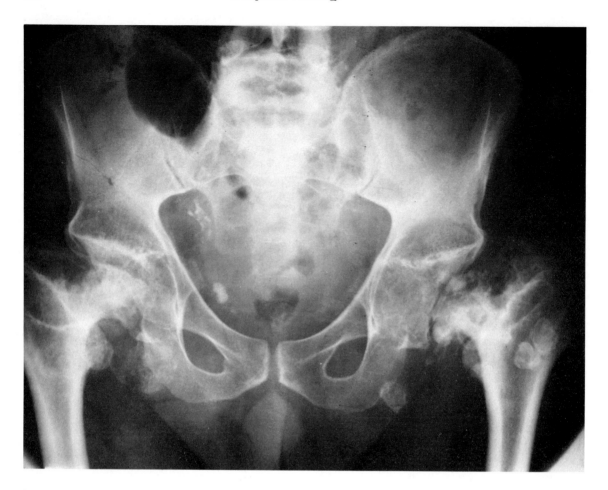

Figure 4.6

Cretinism. The patient is an adult but irregularity and fragmentation of the femoral heads has persisted. The longstanding nature of the disease may be seen particularly at the left acetabulum which is full of new bone as a result of early fragmentation of the adjacent epiphysis.

Table 4.2   Diseases occurring with Wormian bones.

Disease	*Bone density*	*Pathological fractures; Bowing*	*Skeletal maturity*
Hypothyroidism	Normal	None	Delayed
Osteogenesis imperfecta	Reduced	Present	Normal
Hypophosphatasia	Reduced	Present	Delayed
Cleidocranial dysostosis	Normal	None	Slight retardation of growth
Pyknodysostosis	Increased	Present	Small stature

cleidocranial dysplasia, in which skeletal maturity is not retarded, and is *increased* in pyknodysostosis (Table 4.2).

Hypogonadism and hypopituitarism

In hypogonadism and hypopituitarism there is delay in skeletal maturation and fusion, which is associated with osteoporosis.

Steroid excess

Steroid excess, whether iatrogenic or adrenal in origin, causes a delay in skeletal maturation, which is often gross. This is associated with osteoporosis and pathological fractures, vertebral collapse with callus formation (Figure 1.12) and avascular necrosis (Figure 4.8). There are no Wormian bones. Clinically the condition does not resemble osteogenesis imperfecta.

Rickets

Rickets involves some delay in epiphyseal maturation, associated with an abnormal bone texture, metaphyseal irregularity and splaying, and widening of the growth plate (Figure 4.9). Fusion of the ischiopubic synchondrosis, which normally occurs at about seven years of age, may be retarded in conditions where fusion in general is retarded, for example, cretinism. However, Looser's zones are commonly found at that site and should be diagnosed after ten years of age if lucency persists locally.

Skeletal maturity is often delayed in children with severe cardiac, renal or gastro-intestinal disease, or in those with malnutrition, and growth arrest lines may be seen. Severe haemolytic anaemias also retard maturation.

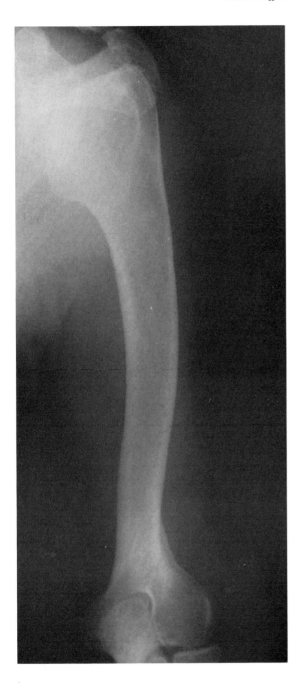

Figure 4.7

Cretinism with humerus varus. Abnormal growth of the epiphysis has resulted in a telephone receiver appearance.

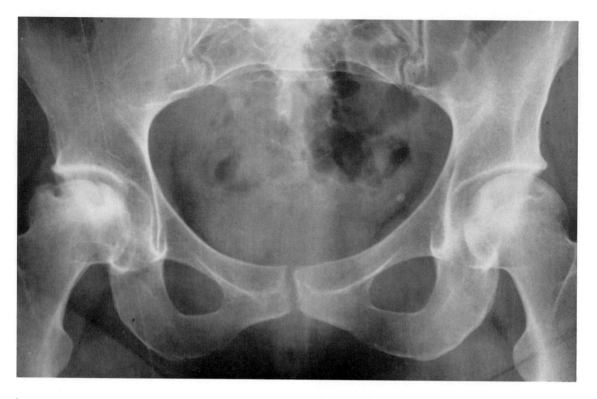

Figure 4.8

In avascular necrosis following
steroid therapy, structural failure
is quite advanced at the right
femoral head with collapse of
sclerotic bone. In the left femoral
head an avascular area is
surrounded by a sclerotic zone of
creeping substitution. Collapse
will occur here too.

**Table 4.3   Causes of accelerated
skeletal maturity.**

Hyperthyroidism

Hypergonadism

Hyperpituitarism—gigantism

Fibrous dysplasia

Adrenogenital syndrome

Homocystinuria

Neurofibromatosis

Still's disease and other causes of increased
    blood flow, eg. in infection (often localized)

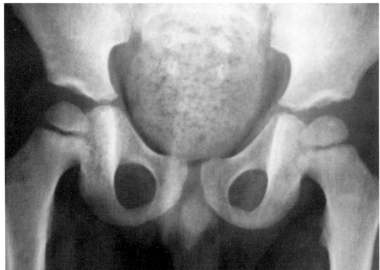

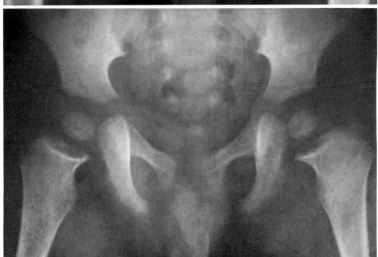

Figure 4.9

Normal epiphyses and rachitic epiphyses. The upper radiograph shows the normal width of the epiphyseal plate, while the lower shows a widened epiphyseal plate. This change is typical of rickets. The bone density elsewhere is diminished.

Causes of acceleration in skeletal maturity (Table 4.3)

Hyperthyroidism

This is rare in children but is associated with accelerated skeletal maturation and osteoporosis.

Hyperpituitarism

This causes an excess of growth hormone, and produces gigantism before skeletal fusion, and acromegaly after it. An adult giant has a different appearance to an acromegalic. Overgrowth in gigantism occurs when epiphyseal plates are open and leads to excessive longitudinal and

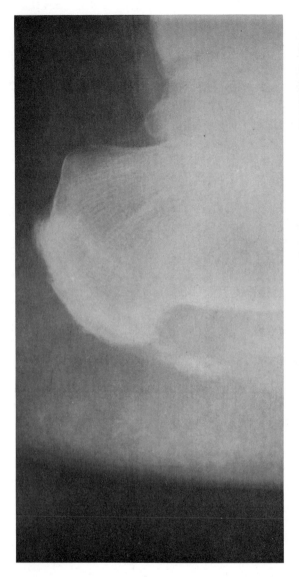

Figure 4.10

Acromegaly. Much new bone is seen on the posterior aspect of the calcaneum and the heel pad thickness is increased.

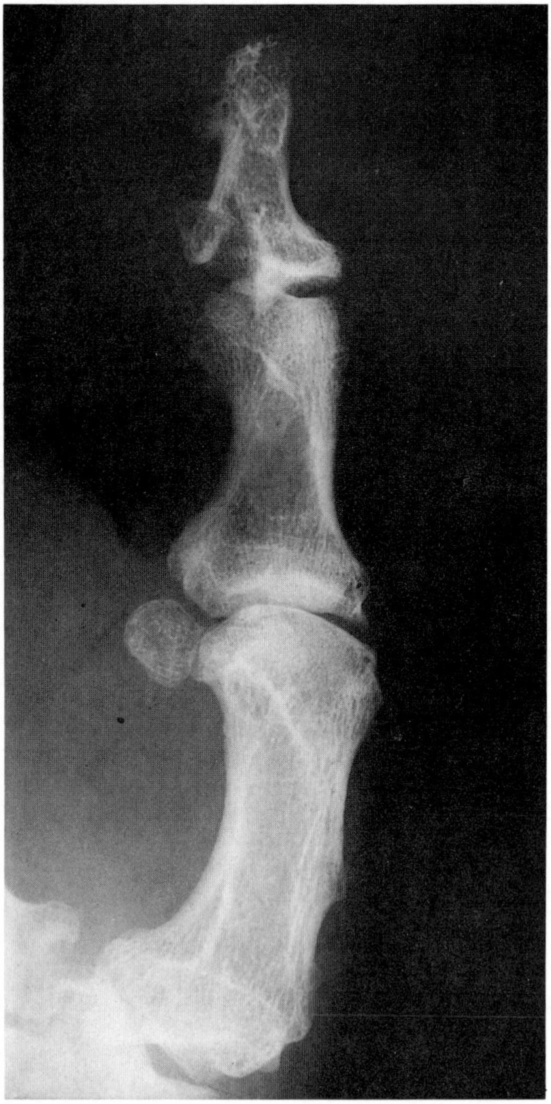

Figure 4.11

In acromegaly, an increase in growth hormone thickens the cartilages so that the joint spaces appear widened. Muscle insertions become more prominent, and secondary osteoarthritis often supervenes. The sesamoids are often enlarged and this can be measured using the sesamoid index.

transverse growth. Acromegalics cannot increase bone length, but soft tissues such as heel pads (Figure 4.10) and intervertebral discs are enlarged, as are joint cartilages, leading to an increase in height. Bones also broaden, particularly at muscle insertions (Figure 4.11). Bone may be resorbed so that cortical thinning, osteoporosis and vertebral scalloping may result. (For other causes of vertebral scalloping, see Table 7.5.)

Fibrous dysplasia

This may be associated with endocrine abnormalities. Albright's syndrome associates fibrous dysplasia with skin pigmentation and precocious sexual development, usually in females. Growth discrepancy in fibrous dysplasia may be due to the fibrous lesion in a bone. Other endocrine anomalies in fibrous dysplasia, Cushing's syndrome, thyrotoxicosis and hyperpituitarism, can also result in altered skeletal maturity and growth.

Precocious sexual development occurs in neurofibromatosis, in which there is also skin pigmentation although in a different form to that of fibrous dysplasia. Other endocrine abnormalities may also be found, but overgrowth of bones in neurofibromatosis is not usually endocrine in origin but part of the dysplasia and not confined to the epiphyses.

Large epiphyses are also found in homocystinuria, fibrodysplasia ossificans progressiva and the Laurence–Moon–Biedl syndrome.

Increase in epiphyseal maturation due to local hyperaemia

This occurs in any condition in which blood flow is increased locally. Epiphyseal growth is advanced and premature fusion may result, so that an initial gain in length is followed by eventual shortening.

Premature fusion

Premature fusion at epiphyses is rarely generalized but is more usually due to local disease. It usually follows infection (Figure 4.12), trauma (Figure 4.13) or irradiation to the growth plate (Figure 4.14).

If the entire growth plate is destroyed, there will be growth arrest across the entire epiphysis. If only part of the growth plate is damaged, then growth around it moves away from the fused part, producing a deformed or 'V'-shaped bone end known as the 'chevron' sign. This appearance also occurs in achondroplasia (Figure 4.15), and in scurvy following fractures through the translucent metaphyseal zone at the knees.

Generalized changes at epiphyses—diseases of joints

Hyperaemia around epiphyses is seen with simple or tuberculous infections, juvenile chronic arthritis and other collagen diseases, haemophilia, and occasionally with tumours. All these diseases have at least one common feature, that is, the joints are affected by changes at both articular surfaces within the confines of the joint capsule, and at the synovium (Tables 4.4 and 4.5).

Rheumatoid erosions

The distribution of erosions is shown in Figure 4.16. Abnormal joints are symmetrically affected and show local soft tissue swelling and osteoporosis. Erosions are the definitive change in rheumatoid arthritis. They occur initially in the para-articular regions, at the cartilage/synovium interface (Figure 4.17). Cartilage destruction results in joint space narrowing (Figure 4.18), followed by erosion of articular surfaces (Figure 4.19). Reactive sclerosis can occur but overall bone density is diminished (Figure 4.20). New bone proliferation is not a prominent feature of rheumatoid arthritis, and erosions do not fill in. Secondary osteoarthritis occurs. Malalignment at joint surfaces is the result of bone destruction and local soft tissue changes, ligamentous laxity and tendinous attrition (Figure 4.21). Neurotrophic or 'cup and pencil' deformities are also seen.

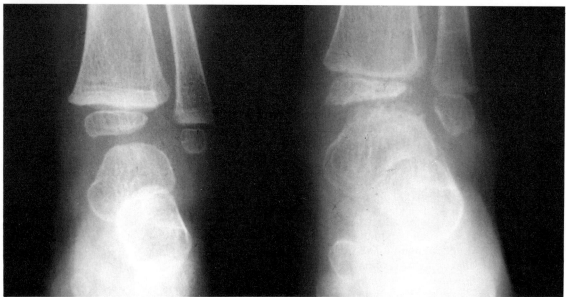

a

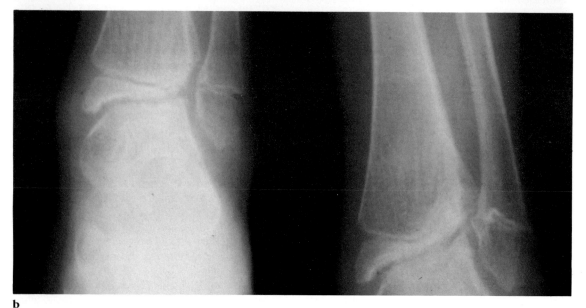

b

Figure 4.12

Premature fusion in osteomyelitis. This series of radiographs was obtained over three years. The initial radiograph (year 1) shows diffuse soft tissue swelling around the ankle joint (**a**). The second (year 2) shows irregularity of the head of the talus and of the adjacent distal tibial epiphysis. The joint space is narrowed, indicating cartilaginous destruction. Subsequently (year 3), there is evidence of failure of growth of the lateral aspect of the dista tibial epiphysis which is associated with a parallel overgrowth of the adjacent talus (**b**). The final radiograph (year 4) shows premature fusion of the growth plate of the distal tibia laterally and of the adjacent fibula, with marked tibio-talar slant and a narrow and irregular joint line, which characterizes an infective aetiology.

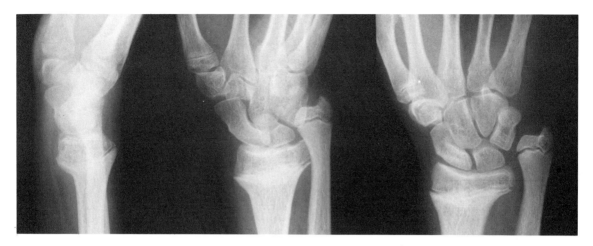

Figure 4.13

Premature fusion secondary to trauma is relatively common and follows compression of the growth plate of the distal radius. The growth plate is fused centrally but is still open laterally, so that peripheral growth can still occur. A chevron deformity results.

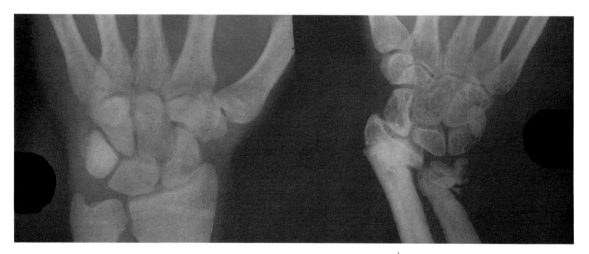

Figure 4.14

Premature fusion following radiation. The left wrist is normal but on the right there is hypoplasia of the distal ulna associated with premature fusion and sclerosis around the epiphyseal plate.

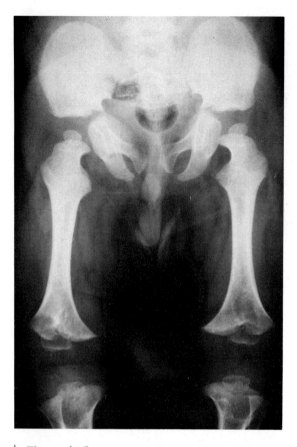

Figure 4.15

Achondroplasia. A chevron deformity occurs as a normal phenomenon at the distal femur.

Table 4.4   Causes of widespread changes in epiphyseal shape.

Osteoarthritis

Rheumatoid arthritis, juvenile rheumatoid arthritis, psoriatic arthritis

Hypothyroidism

Haemophilia

Following avascular necrosis

Acromegaly

Rickets

Dysplasias of bone

Achondroplasia

Pseudoachondroplasia

Dysplasia epiphysealis multiplex (Fairbank)

Dysplasia epiphysealis hemimelica (Trevor)

Spondyloepiphyseal dysplasia

Mucopolysaccharidoses

Enchondromatosis

Table 4.5   Generalized changes at epiphyses—diseases of joints.

Seronegative and seropositive arthritides

Rheumatoid arthritis

Psoriasis

Reiter's syndrome

Ankylosing spondylitis

Enteropathic spondylarthritides

Juvenile rheumatoid arthritis

Osteoarthritis

Septic arthritis

Gout

Haemophilia

Synovial tumours

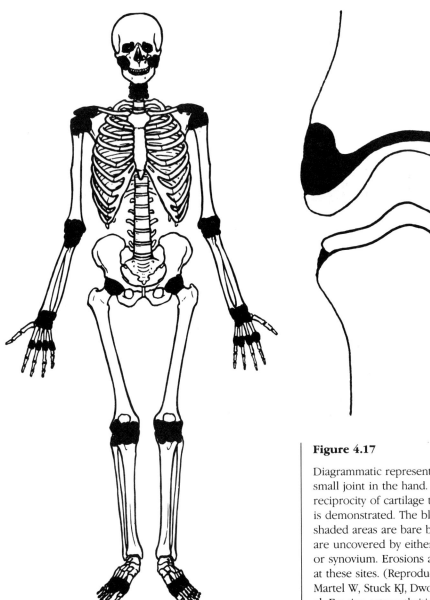

Figure 4.16

Distribution of rheumatoid disease (shaded areas).

Figure 4.17

Diagrammatic representation of a small joint in the hand. The reciprocity of cartilage thickness is demonstrated. The black shaded areas are bare bone and are uncovered by either cartilage or synovium. Erosions arise first at these sites. (Reproduced from Martel W, Stuck KJ, Dworin AM et al, Erosive osteoarthritis and psoriatic arthritis: a radiologic comparison in the hand, wrist and foot, *American Journal of Roentgenology* (1980) **134**: 125–35, with permission.)

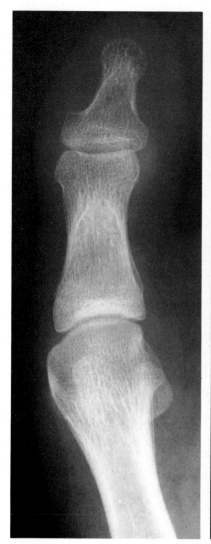

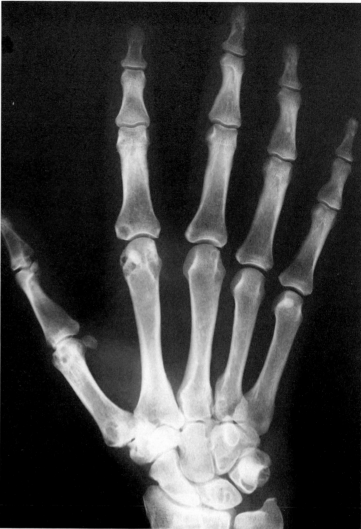

Figure 4.18

In this patient with rheumatoid arthritis, there is soft tissue swelling around the great toe metatarsophalangeal joint. Fine lamellar periosteal reactions can be seen along the metatarsal and phalangeal shafts. The metatarsophalangeal joint is narrower than the interphalangeal joint.

Figure 4.19

Rheumatoid arthritis. Narrowing of the thumb and index metacarpophalangeal joints is associated with local erosive change. Further erosions are seen in the carpal bones.

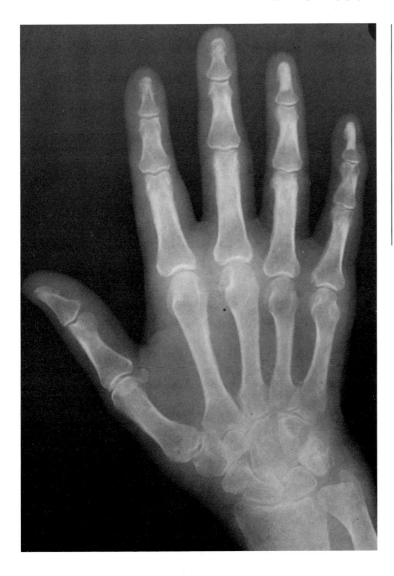

Figure 4.20

In this patient with rheumatoid arthritis, there is soft tissue swelling particularly over the index and middle finger metacarpophalangeal joints and proximal phalanges. Bone density is reduced overall. The distal phalanges, however, show terminal phalangeal sclerosis, which is associated with, and often pre-dates, the onset of an erosive arthritis. Erosive change is also present at the fourth and fifth metacarpophalangeal joints.

Psoriatic arthritis

The distribution of lesions in this disease is shown in Figure 4.22. Typical psoriatic arthritis is found in only 30 per cent of patients with both psoriasis and arthritis. The combination of diseases occurs in 5–20 per cent of psoriatics, and 70 per cent of these have either rheumatoid-like changes or a mixed pattern.

Soft tissue swelling is seen. Density at affected joints is usually preserved, but this is not inevitable. Increase in the density of affected digits occurs in the presence of marked periostitis ('sausage' digit) (Figure 4.23).

Erosions at affected joints, particularly the great toe and distal phalanges, occur on the articular surfaces rather than at joint margins, and are associated with marked local new bone formation. At distal phalangeal bases a 'gull's

Figure 4.21

(**a**) End-stage rheumatoid arthritis with radiocarpal fusion. Cup and pencil deformities with bone resorption are present at the metacarpophalangeal joints, while the interphalangeal joints are fused. There is overall demineralization and soft tissue wasting. (**b**) The resorption of bone around the glenohumeral joints is almost neuropathic. The bone surfaces are no longer in alignment, and are smooth and sclerotic. Also, there is erosion of the upper surfaces of the third, fourth and fifth ribs. This phenomenon is probably related to muscle wasting and scapular attrition.

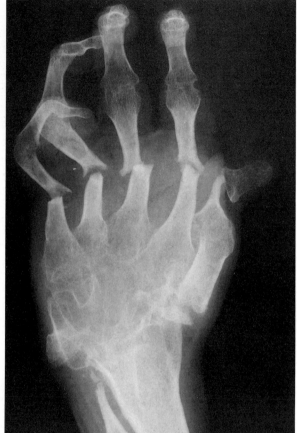

a

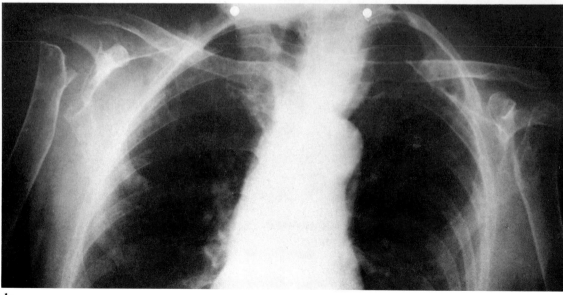

b

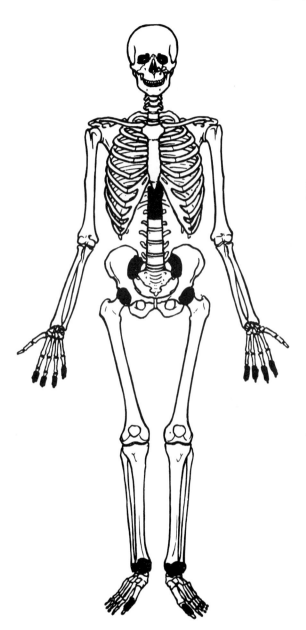

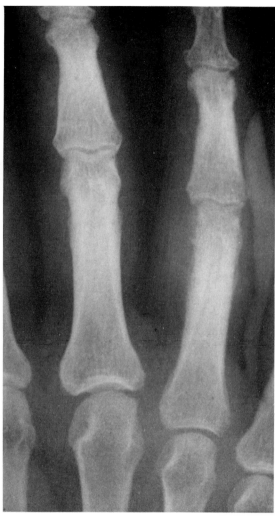

Figure 4.23

In this psoriatic patient, swelling of the ring finger is associated with a periostitis of the proximal and middle phalanges and an overall increase in bony density.

Figure 4.22

Distribution of lesions in psoriasis (shaded areas).

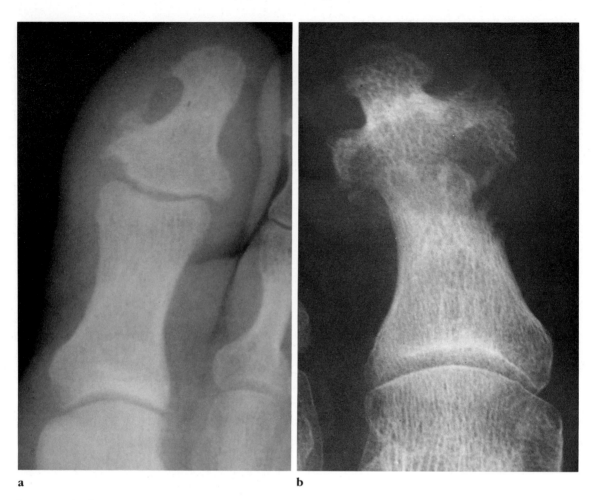

a   b

Figure 4.24

Psoriasis. (**a**) Soft tissue swelling is seen over the great toe and the erosions at the bases of the distal phalanges are on the articular, rather than the periarticular surface, producing a gull's wing appearance (**b**). (**c**) The distal interphalangeal joints are involved in this condition. Bone density is often preserved. Erosions proceed along the bases of the distal phalanges and there is splaying of bone locally. Despite the erosive change, the joints may be increased in width or, alternatively, fused. These changes are totally unlike those seen in rheumatoid arthritis, both in appearance and distribution. There is also a neurotrophic change at the distal and middle phalanges, with longitudinal and concentric bone resorption, producing a 'licked candy stick' appearance.

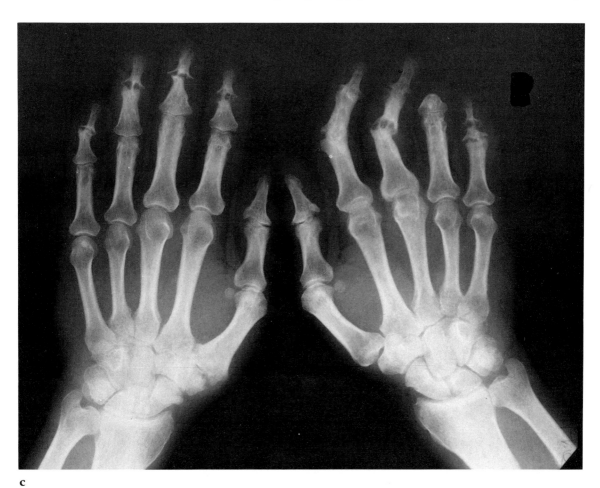

c

Figure 4.24 *continued*

wing' appearance results (Figure 4.24). Bony proliferation at erosions is a feature of psoriatic arthritis, and occurs at joints and also at musculo-tendinous and ligamentous insertions into bone, known as the entheses (Figure 4.25). Changes at major joints are similar to those seen in rheumatoid disease.

Reiter's syndrome

This disease involves soft tissue swelling around affected joints but the changes are asymmetrical, unlike those seen in rheumatoid arthritis. Meta-tarsophalangeal joints are involved, and the feet are more often involved than the hands. New bone formation is prominent (Figure 4.26).

Ankylosing spondylitis and enteropathic spondylarthritis

Peripheral joint disease is not prominent but may precede the spinal changes, particularly in children. Rheumatoid-type change can be followed by fusion of affected joints.

Osteoarthritis

The distribution of lesions in osteoarthritis is shown in Figure 4.27. Primary osteoarthritis has no obvious underlying aetiology whereas secondary disease usually follows articular malalignment, for example, after congenital anomalies or

Figure 4.25

Psoriasis. The left sacroiliac joint
is eroded laterally with
underlying reactive sclerosis. The
left hip joint is narrowed,
particularly superomedially, and
the articular surfaces are
irregular. There is no reactive
new bone formation. Erosions
are seen at the musculo-
tendinous insertions on the
ischium.

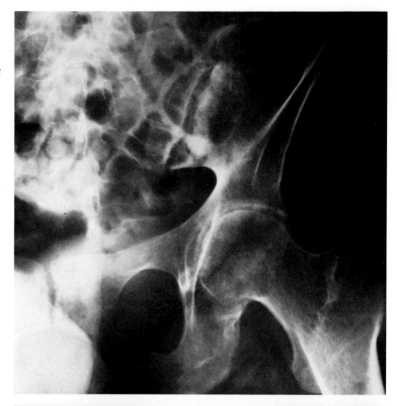

Figure 4.26

Reiter's syndrome. New bone
formation on the inferior and
posterior aspects of the
calcaneum is fluffy and associated
with erosive change at the tendo
Achillis insertion.

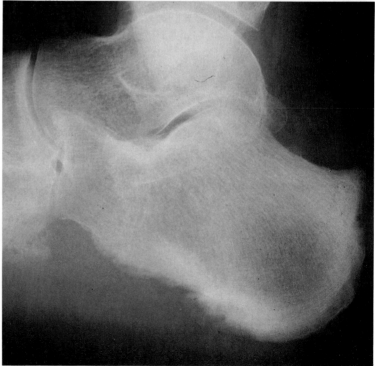

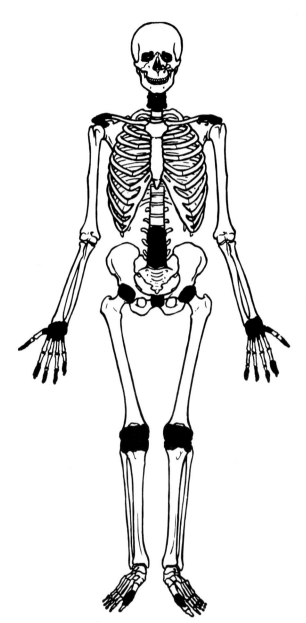

Figure 4.27

Distribution of osteoarthritis (shaded areas).

acquired, traumatic or infective lesions. Soft tissue swelling around the affected joints reflects underlying new bone proliferation, particularly at the distal interphalangeal joints (Figure 4.28). Bone density is unaffected by this condition, which is not associated with significant hyper-aemia. Joint narrowing due to cartilage loss occurs primarily at areas of maximal stress, for example, the weight-bearing areas, and is follo-wed by loss of articular bone (Figure 4.29). However, bone is laid down in the non-weight-bearing areas of joints and often in subarticular regions (Figure 4.30). Marginal osteophytes are characteristic features.

Juvenile chronic arthritis

In juvenile chronic arthritis, 90 per cent of patients are seronegative. The remaining seropo-sitive patients have an erosive pattern of disease similar to adult rheumatoid arthritis. Usually, the erosions are not prominent, which may be because the ossific nuclei of the epiphyses are protected by a thick cover of cartilage. Soft tissue swelling and osteoporosis are seen and bone growth is accelerated because of local hyper-aemia (Figure 4.31). Epiphyses become enlarged and abnormal in shape, often angular and squared rather than round and smooth. Overgrowth results in joint space narrowing (Figure 4.32) and premature fusion at growth plates results in small stature, which is often compounded by corticosteroid administration (Figure 4.33).

Because the bony changes in juvenile chronic arthritis are due to synovial disease, they are similar to those seen with two other diseases, tuberculosis (Figure 4.34) and haemophilia (Figure 4.35), in which identical epiphyseal modelling abnormalities are seen. In haemophilia a deepened intercondylar notch occurs due to bleeding into the cruciate ligament origins (Figure 4.35); however, this deepening may be a reflection of condylar overgrowth. In both haemophilia and tuberculosis, cartilage and bone destruction can occur because of synovial pro-liferation.

Table 4.6 shows that spinal changes and sacroiliitis are features of seronegative arthriti-des. Rheumatoid arthritis only occasionally

Figure 4.28

Osteoarthritis. Involvement of
the middle and distal
interphalangeal joints is shown
with joint space narrowing and
sclerosis of the articular surfaces.
At the distal interphalangeal
joints particularly there is
proliferation of new bone
around the joints.

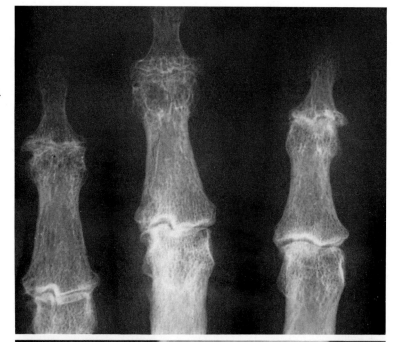

Figure 4.29

In this patient with osteoarthritis,
the joint space of the hip is
narrowed superiorly and the
subjacent articular surfaces show
reactive sclerosis. New bone
formation is seen laterally on the
acetabular margin and femoral
head. Drift of the femoral head
occurs in a lateral direction and
new bone fills in the medial
aspect of the acetabular fossa.

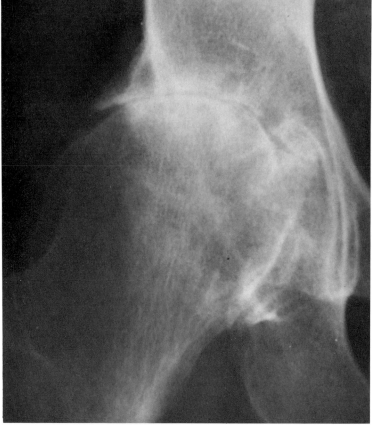

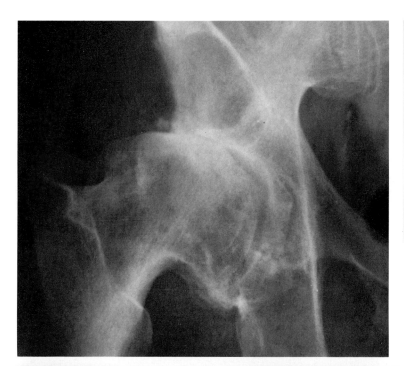

Figure 4.30

Progression of osteoarthritis in the previous patient. The femoral head has migrated further laterally and has lost volume superiorly in the weight-bearing area. However, new bone has formed medially on the femoral head and to a greater extent on the acetabulum, so that the new medial joint space appears separate from the old, which is still discernible. There is a large cyst in the superior aspect of the acetabulum.

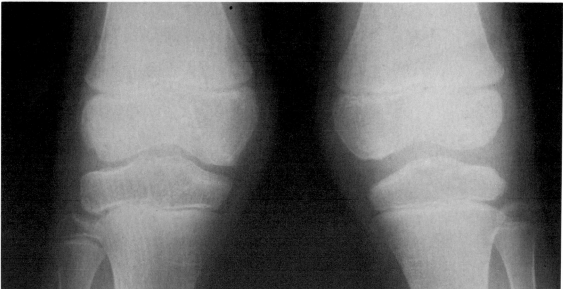

Figure 4.31

Juvenile chronic arthritis. The right knee shows overgrowth of its epiphyses with a resultant apparent narrowing of the joint space. The overgrowth is not smooth and is associated with angularity rather than roundness of articular margins. This feature follows synovial hyperplasia and hyperaemia in this disease. Growth arrest lines are also seen, superimposed on osteoporosis.

Figure 4.32

In this patient with juvenile
chronic arthritis, changes affect
the left knee with resultant
overgrowth of all the epiphyses,
including that for the proximal
fibula. The overgrown epiphyses
have angular margins.

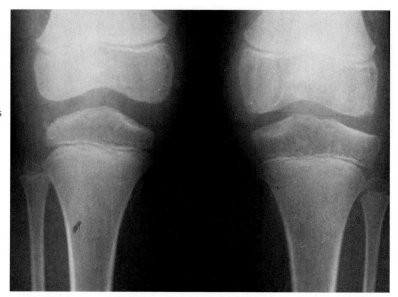

Figure 4.33

In this extreme case of juvenile
chronic arthritis, both knees are
affected after five years of illness.
There is osteoporosis, which is
probably compounded by
steroid administration, and
marked muscle wasting.
Overgrowth of epiphyses results
in bulbous and angular articular
surfaces. The only remaining
trabeculae are along the lines of
stress.

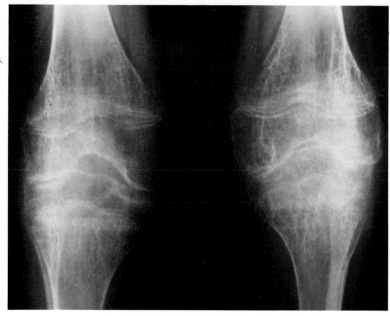

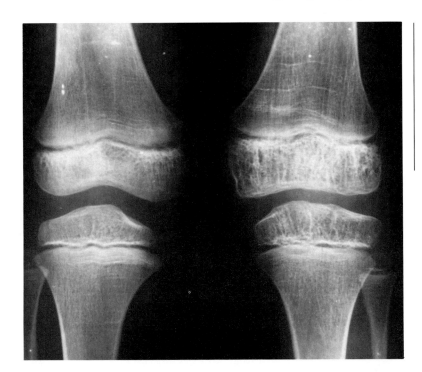

Figure 4.34

Synovial tuberculosis. The left knee is affected and the appearances are basically identical to those seen with juvenile chronic arthritis. There is overgrowth of epiphyses, which are squared, and stress trabeculae; growth arrest lines are prominent.

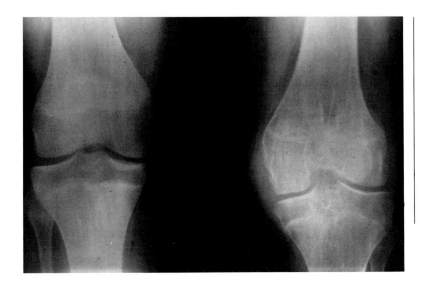

Figure 4.35

Haemophilia. The affected limb shows soft tissue swelling around the joint and quadriceps wasting when compared to the normal side. There is an effusion or blood in the joint. The bones are demineralized and increased in length, and the joint space is narrowed, which is partly due to overgrowth of epiphyses. The intercondylar notch appears deepened, and stress trabecular lines are prominent.

Table 4.6   Distribution of changes in arthritis

Condition	Hands	Feet	Hips	Knees	Shoulders
Osteoarthritis	DIP CMC	Hallux MTP	++	++	—
Rheumatoid arthritis	MCP Carpus	MTP	+	++	+
Reiter's syndrome	Occasional	Hallux MTP + IP	Occasional	Occasional	Occasional
Psoriatic arthritis	DIP	DIP	Occasional	Occasional	Occasional
Ankylosing spondylitis Enteropathic spondylarthritis	Occasional	Occasional	Occasional	Occasional	Occasional
Juvenile chronic arthritis	All over	All over	+	+	+

CMC = Carpometacarpal   MTP = Metatarsophalangeal
DIP = Distal interphalangeal   MCP = Metacarpophalangeal
 IP = Interphalangeal

Figure 4.36

Cervical spine in rheumatoid arthritis. The space between the odontoid peg and the arch of the atlas is increased. Disc spaces are narrow and irregular from C2 downwards. Subluxation is present. The facet joints are eroded and the spinous processes thin and tapered. Vertebral body fusion is also present in the mid-cervical spine.

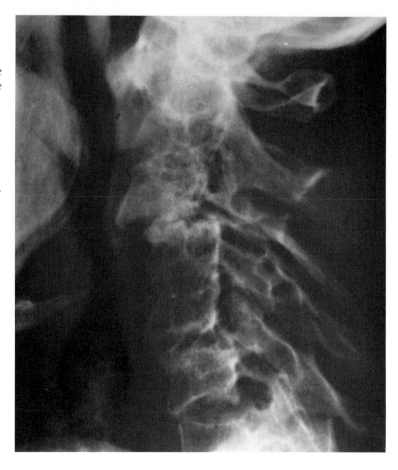

causes sacroiliitis, which is often unilateral. Spinal changes below the upper cervical spine are infrequent in rheumatoid arthritis but they may result in fusion locally (Figure 4.36). Psoriasis is associated with joint disease to a greater extent than Reiter's syndrome, although both have a form of spinal ankylosis which may differ slightly in appearance from the classical 'bamboo spine' of ankylosing spondylitis (Figure 4.37), and a sacroiliitis which may be unilateral. An enthesopathy is prominent in the seronegative spondylarthropathies, but is less common in rheumatoid arthritis. In ankylosing spondylitis, spinal and sacroiliac changes predominate over joint changes. Erosions are prominent at the entheses in all the seronegative disorders.

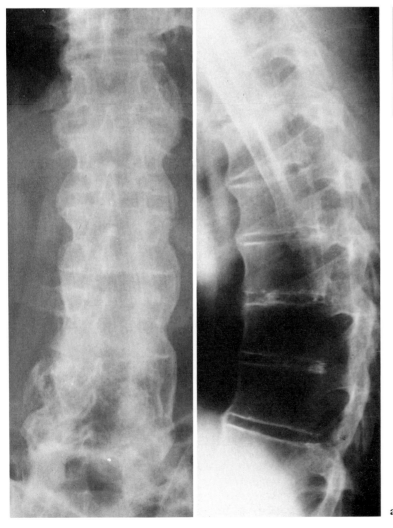

a

Figure 4.37

(**a**) Reiter's disease. Paraspinal new bone can be seen around the discs, but is not attached to the vertebral margin. A floating or non-marginal syndesmophyte is more typical of Reiter's disease.

Figure 4.37 continued

(**b**) Ankylosing spondylitis. There is symmetrical fusion of the sacroiliac joints. A bamboo spine is present. There is paraspinal ossification, which is marginal in some places and non-marginal in others. Ossification of the interspinous ligaments is seen.

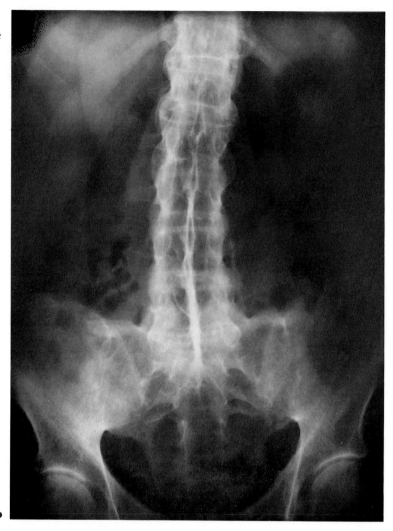

b

Septic arthritis

Joint effusions and osteoporosis are followed by cartilage destruction and joint narrowing (Figure 4.38), and the epiphyses overgrow in children. If the metaphysis is intracapsular, the focus of inflammation originating there may have entered the joint laterally through the metaphyseal cortex. When the epiphyseal plate is open it acts as a barrier to the direct spread of infection from the metaphysis into the epiphysis and joint (Figure 4.39).

Osteoporosis in subarticular regions may initially allow the thinned cortex to appear prominent, but the cortex then becomes destroyed, and bone destruction follows. Affected joints show increased uptake on isotope scanning, and aspiration of pus from an affected joint may be

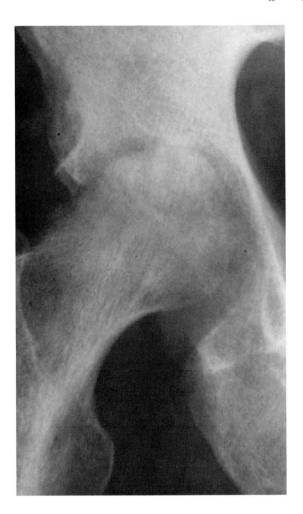

Figure 4.38

Septic arthritis. The hip joint shows quite marked surrounding osteoporosis. The articular cortex is no longer visible and the joint is narrowed, particularly superiorly.

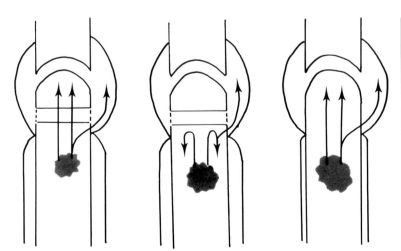

Figure 4.39

The shaded area in the metaphysis represents a focus of osteomyelitis. From 1–16 years of age the epiphyseal plate acts as a barrier to infection but, if the metaphysis is intracapsular, the joint can still be affected.

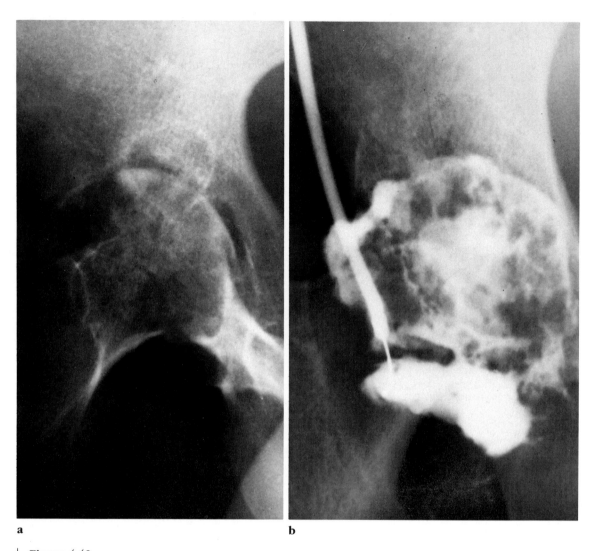

a   b

Figure 4.40

Tuberculosis of the hip. (**a**) The joint space is narrow and irregular, and destruction of bone is seen on both sides of the joint. (**b**) Arthrography. Following aspiration of pus, contrast is injected into the joint. The synovium is irregular, erodes the underlying bone and the capsule is contracted.

followed by arthrography, demonstrating abnormal synovium and the destruction of cartilage and bone (Figure 4.40).

Synovial tumours

These are uncommon and may be benign or malignant. They erode bone on both sides of the joint but, unlike rheumatoid disease, infection or haemophilia, do not necessarily destroy articular cartilage or subcartilaginous bone, so that the scalloping is para-articular (Figure 4.41). The

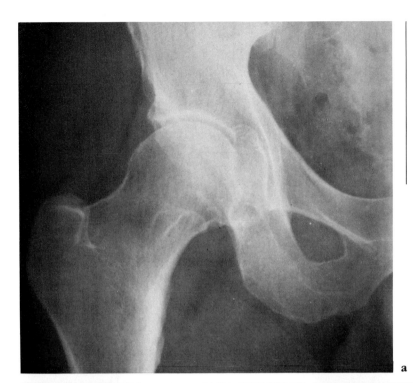

a

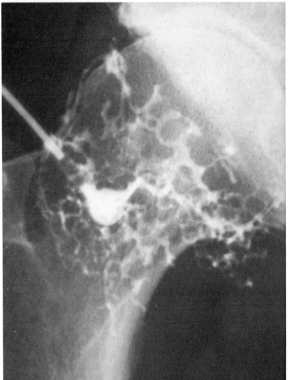

b

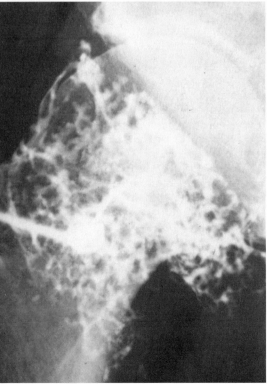

Figure 4.41

Pigmented villonodular synovitis. (**a**) Well-demarcated erosions are seen on the medial aspect of the femoral neck and in the medial wall of the acetabulum. Superiorly the joint space is intact. (**b**) After injection, contrast is shown around the proliferating synovium. The cartilage-covered areas are spared.

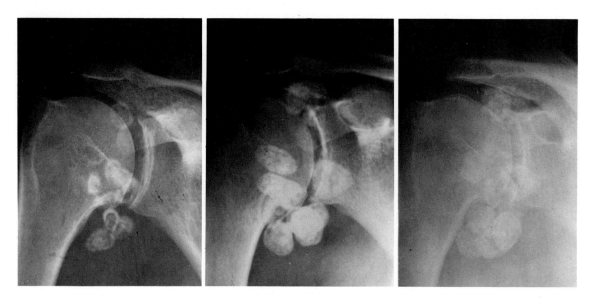

Figure 4.42

Synovial osteochondromatosis.
Multiple, calcified loose bodies
are growing in this patient.

scalloped margins are well defined if the tumour
is benign, for example, pigmented villonodular
synovitis or synovial osteochondromatosis. Multiple (more than four), apparently loose bodies
are a feature of synovial osteochondromatosis
(Figure 4.42).

The malignant synovioma invades underlying
bone resulting in irregular destruction of the
cortex which is not as well-defined as with
pigmented villonodular synovitis.

Gout

Eccentric soft tissue swelling around joints,
which may calcify, is associated with deep
erosions which undercut the cortex, often some
distance from the joint margin (Figure 4.43).
Large, curved bony spurs are seen at the margins
of erosions. Distribution may be random but gout
classically affects the metatarsophalangeal joint
of the big toe. Bone density is preserved, and
chondrocalcinosis is common. (For a list of
causes of chondrocalcinosis, see Table 1.10.)

Abnormal epiphyseal contours in children

Perthes' disease

Perthes' disease is the commonest cause of
flattening and irregularity of the femoral head in
children. In the early phase, hip pain is associated
with widening of the joint space, and an isotope
bone scan may show diminished or no uptake in
the femoral head. When the disease becomes
established, there is fissuring beneath the articular cortex and loss of its normal contour, which
are often best seen with a 'frog' lateral view,
which demonstrates the anterosuperior aspect of

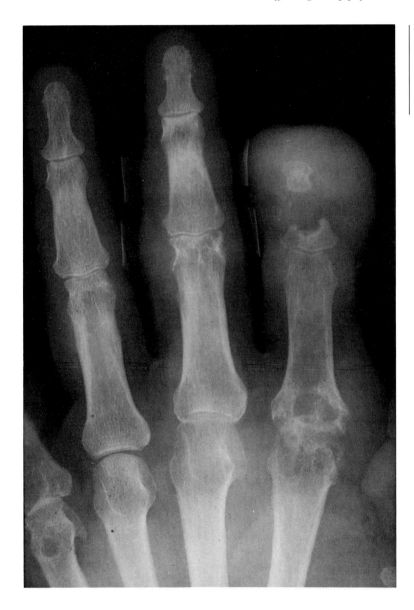

Figure 4.43

Gout. There is massive soft tissue swelling around the affected digits. Large, punched-out cystic defects are shown. On occasion, the gouty tophi calcify.

the head (Figure 4.44). This part is often the first and more severely affected, but as the disease becomes established the ossific nucleus becomes flattened, fragmented and fissured to varying degrees. Cystic changes also occur in the metaphysis. Arthrography reveals that the cartilaginous portion of the head is only slightly altered (Figure 4.45) by being mildly flattened and laterally displaced from the acetabulum. Although in 50 per cent of cases the change is bilateral, it is only very rarely symmetrical. No other joints will be affected. The outline of a flattened ossific nucleus reforms with healing, but residual deformity remains, the extent of

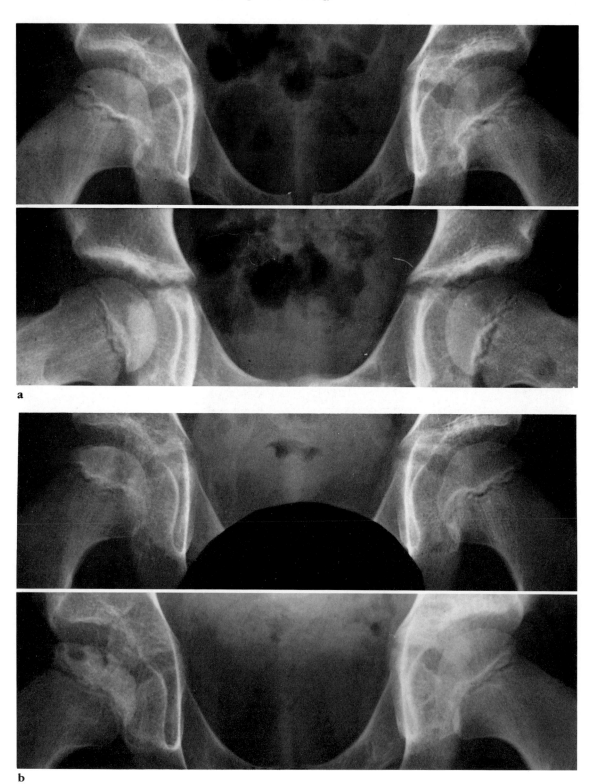

a

b

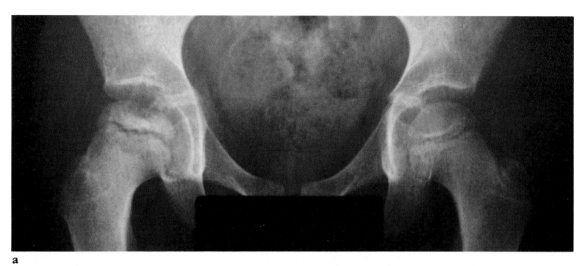

a

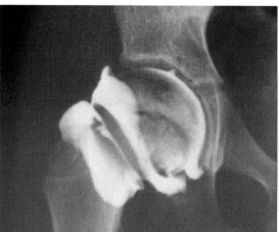

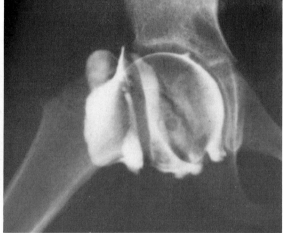

b

Figure 4.44

Perthes' disease. (**a**) In the right hip, a crescentic rim of radiolucency is seen beneath the anterosuperior aspect of the femoral head on both the anteroposterior and frog lateral views. The disease develops from here. (**b**) Examination two (*top*) and eight (*bottom*) months later shows progressive flattening and condensation of the femoral head.

Figure 4.45

Perthes' disease. (**a**) Prior to arthrography the femoral head appears flattened, sclerotic and fissured. (**b**) The cartilaginous dome, containing the flattened ossific nucleus, has a more normal appearance at arthrography. Pooling of contrast is seen medially in the film taken in abduction. This indicates that joint incongruity is maximal in this position.

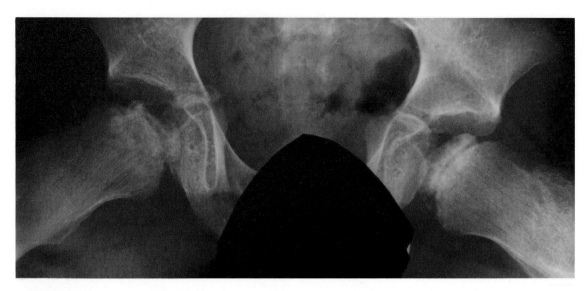

Figure 4.46

Dysplasia epiphysealis multiplex.
Bilateral and symmetrical
Perthes-like changes are seen in
the femoral head.

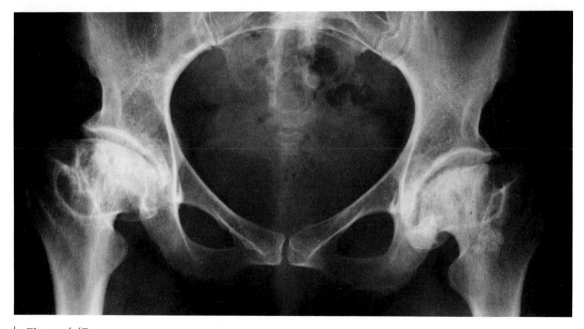

Figure 4.47

Dysplasia epiphysealis multiplex.
In adulthood, flattening of the
femoral head results in
secondary degeneration.

which depends on the initial extent of the avascular process.

Flattened, or fragmented and irregular femoral capital ossific nuclei are also found in cretinism and dysplasia epiphysealis multiplex (Figure 4.46).

Dysplasia epiphysealis multiplex (Fairbank's disease)

This produces flattened epiphyses at the hip which persist through adolescence and adult life. Changes, ranging from minor to severe, vary from patient to patient, and are associated with premature degeneration (Figure 4.47). The abnormalities are symmetrical, unlike those seen in Perthes' disease, and also affect other major joints. At the shoulder, humerus varus and epiphyseal hypoplasia are similar in appearance to a telephone receiver (Figure 4.48). At the knees, the femoral condyles may be hypoplastic or even absent (Figure 4.49), and changes are also seen in the spine which resemble widespread Scheuermann's disease with end-plate irregularity (Figure 4.50) and minor platyspondyly. At the ankle, a characteristic tibio-talar slant is seen. The plafond of the ankle joint, which is the distal tibial articular surface, is no longer

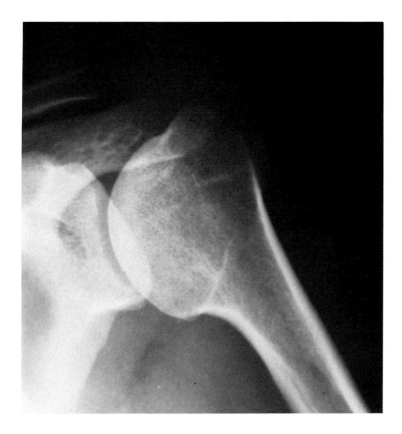

Figure 4.48

Dysplasia epiphysealis multiplex. Hypoplasia of the humeral head results in a varus deformity which has been likened in appearance to a telephone receiver.

Figure 4.49

Hypoplasia of the femoral condyles is a variable but prominent feature of dysplasia epiphysealis multiplex. There is also irregularity of the proximal tibial and fibular epiphyses in this patient.

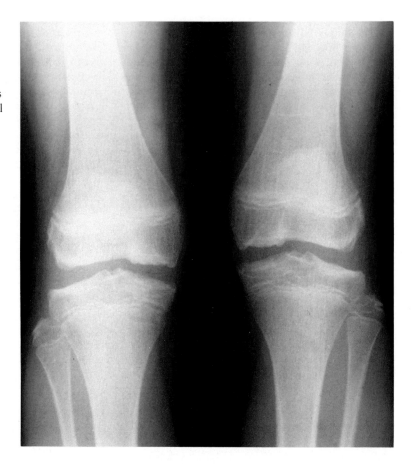

parallel to the weight-bearing plane but slopes, with hypoplasia of part of the distal tibial epiphysis and overgrowth of the adjacent talus (Figure 4.51) (Table 4.7).

Cretinism

Cretinism presents with symmetrically flattened and fragmented femoral heads in the presence of delayed skeletal maturity (Figure 4.3). With

Table 4.7   Causes of tibio-talar slant.

Multiple epiphyseal dysplasia

Haemophilia

Mucopolysaccharidoses

Dysplasia epiphysealis hemimelica

Asymmetrical epiphyseal plate fusion, eg, following
   infection or trauma in childhood

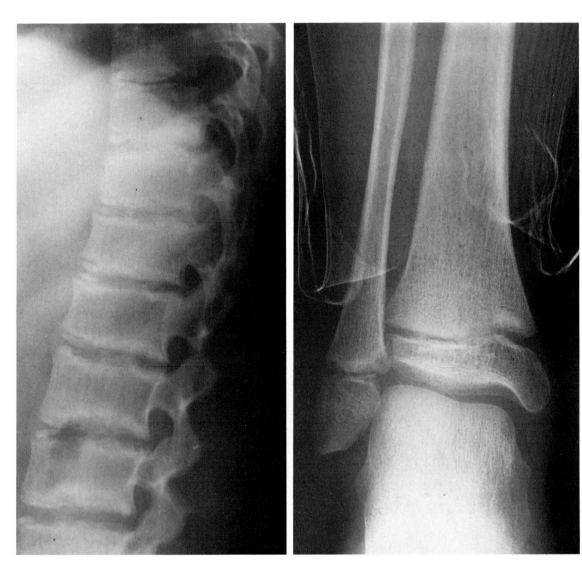

Figure 4.50

Dysplasia epiphysealis multiplex.
Changes in the spine include
platyspondyly and end-plate
irregularity resembling
Scheuermann's disease.

Figure 4.51

Dysplasia epiphysealis multiplex.
There is a tibio-talar slant. The
upper surface of the talus is no
longer parallel to the weight-
bearing plane.

growth and treatment, epiphyseal fusion takes place but the femoral head may remain fragmented. Again, changes may be seen in the other major joints, and humerus varus is present. The vertebral bodies may be hypoplastic.

None of these three conditions is seen in the neonate. Radiologically, Perthes' disease is probably the last to occur at about 6–8 years of age. Cretinism will be evident earlier, while multiple epiphyseal dysplasia may not present clinically until adult life, often with joint pain. Earlier presentation is due to dwarfism in severe cases.

Spondyloepiphyseal dysplasia tarda

This is a rare condition with a minor incongruity of the hips due to a femoral head dysplasia which can resemble a mild case of multiple epiphyseal dysplasia and result in premature osteoarthritis (Figure 4.52). There are spinal changes particularly in the tarda form, which distinguish these lesions. The spinal abnormality consists of a heaping up of bone primarily posteriorly on the end-plates, which is associated with severe discal degeneration (Figure 4.53).

Figure 4.52

Spondyloepiphyseal dysplasia tarda. Minor incongruity at the hip joints results in gross secondary degenerative changes at the hips. The diagnosis is made on inspection of the lumbar vertebral bodies which show a central hump on the anterior view.

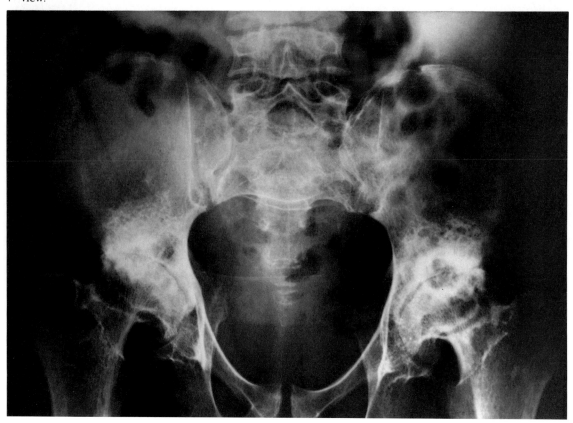

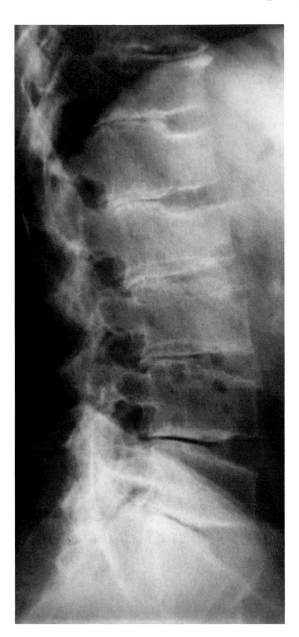

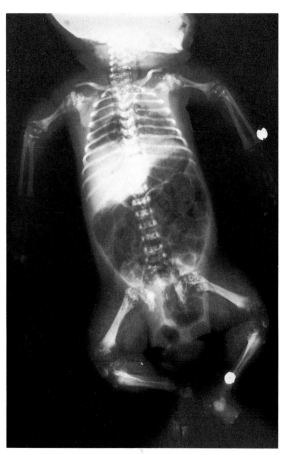

Figure 4.54

This child with chondrodystrophia calcificans congenita survived for a short time after birth. Inguinal hernias are visible as well as gas in the pericardial sac. The lung fields are almost totally opaque. There is gross short-limbed dwarfism and the epiphyses are fragmented and stippled. Similar changes are seen in the tracheal cartilages. There is platyspondyly and vertebral defects.

Figure 4.53

Anterior defects in the lumbar vertebral bodies with a characteristic posterior hump are seen in this patient with spondyloepiphyseal dysplasia tarda.

Chondrodystrophia calcificans congenita (stippled epiphyses)

This occurs in mild and severe forms. Both show punctate calcification of cartilages at birth, particularly at the epiphyses, but also in the trachea (Figure 4.54). The mild form may develop into a dysplasia similar or identical to multiple epiphyseal dysplasia. Cleft vertebrae are seen in the severe form in association with a gross form of short-limbed dwarfism which is markedly rhizomelic.

Dysplasia epiphysealis hemimelica (Trevor's disease)

First described by Trevor as a disease localized to the ankle (tarso-epiphyseal aclasia), Fairbank showed that the other major joints were also involved. Changes are unilateral and maximal on one side of the epiphysis. The most prominent feature is a cartilage-capped exostosis arising on one half of the epiphysis. An epiphyseal lesion never occurs in multiple exostoses. At the talus, a lateral osteochondroma causes a lateral defect at the plafond of the tibia, so that a form of tibiotalar slant is produced (Figure 4.55). Other local

Figure 4.55

Dysplasia epiphysealis hemimelica. The left ankle appears normal; however the right has overgrowth of bone, particularly at the medial malleolus, resulting in a tibiotalar slant. There is also overgrowth of the distal fibular epiphysis.

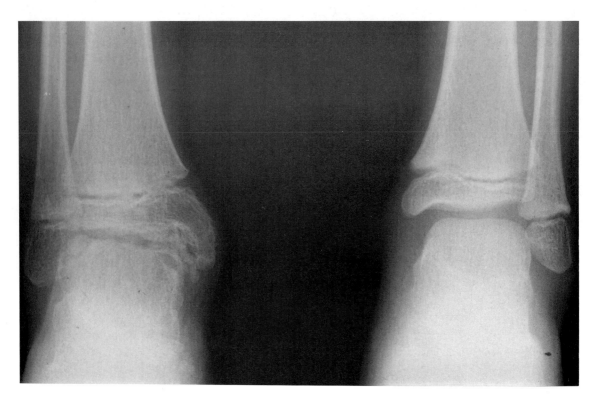

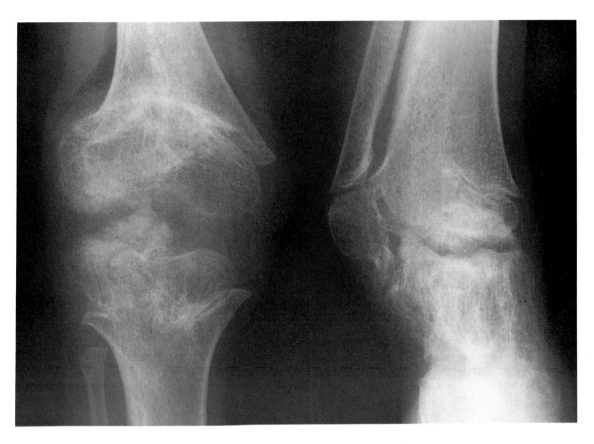

growth anomalies may be present, with over-growth of other epiphyses (distal fibular) and fusion between the local long bones. Similar osteochondromas are seen at all the major joints (Figure 4.56).

Mucopolysaccharidoses

These are a complex group of heterogeneous conditions.

In MPS I-H (Hurler's syndrome) changes are progressive during infancy and eventually the entire skeleton is affected. The ring epiphyses in the carpus and tarsus become progressively irregular and fragmented, the proximal metacarpals taper (Figure 4.57), and the phalanges become bullet-shaped. The mandibular condyles

Figure 4.56

Dysplasia epiphysealis hemimelica. In this patient a chevron sign is seen at the distal femur and proximal tibia, with a large osteochondromatous excrescence on the lateral tibial plateau. Premature fusion at one part of the epiphyseal plate at the ankle results in a tibio-talar slant. Articular irregularity due to osteochondromatous lesions is prominent. The fibular epiphysis is overgrown and has fused with the distal tibia.

Figure 4.57

MPS I-H. There is overall
demineralization and thin
cortices are apparent. The distal
radius and ulna slope towards
each other, and the proximal
aspects of the metacarpals are
pointed. Overall, the bones are
broadened, and the phalanges
resemble bullets.

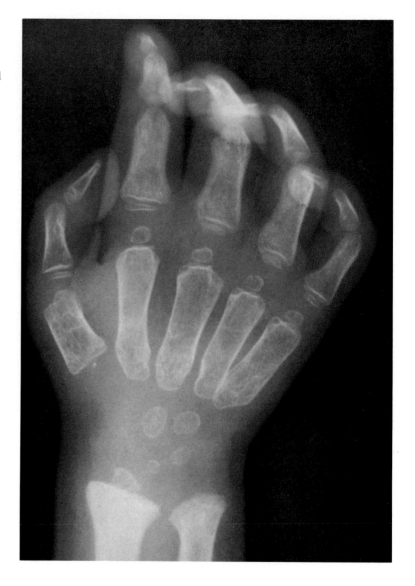

become irregular and hypoplastic with an
upward concavity (Figure 4.58). It is probable
that this condylar defect is specific for mucopolysaccharidoses. The ankle also shows a tibio-talar
slant, but with overgrown, hyperplastic epiphyses (Figure 4.59) and the metaphyses and

diaphyses are also broad. A similar V deformity
is also seen at the distal radius and ulna.

The skull shows enlargement with a J-shaped
sella. The ribs become paddle-shaped with a
posterior constriction (Figure 4.60) and the
spine has a thoracolumbar hook associated with

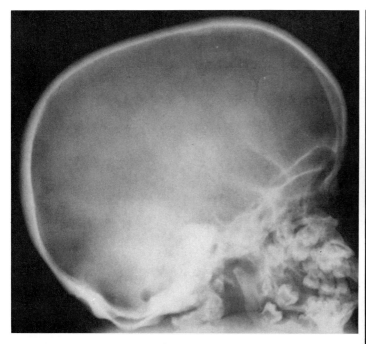

Figure 4.58

The skull in MPS I-H.
Enlargement of the pituitary fossa
is seen. It is described as omega-
shaped. The condyle of the
mandible is hypoplastic, and the
odontoid peg is similarly
underdeveloped.

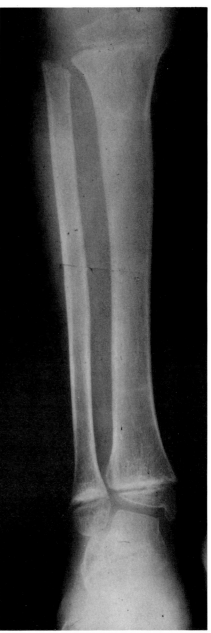

a kyphos, probably due to local postural instability.

MPS IV (Morquio–Brailsford syndrome) is
perhaps the next best known, but is extremely
rare (see Chapter 7, page 360).

Fragmentation of epiphyses and apophyses

Fragmentation of epiphyses or apophyses may be
generalized or unifocal, and occurs in many
different diseases, although often the end appearances are identical. Therefore, the femoral heads
in Perthes' disease, cretinism and multiple

Figure 4.59

In this patient with MPS I-H, a
tibio-talar slant is visible at the
ankle and the paired long bones
show undertubulation. The
proximal metaphyses show an
abnormal slant.

Figure 4.60

This chest X-ray in an MPS I-H patient shows that the ribs are constricted posteriorly and broadened anteriorly. The distal clavicles are pointed.

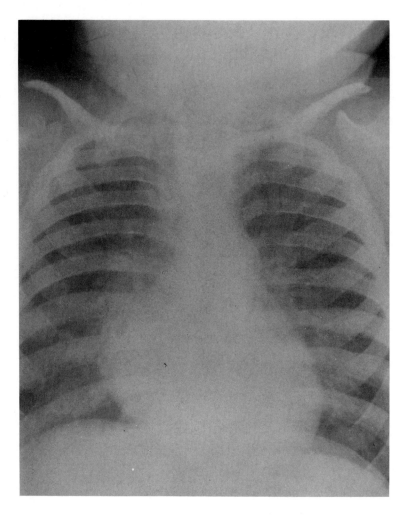

epiphyseal dysplasia may all be similar in appearance. The causes of epiphyseal fragmentation vary. Perthes' disease may be due to a rise in intracapsular pressure causing vascular occlusion in the ligamentum teres, while fragmentation at the second metatarsal head and tibial tuberosity are due to trauma (Tables 4.8 and 4.9).

Causes of widespread epiphyseal fragmentation

Cretinism

There is multiple joint involvement with flattening and fragmentation, and skeletal growth and maturity is retarded. Beaking at the thoracolumbar junction of the spine is due to diminished tone. Bone density is normal or increased.

Cushing's syndrome and steroid excess

There is generalized osteoporosis in these conditions. Spinal collapse is associated with callus. Resorption of bone in subarticular regions of joints results in a local rim of radiolucency beneath the articular cortex, which is crescentic in the femoral head. Structural failure with collapse of joint surfaces then follows in weight-bearing areas (Figure 4.61).

Table 4.8   Causes of widespread epiphyseal fragmentation.

Cretinism

Cushing's syndrome

Steroid excess

Alcoholism

Renal failure, dialysis

Systemic lupus erythematosus

Gaucher's disease

Sickle-cell disease

Pancreatic disease

Caisson disease

Hodgkin's disease

Multiple epiphyseal dysplasia

Dysplasia epiphysealis hemimelica

Chondrodystrophia calcificans congenita

Table 4.9   Local causes of epiphyseal fragmentation in the hip.

Perthes' disease

Following treatment for congenital dislocation of the hip and slipped epiphysis

Following dislocations, fractures and surgery

Following local irradiation

All the causes of generalized fragmentation

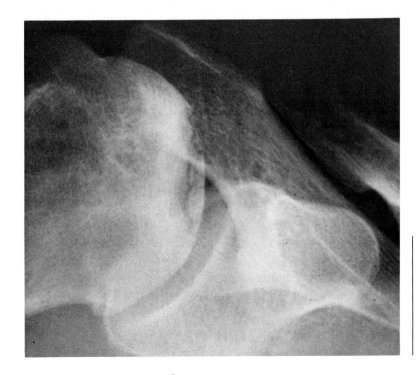

Figure 4.61

Avascular necrosis following steroid therapy. A crescentic rim of density is seen beneath the fragmented articular cortex. Overall, the head shows reactive sclerosis and there is structural failure.

Figure 4.62

Systemic lupus erythematosus.
Avascular necrosis is seen at the
left femoral head which shows
early structural failure. A dense
zone of creeping substitution is
visible around the infarcted area.

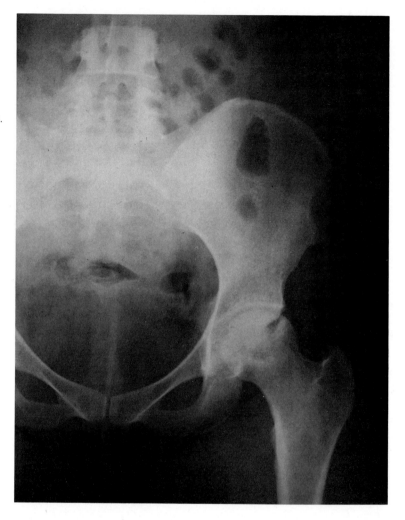

Patients with systemic lupus erythematosus
show similar changes but they are often receiving steroids. Patients with rheumatoid arthritis
can also show articular collapse, and these
changes are compounded in steroid therapy by
the concomitant euphoria and diminution of pain
induced by the drug (Figure 4.62). Following
collapse of the cortex and subarticular area,
there may be a local increase in bone density due
to trabecular compression, as well as dystrophic
calcification in necrotic tissue.

Renal disease, pancreatitis and alcoholism

Similar changes are also seen at the hips and,
particularly, the shoulders in patients with renal
disease who are often receiving steroids or
dialysis.

Infarcts and avascular necrosis in pancreatitis
may be due to fat emboli, and alcoholism may

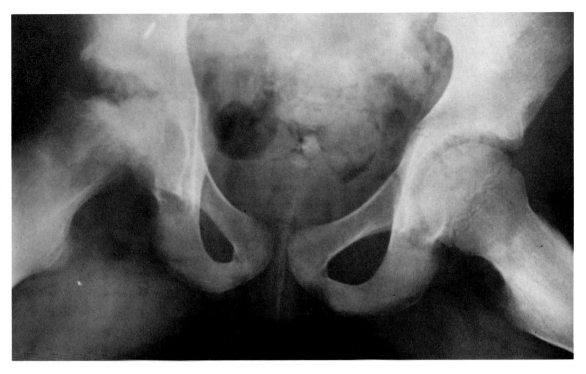

Figure 4.63

There is a generalized increase in density and avascular necrosis of the right femoral head in this patient with sickle-cell disease.

cause avascular necrosis by inducing pancreatitis, hepatic failure and elevated steroid levels (see Chapter 1, page 5).

Caisson disease

Avascular necrosis and infarction in caisson disease result from nitrogen emboli. Cortical infarcts can occur, but a ring of serpiginous sclerosis in the subarticular bone—the zone of creeping substitution—is more typical and represents the edge of revascularization around the infarcted area of bone (Figure 3.28). These changes can occur beneath all major joints, and

may also be seen following chemotherapy and radiotherapy, for example, in Hodgkin's disease. The avascular areas also suffer structural failure, leading to collapse of articular surfaces.

Gaucher's and sickle-cell diseases

Changes of avascular necrosis also occur in Gaucher's disease and sickle-cell disease. Avascular necrosis at the hips in a negro child is usually due to sickle-cell disease rather than Perthes' disease (Figure 4.63). Cortical infarcts occur in both diseases, but Erlenmeyer flask changes are more usual in Gaucher's disease, and generalized osteosclerosis is more common in sickle-cell anaemia. The joint space does not narrow until secondary osteoarthritis supervenes.

Causes of a mushroom-shaped femoral head

Avascular necrosis of the femoral head in children follows vigorous treatment for congenital dislocation of the hip, pinning of the head for slipped epiphysis (Figure 4.64), sickle-cell anaemia and Gaucher's disease. It may also follow trauma and surgery to the femoral head and neck in adults. Infection in childhood may destroy the femoral head either partially or totally. The ossific nucleus may disappear permanently, or a deformed flattened head may result (Figure 4.65). Premature fusion of the growth plate results in local shortening (Table 4.10).

Figure 4.64

Avascular necrosis of the femoral head. (**a**) The initial radiograph shows congenital dislocation. (**b**) An iliac osteotomy is pinned, and the pins protrude into the femoral head. (**c**) Avascular necrosis results.

a

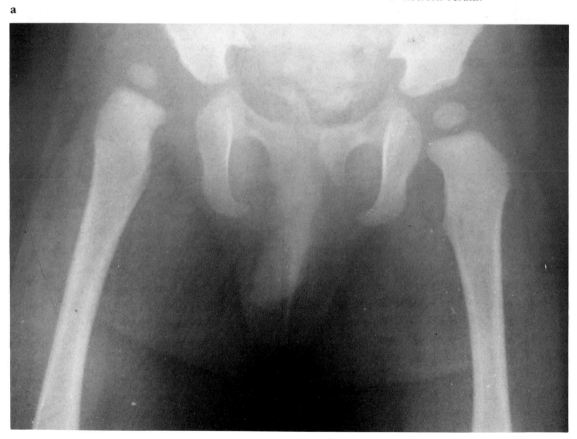

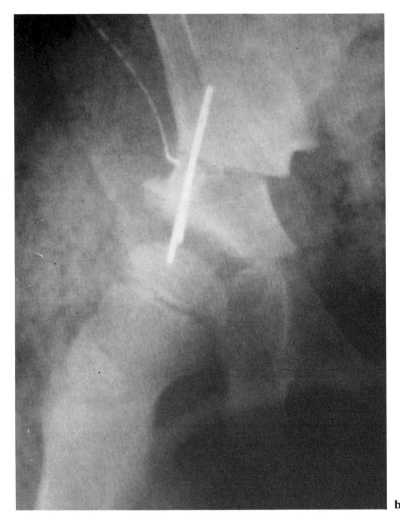

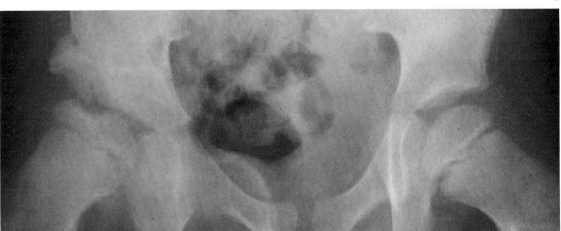

Figure 4.64 *continued*

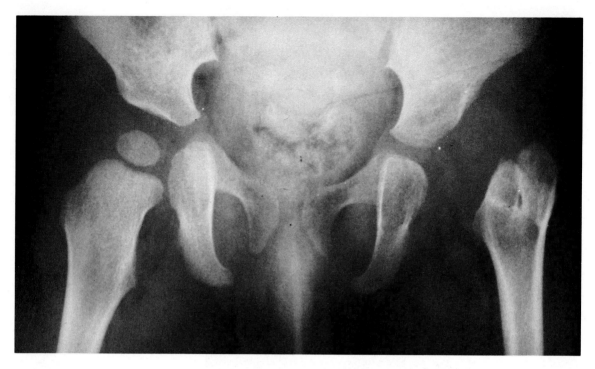

Figure 4.65

Infantile septic arthritis. The left femoral head has failed to appear and healed metaphyseal defects are seen in this patient following septic arthritis in early childhood.

Table 4.10   Causes of a mushroom-shaped femoral head.

Perthes' disease and other causes of avascular necrosis in childhood

Congenital dislocation of the hip complicated by avascular necrosis

Slipped epiphysis

Osteomyelitis

Avascular necrosis in adult life

Secondary osteoarthritis

Perthes' disease

In Perthes' disease, the femoral head ends up flattened in a mildly dysplastic acetabulum. The joint space is preserved for many years. The head is slightly uncovered laterally and the medial aspect of the acetabulum is essentially normal (Figure 4.66).

Congenital dislocation of the hip

Lateral uncovering of the head is more marked than in Perthes' disease and the medial wall of the acetabulum is much thicker, due to the absence of the stimulus of a normal head against it (Figure 4.67). Again, the joint space narrows when secondary osteoarthritis supervenes. Avascular necrosis superimposed on congenital dislocation of the hip can cause gross flattening of the femoral head (Figure 4.64).

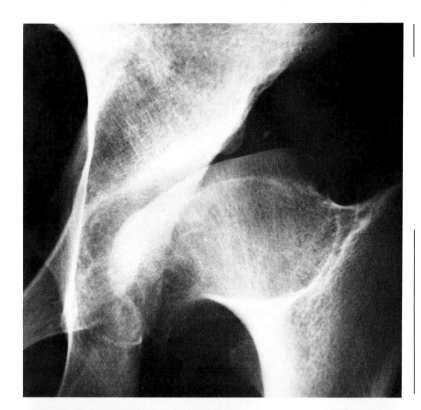

Figure 4.66

Old Perthes' disease.

Figure 4.67

Congenital dislocation of the hip. The right hip is normal, but the left acetabulum is dysplastic and shows internal new bone formation. The femoral head is uncovered laterally, where it is slightly bulbous, but is flattened where it bears weight. Secondary osteoarthritic changes have supervened.

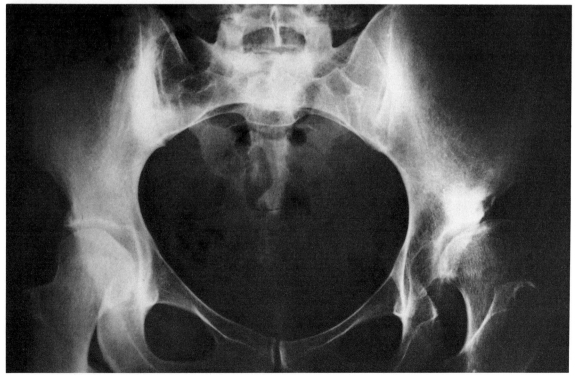

Figure 4.68

Slipped upper femoral epiphysis.
The slip is both medial and
posterior.

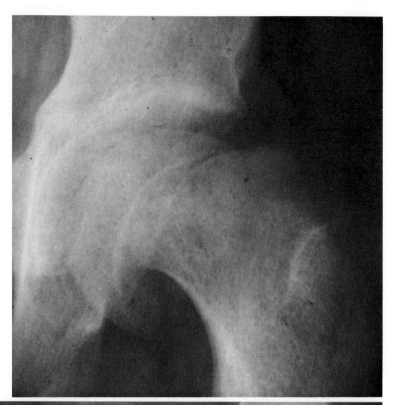

Figure 4.69

Slipped upper femoral epiphysis.
The anteroposterior radiographs
do not show obvious slip but
there is asymmetry of the
epiphyseal plates. On the right, a
normal appearance is seen but,
on the left, the margins of the
plate are poorly defined. The left
femoral head has also lost height,
indicating a posterior slip. The
lateral view demonstrates the
left-sided slip.

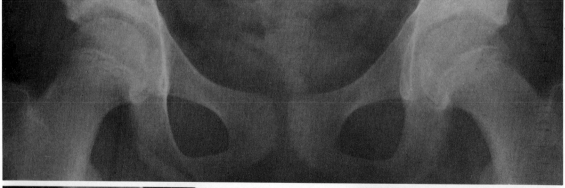

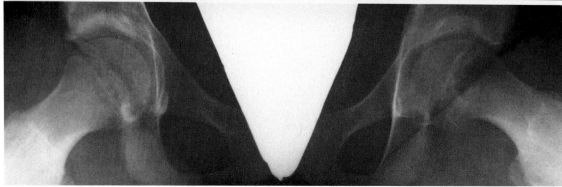

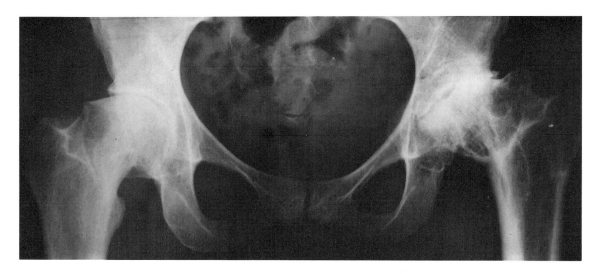

Figure 4.70

Slipped upper femoral epiphysis.
This patient has bilateral slipped
epiphyses with quite marked
degeneration of the left hip.

Slipped epiphysis

In slipped epiphysis, the femoral head usually
slips inferomedially, and the contour seems
deficient superolaterally. The femoral neck is
displaced laterally by the head and the medial
acetabulum is normally formed. Secondary
osteoarthritis supervenes (Figures 4.68, 4.69 and
4.70).

Infection

With infection, the joint space may be narrowed
or widened, but bone is destroyed on either side
of the joint. Again, secondary osteoarthritis
supervenes.

Classical osteoarthritis

In classical osteoarthritis, loss of cartilage and
bone occurs, particularly at the dome of the

femoral head on the anteroposterior view. This
causes the head to migrate laterally and new
bone is laid down internally on the medial
acetabulum, and laterally as retaining osteophytes on the acetabulum and femoral head (Figure
4.29). The acetabulum also becomes dysplastic
and secondary cystic change is often followed by
articular collapse (Figure 4.71).

Common sites of osteochondritis (Table 4.11)

The tibial tubercle

This occurs in adolescents, often those with a
history of sporting activity. Traction causes
fragmentation of the tibial tubercle. Pain and soft
tissue swelling are essential features of the
diagnosis (Figure 4.72).

Figure 4.71

Osteoarthritis. (**a**) There is cyst
formation in the femoral head.
The superior joint space is
narrowed, and new bone
formation is seen medially and in
the acetabulum. (**b**) The cysts at
the femoral head and acetabulum
collapse with weight-bearing.
Protrusio of the acetabulum and
a 'bird's beak' appearance of the
femoral head result.

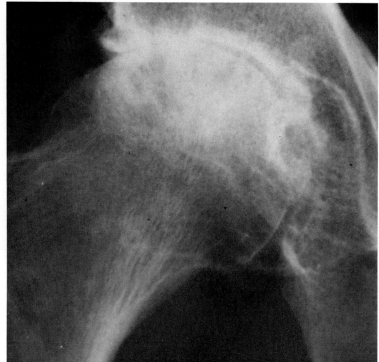

a

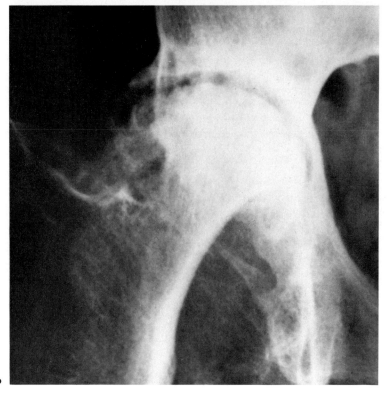

b

Table 4.11 Common sites of osteochondritis.

Disease	Cause	Site
Perthes'	Primary aseptic necrosis	Femoral head
Kohler	? Primary aseptic necrosis ? Necrosis following fracture	Tarsal navicular
Freiberg	? Primary aseptic necrosis ? Necrosis following fracture	Metatarsal head
Kienbock	? Primary aseptic necrosis ? Necrosis following fracture	Lunate
Osgood–Schlatter	Necrosis following partial avulsion of patellar tendon	Tibial tubercle
Sinding–Larsen	Necrosis following partial avulsion of patellar tendon	Lower pole of patella
Sever	Necrosis following partial avulsion of tendo Achilles	Calcaneal apophysis
Calvé	Eosinophilic granuloma	Vertebral body
Scheuermann	Disc herniation through defective end-plate	Ring-like epiphysis of vertebra

Adapted from Catto M, *Aseptic necrosis of bone*, (Excerpta Medica: Amsterdam 1976) with kind permission.

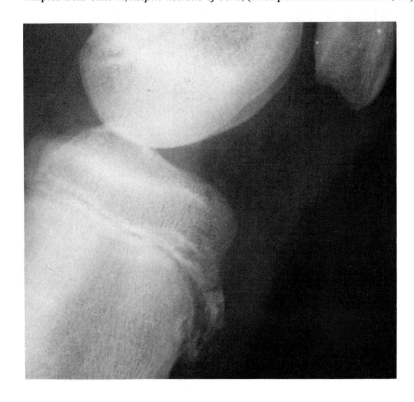

Figure 4.72

Osgood–Sclatter's disease. Fragmentation of the tibial tubercle is associated with overlying soft tissue swelling in this painful lesion.

Figure 4.73

Osteochondritis of the second metatarsal head (Freiberg's disease). Collapse and sclerosis of the epiphysis is shown. The adjacent phalangeal base soon remodels to correspond to the altered appearance of the metatarsal head.

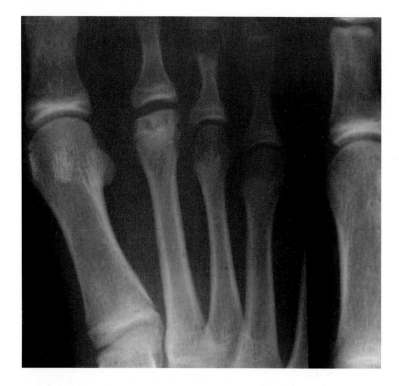

Figure 4.74

Osteochondritis of the tarsal navicular (Kohler's disease). Flattening and fragmentation with sclerosis are features of this disorder, which is self-limiting.

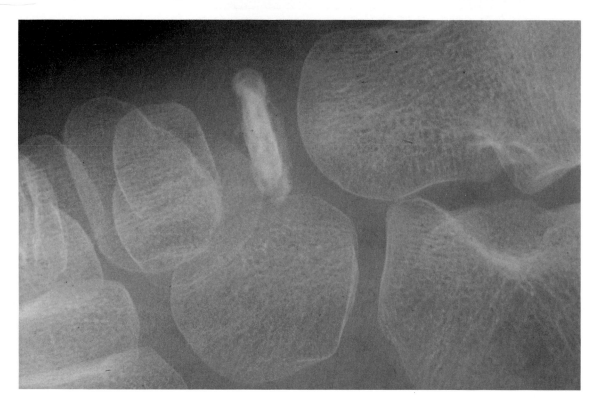

The metatarsal head

The second metatarsal head is usually involved in adolescent girls. The epiphysis flattens and fragments and, after epiphyseal fusion and healing, a flat, broad head results, often accompanied by local degeneration (Figure 4.73).

The tarsal navicular

The affected bone becomes flattened, sclerotic and fissured, but the adjacent joint spaces are not narrowed. The lesion is painful, but the bone usually reverts to normal (Figure 4.74).

Tumours appearing in the epiphyseal region are listed in Table 3.5.

5 | Abnormalities in the region of the metaphysis

The metaphysis is the part of the immature skeleton which is just proximal to the growth plate, where it is generally transverse, at right angles to the shaft, but is occasionally curved, for example, beneath the iliac crest apophysis. The contour matches that of the epiphysis and is slightly undulant. The margin at the growth plate is sharply defined, sclerotic and usually less than 1 mm wide. This sclerosis represents the zone of provisional calcification. The metaphysis as a whole widens smoothly to the growth plate until it matches the epiphysis in width, and the contours of epiphysis and metaphysis are contiguous.

Metaphyseal changes may be generalized or localized to one, or a few metaphyses. Metaphyseal abnormalities may affect the growth plate and epiphysis and, conversely, changes at epiphyses may affect more proximal parts of the bone. In some conditions, particularly the dysplasias, changes occur in both the epiphyses and metaphyses.

Table 5.1 Generalized transverse bands of metaphyseal lucency.

Normal appearance in neonates

Immobilization

Systemic disease

Leukaemia

Neuroblastoma

Cushing's syndrome

Scurvy

Rickets

Syphilis

Rubella

Transverse bands of metaphyseal lucency

In all conditions in Table 5.1, many metaphyses are usually affected by a band of radiolucency extending across the entire metaphyseal width.

Immobilization and systemic disease

Disuse of part or all of a limb may cause radiologically demonstrable osteoporosis which may be generalized or localized. Patients, particularly children, who are immobilized because

266

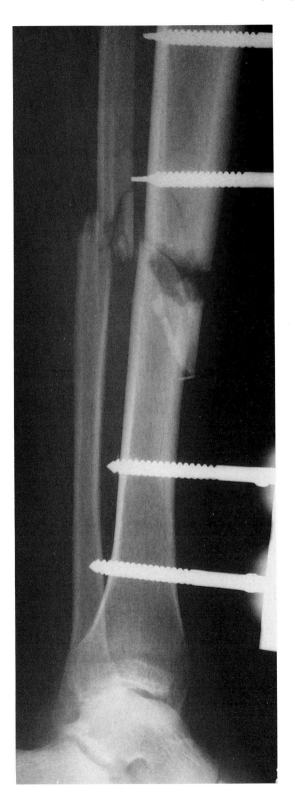

Figure 5.1

Metaphyseal osteoporosis due to immobilization following a fracture of the midshaft of the tibia and fibula. Surgery and immobilization have resulted in a band of lucency at the distal metaphysis of the tibia, extending to the scar of the epiphyseal plate which is rendered more prominent.

of major illness, lose bone density generally, but the appendicular skeleton is more severely affected than the axial. At the metaphysis, a translucent band of demineralization, 2–4 mm deep, develops beneath the zone of calcification, and extends across the entire metaphysis (Figure 5.1). This zone of lucency may be demarcated more clearly than that seen with widespread malignancy in children, which tends to be poorly defined and often associated with marginal cortical erosions.

Leukaemia and neuroblastoma

In leukaemia and neuroblastoma, the band of metaphyseal radiolucency tends to be deeper, more irregular and usually associated with a more obviously aggressive osteolytic process elsewhere (Figure 5.2). Focal areas of medullary and cortical destruction, and sutural widening of the skull are seen in these conditions.

Scurvy and rickets

These are often described together but their radiological appearances are dissimilar. In scurvy, a prominent metaphyseal band of

Figure 5.2

Leukaemia. There is generalized
loss of bone density which is
accentuated at the metaphyses
and a band of lucency extends
across the entire metaphyseal
region.

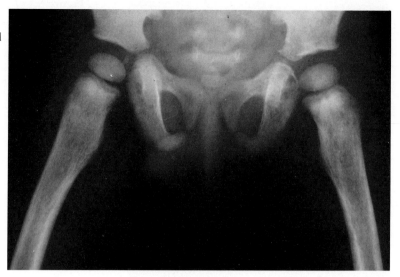

lucency is associated with generalized demineralization which makes the cortical margins prominent. This change occurs particularly at the ring
epiphyses in infants. The zone of translucency
(Trummerfeld zone) at the metaphysis may
fracture transversely, particularly at the distal
femur, which bears the child's weight when it is
crawling (Figure 5.3). This leaves lateral bone
spurs known as Pelkan's spurs.

In rickets, there is loss of metaphyseal density
due to the presence of excess non-mineralized
osteoid, so that the metaphysis becomes irregular across its entire surface and the epiphyseal
plate appears to widen. The metaphysis also
becomes splayed because of local softening
(Figure 5.4).

Congenital syphilis

Congenital syphilis in the neonate is rare in the
UK but involves gross, irregular bone destruction
often associated with cortical erosions at the
metaphyses, which may fracture. The presence
of a periostitis causes an appearance which may
resemble leukaemia and neuroblastoma, but
bone density in congenital syphilis is often
increased (Figure 5.5). In the skull, there is no
sutural splaying and the changes are more
typically those of a focal osteomyelitis.

Rubella

Rubella as a result of uterine infection in non-
immune mothers, produces skeletal changes
which are usually maximal around the knee. The
metaphysis becomes slightly broadened and
frayed, and characteristically shows alternating
bands of lucency and density perpendicular to
the growth plate—the 'celery stick' appearance
(Figure 5.6). Occasionally, more conventional
transverse bands of lucency are found. These
changes regress with growth.

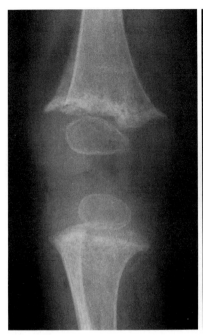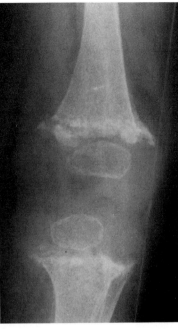

Figure 5.3

Scurvy. A fracture has occurred through the metaphyseal lucency, leading to marginal spurs and subperiosteal new bone. Osteoporosis is prominent in the epiphyses at the knee.

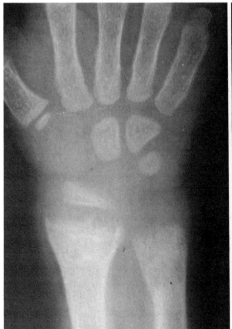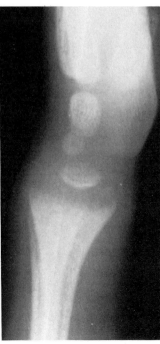

Figure 5.4

In this patient with rickets, the metaphysis is splayed and irregular and the epiphyseal plate increased in width. Bone density is reduced generally.

Figure 5.5

In this patient with congenital syphilis, the shafts of the long bones show increased density and periostitis. The metaphyses show irregular margins and irregular bands of lucency extending across the entire width of the bone.

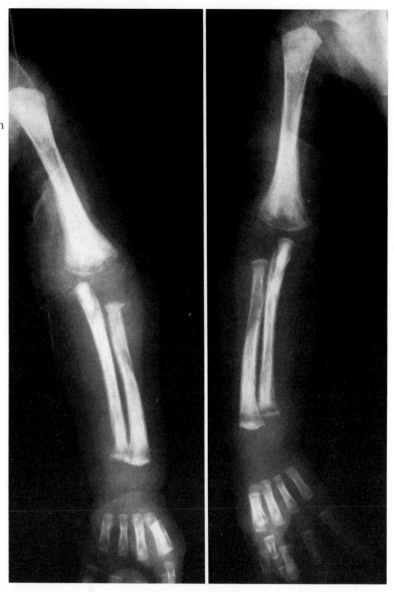

Focal areas of metaphyseal destruction

Destructive metaphyseal lesions do not always traverse the entire width of the bone; occasionally there may be focal destructive lesions, resembling 'bites' (Table 5.2).

Between 1 and 16 years of age, the metaphysis is the site of end-arteries and therefore the focus

Table 5.2   Causes of metaphyseal bites.

Simple osteomyelitis

Tuberculous osteomyelitis

Chronic granulomatous disease

Eosinophilic granuloma

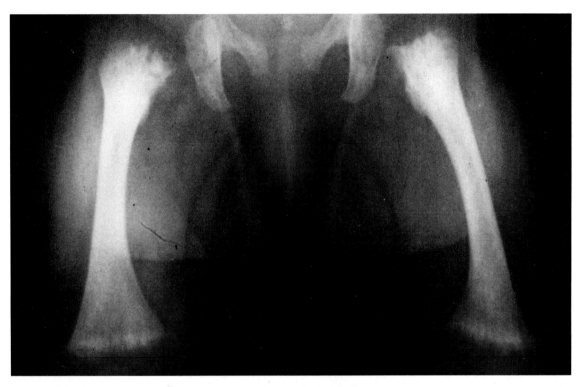

Figure 5.6

Rubella. Vertical lucencies at the
metaphyses give a celery stick
appearance.

Figure 5.7

Osteomyelitis. A fairly well-
localized metaphyseal focus of
destruction is visible and cortical
sequestration is evident.

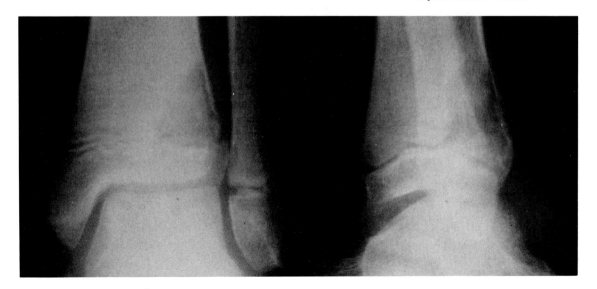

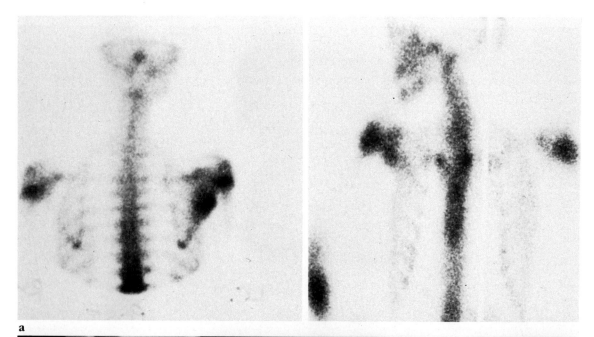

a

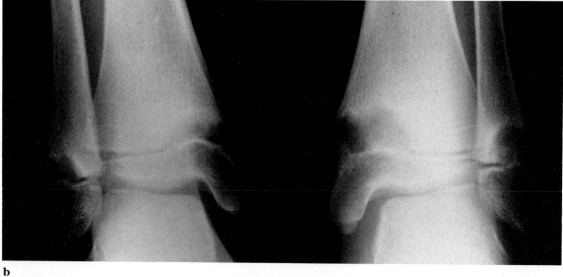

b

Figure 5.8

Chronic granulomatous disease.
(**a**) The radioisotope bone scan
shows widespread foci of
increased uptake with expansion
of bone. The changes are mainly
metaphyseal. (**b**) Partial
metaphyseal defects are present
and are well defined at both
distal tibiae and fibulae.

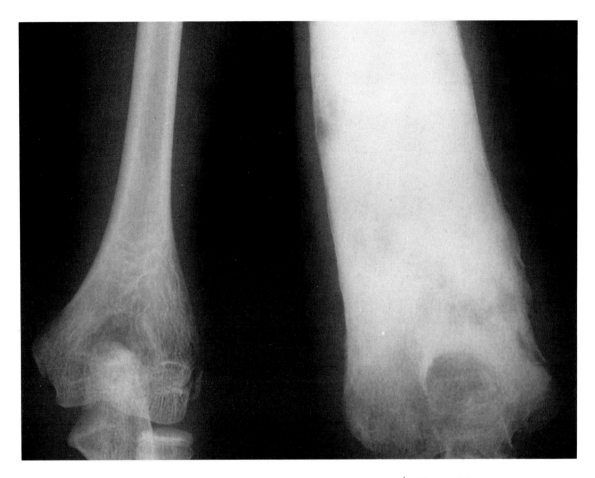

Figure 5.9

In chronic granulomatous disease, the entire bone may become involved. In this patient with longstanding disease, the appearances of bone expansion, sclerosis and periostitis are those of a chronic infection. The normal humerus is shown for comparison.

for septic emboli. In the chronic stage of infection, a well-demarcated lytic defect extends to the epiphyseal plate over part of the metaphysis, which is seen as a solitary lesion in simple infections (Figure 5.7). In children with immune defects, such as the 'lazy leucocyte' syndrome or chronic granulomatous disease, the lesions may be multiple (Figure 5.8). Chronic granulomatous disease eventually results in reactive sclerosis and expansion of bone which extend proximally for some distance into the diaphysis. The original metaphyseal focus of destruction may be obscured (Figure 5.9).

Multiple metaphyseal foci of destruction may be seen in eosinophilic granuloma and tuberculosis which are often associated with lytic defects elsewhere (Figure 5.10).

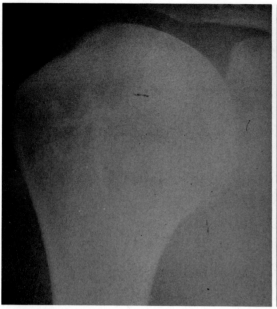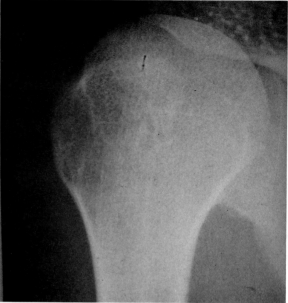

Figure 5.10

Tuberculosis of the greater tuberosity. This is a recognized site of osseous tuberculosis associated with cystic rarefaction of bone. Similar changes are seen at the greater trochanter.

Conditions causing an increase in density at the metaphysis

The normal zone of provisional calcification at the metaphysis is seen as a dense line, less than 1 mm thick. Occasionally the metaphyseal density may be thicker, particularly in the neonate. The conditions causing an increase in density at the metaphysis are listed in Table 5.3.

Table 5.3   Causes of metaphyseal density.

Normal in neonates
Growth arrest lines
Heavy metal poisoning
Healing rickets
Healing leukaemia
Healing scurvy
Osteopetrosis
Chronic infection and chronic granulomatous disease

Lead poisoning

In the acute phase of lead poisoning in children, the only manifestation may be suture diastasis due to cerebral oedema, and there may be particulate densities in the gut representing ingested paint. However, chronic lead ingestion causes a dense band of metaphyseal density, which is seen at all metaphyses, including the proximal fibula, which is not usually dense under normal physiological conditions. Inhibition of osteoclastic activity by lead also causes under-tubulation of metaphyses (Figure 5.11a).

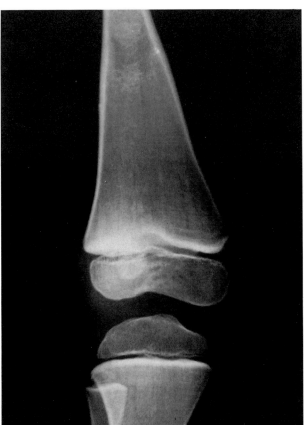

Figure 5.11

(**a**) Lead poisoning. Failure of modelling of the metaphysis is evident, producing an Erlenmeyer flask appearance at the distal femur and proximal fibula. The metaphyses are dense, with a so-called 'lead line'. Fainter bands of metaphyseal density are evidence of previous episodes of lead poisoning and medullary density in the region of maximal undertubulation of the distal tibial diaphyses confirms this. (**b**) Phosphorus poisoning. Poisoning by other heavy metals also results in metaphyseal bands of density.

a

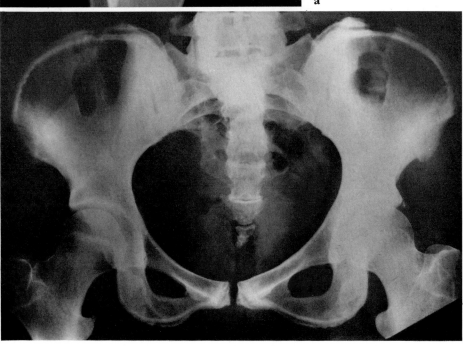

b

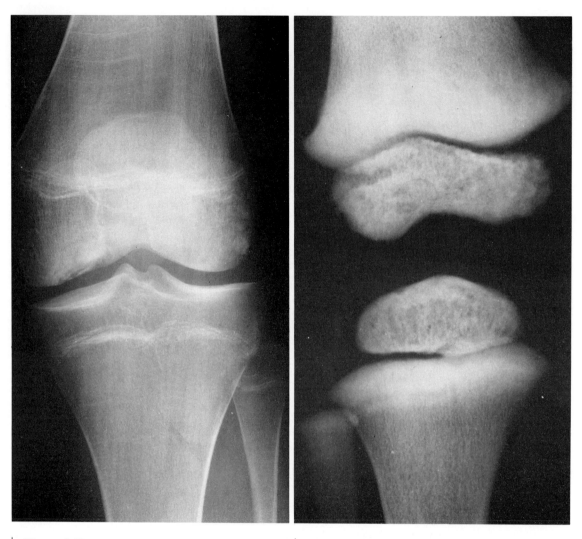

Figure 5.12

Growth arrest lines are
prominent at both knees in this
patient with bilateral
osteochondritis dissecans.

Figure 5.13

A patient with osteopetrosis
involving metaphyseal density
and broadening.

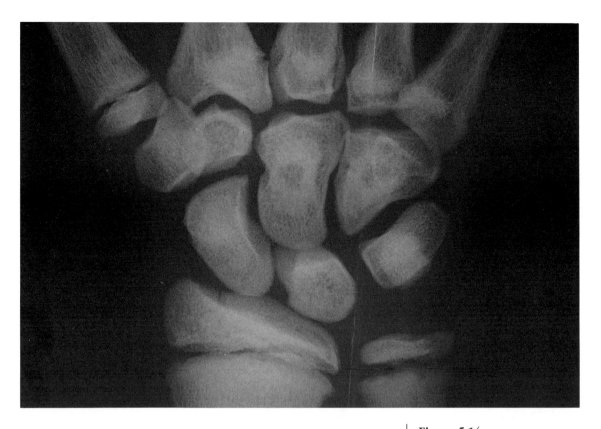

Figure 5.14

Osteopetrosis. A bone-within-a-bone appearance can be seen in the carpus, proximal metacarpals and distal radial and ulnar metaphyses.

Other heavy metals, such as phosphorus, bismuth and arsenic, have a similar effect (Figure 5.11b). Vertebral bodies may be affected, giving a bone-within-a-bone appearance, corresponding to the episodes of heavy metal poisoning.

growth resumes, this dense line is left behind and lies proximally in the shaft. Often a number of these thin transverse bands are seen, indicating separate episodes of growth arrest (Figure 5.12).

Growth arrest lines

These are seen during severe illness and immobilization, when longitudinal growth behind the epiphyseal plate ceases, but local calcium deposition continues, so that the zone of provisional calcification becomes particularly dense. When

Osteopetrosis

Alternating bands of dense and normal bone are seen in the epiphysis, metaphysis and diaphysis. The bands of increased density vary in thickness, but are never as thin as growth arrest lines (Figures 5.13 and 5.14).

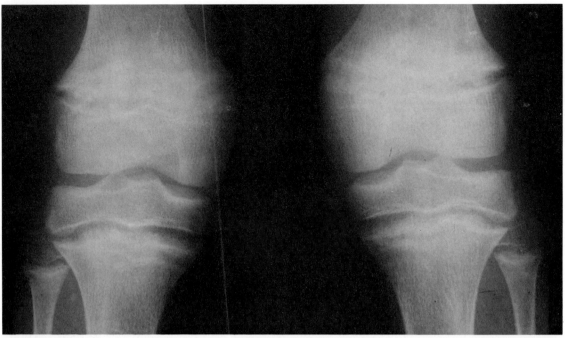

a

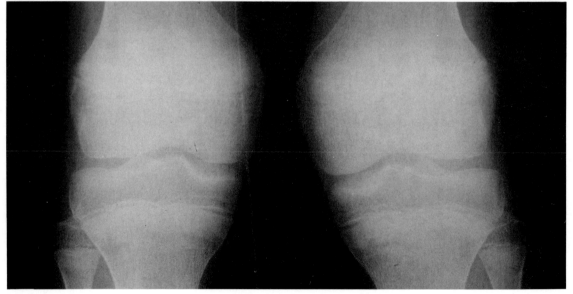

b

Figure 5.15

Healing rickets. The initial radiograph (**a**) shows changes of rickets, with widened epiphyseal plates and irregular metaphyses, although healing is probably taking place. Growth arrest lines are visible. After healing (**b**), marked metaphyseal density is seen, and the growth plate is normal in width.

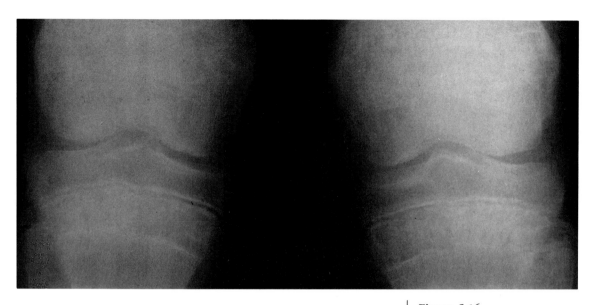

Figure 5.16

Skeletal fusion at maturity in rickets. Skeletal fusion is not particularly delayed. The metaphysis fills with coarse and irregular woven bone, and the epiphyseal plate then fuses.

Healing rickets

The poorly mineralized and irregular metaphysis gradually ossifies with treatment, producing an appearance of woven rather than well-formed bone (Figure 5.15). The adjacent epiphyseal plate narrows to a more normal width, and the epiphysis and subperiosteal region become more clearly defined. When epiphyseal fusion occurs in rachitic patients, the previously widened epiphyseal plate is obliterated by a band of coarsely trabeculated woven bone (Figure 5.16).

Conditions causing metaphyseal broadening (Table 5.4)

The Erlenmeyer flask used in simple chemical experiments is cone-shaped, and a similar shape is found, particularly at the distal ends of long bones, in conditions in which marrow hypertrophy or infiltration occur (see Chapter 1, page 58).

Healing leukaemia

In healing leukaemia there is an increase in general bone density, and healing may occur in the destructive metaphyseal lesions, occasionally resulting in local sclerosis. Ten per cent of leukaemic patients are osteosclerotic in the acute phase.

Thalassaemia

Thalassaemia is associated with the most severe form of anaemia and therefore presents with the most marked marrow hypertrophy and bone expansion. Bone density is reduced and the cortex thinned, particularly at the metaphyses, where it may be breached by masses of marrow

Table 5.4   Conditions causing metaphyseal broadening.

Erlenmeyer flask appearance

Haemolytic anaemias:	Thalassaemia ⎫ Sickle-cell disease ⎬	Associated with marrow hyperplasia ⎫
Storage disease:	Gaucher's disease	Associated ⎬ with infarcts

Rickets	
Hypophosphatasia—generally more severe in appearance than rickets' ⎫	Associated with metaphyseal
Metaphyseal dysostosis—generally less severe in appearance than rickets ⎬	irregularity

Enchondromatosis ⎫	Associated with multiple
Diaphyseal aclasia ⎬	tumours of cartilaginous origin
Osteopetrosis ⎫	Associated with increased
Lead poisoning ⎬	metaphyseal density
Perthes' disease	At the hip only

(Figure 5.17), but infarcts do not occur. Else-where, changes of marrow hypertrophy are gross, for example, in the skull (Figure 5.18), spine and hands (Figure 1.63). The liver and spleen are enlarged and extramedullary haemo-poiesis may be seen (Figures 1.61 and 5.19).

Sickle-cell disease

In sickle-cell disease, infarcts causing sclerosis, cortical splitting (Figure 5.20) and avascular necrosis at joints (Figure 5.21) complicate the marrow hypertrophy which is less marked than in thalassaemia. The spleen is generally small.

Gaucher's disease

In Gaucher's disease, marrow infiltration expands the bone and thins the cortex. There are

infarcts, avascular necrosis and splenomegaly. Focal areas of osteolysis are seen due to local aggregations of Gaucher cells (Figure 5.22).

Enchondromatosis

In enchondromatosis, multiple radiolucent carti-laginous tumours are present in the diaphyses and metaphyses of tubular bones. The lesions show characteristic punctate calcification, have thin, well-defined margins, scallop the cortices from within, and expand the bone. Smaller bones, such as those in the hand, have the greatest relative enlargement and deformity. The enchondromatous lesions may abut onto the growth plate but do not cross it until after epiphyseal fusion. Occasionally, long strands of lucent cartilage stream backwards from the growth plate in parallel strands (Figure 5.23). Abnormalities of growth also occur in enchon-dromatosis at the wrist, with ulnar shortening

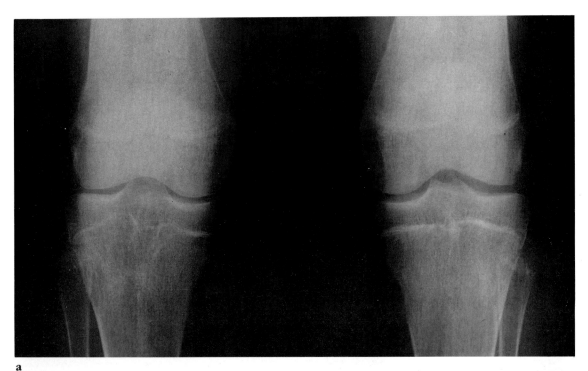

a

b

Figure 5.17

Thalassaemia. (**a**) There is an Erlenmeyer flask appearance, the bones are expanded, the cortices thinned and medullary density is reduced. In places the metaphyseal cortices are breached by soft tissue masses of marrow. (**b**) A close-up view of the metaphysis shows the soft tissue mass breaking through the cortex.

Figure 5.18

The skull of this patient with thalassaemia shows a marked increase in vault thickness with a hair-on-end appearance. The basi-occiput and squamous temporal bones are not involved in this process. The change affects the spine and mandible. The paranasal air sinuses are full of marrow, with the exception of the ethmoids.

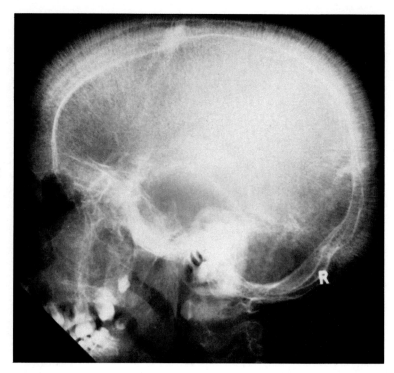

(Figure 5.24), and similar dysplastic changes are seen at the distal radius and ulna in diaphyseal aclasia.

Diaphyseal aclasia (multiple exostoses)

In this condition, the metaphyses of the long bones, particularly at the shoulders, hips, knees and ankles, become progressively irregularly expanded and club-like. Exostoses arise on the expanded metaphyseal regions, grow in size (Figure 5.25), and finally point away from the adjacent joint. The exostosis is surrounded by a lucent cartilaginous cap which ossifies progressively during growth, becoming completely ossified at the time of skeletal maturity (Figure 5.26), (see Chapter 7, page 368).

Osteopetrosis

Osteopetrosis is the result of failed resorption of bone by vascular mesenchyme during growth, which results in the persistence of foetal dense bone and abnormal modelling, particularly at the metaphyses, which show undertubulation (Figure 5.27).

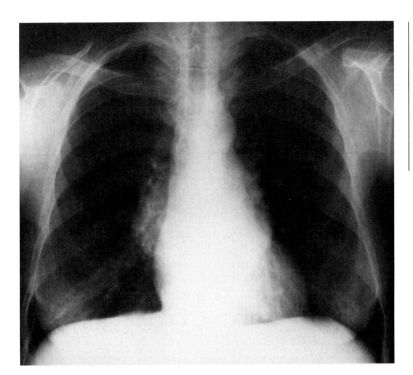

a

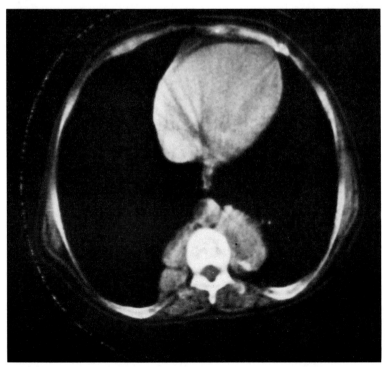

b

Figure 5.19

Thalassaemia. (**a**) The bones are expanded, the cortices thinned, and trabeculation is sparse. These features are particularly prominent in the clavicles. Hilar masses are also seen. (**b**) The CT scan confirms the presence of extramedullary haemopoiesis.

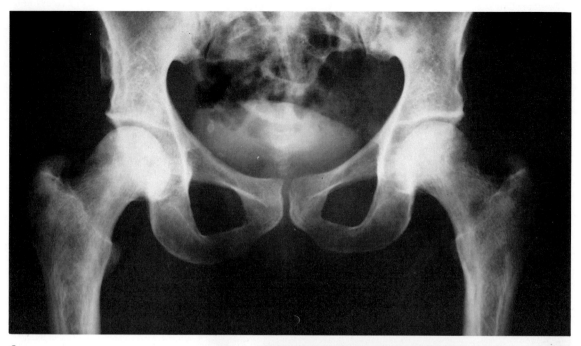

a

Figure 5.20

Sickle-cell disease. (**a**) There is a
generalized increase in bone
density. Cortical splitting is seen
in the proximal femora, and the
femoral heads show avascular
necrosis. (**b**) The femoral shafts
show cortical thickening and
splitting, and there is a
generalized increase in density.

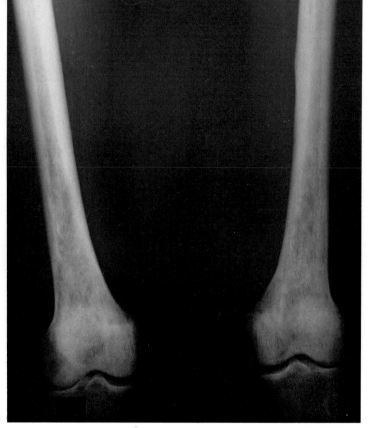

b

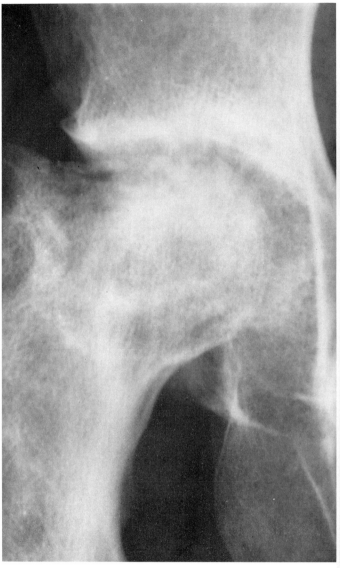

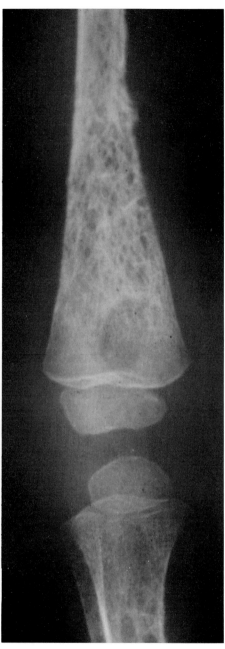

Figure 5.21

Avascular necrosis of the femoral head in sickle-cell disease. The joint space is preserved but the femoral head has collapsed. Infarctive changes are shown with structural failure and splitting-off of a dead cortical fragment. Buttressing is present at the medial cortex of the femoral neck, implying that this process is longstanding.

Figure 5.22

In this patient with Gaucher's disease, there is widespread marrow infiltration due to deposition of Gaucher cells. The cortex is broken through in places.

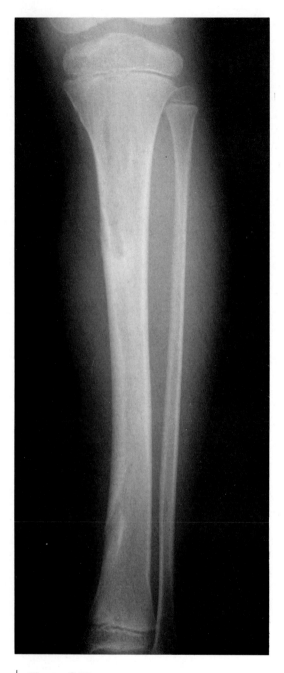

Figure 5.23

Enchondromatosis. Strands of
radiolucent cartilage stream back
from the growth plates
proximally and distally in the
tibia. This is associated with a
minor modelling abnormality.

Lead poisoning

In lead poisoning, inhibition of osteoclastic
activity also results in broadening of metaphyses
in association with local dense lead lines (Figure
5.11a).

Rickets

Rickets is the most common form of metaphyseal
broadening with irregularity (see Chapter 1,
page 37), which results from excess, localized,
soft, non-mineralized osteoid.

Hypophosphatasia

This resembles rickets but radiologically the
disease presents with changes of varying severity.
Neonates are most severely affected with marked
rickets-like changes at metaphyses and minimal
general ossification. The skull vault particularly
shows non-mineralization. In infant and adolescent patients, severe rickets-like changes are
seen, particularly affecting metaphyses (Figure
5.28). In the adult, an Erlenmeyer-flask appearance is seen. All groups show pathological
fractures and demineralization.

Metaphyseal dysostosis

Metaphyseal dysostosis is rare and, of the three
relatively common types (Schmid, McKusick and
Jansen), only Schmid is seen relatively often. The
metaphyses are splayed, broadened and show
irregular mineralization but the epiphyses are
normal, which is not true of rickets and
hypophosphatasia. The long bones are often
shortened (Figure 5.29).

Perthes' disease

Perthes' disease is the eponymous term for
avascular necrosis of the femoral head during

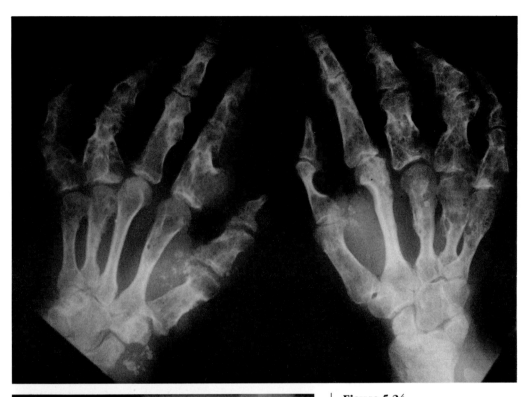

Figure 5.24

This patient with enchondromatosis has numerous enchondral tumours which deform and distort normal anatomy, and are manifest clinically. The ulna is short and the radius overgrown.

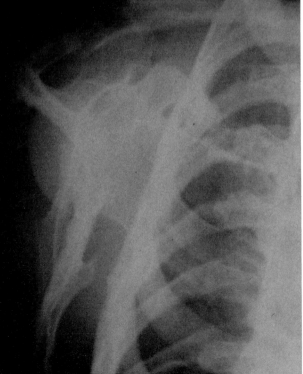

Figure 5.25

Multiple exostoses. Exostoses often arise on the scapula, and patients complain of pain when using the arm.

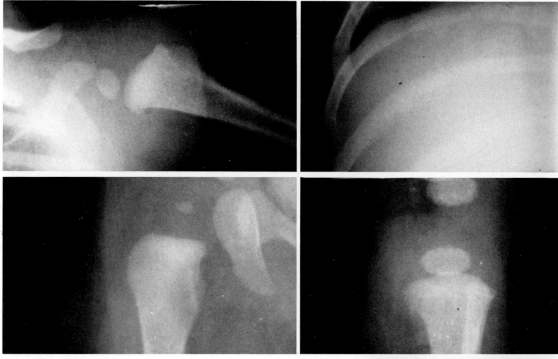

a

Figure 5.26

Growing lesions in multiple
exostoses (diaphyseal aclasia). (**a**)
An initial radiograph taken at
three months of age shows small
metaphyseal spurs. (**b**) At 13
months of age, metaphyseal
broadening and spurring is more
evident. (**c**) At 40 months, the
disease is now gross. (**d**) In the
same patient at ten years of age,
modelling defects are now
prominent.

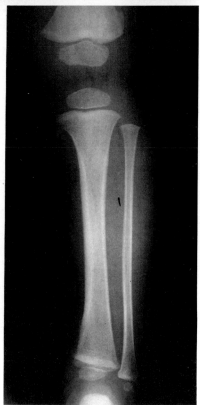

b

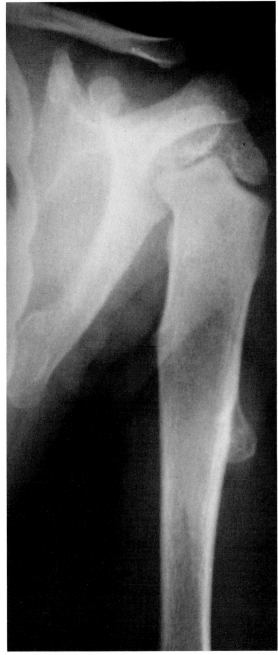

c

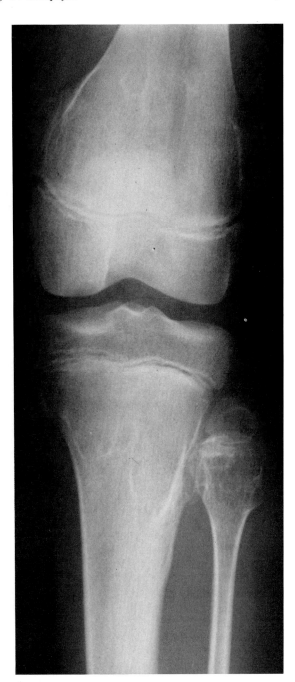

d

Figure 5.27

Osteopetrosis. Metaphyseal
broadening is associated with
increased density; alternating
bands of dense and normal bone
can be seen, producing a bone-
within-a-bone appearance.
Pathological fractures have
occurred in the midshafts of the
radius and ulna.

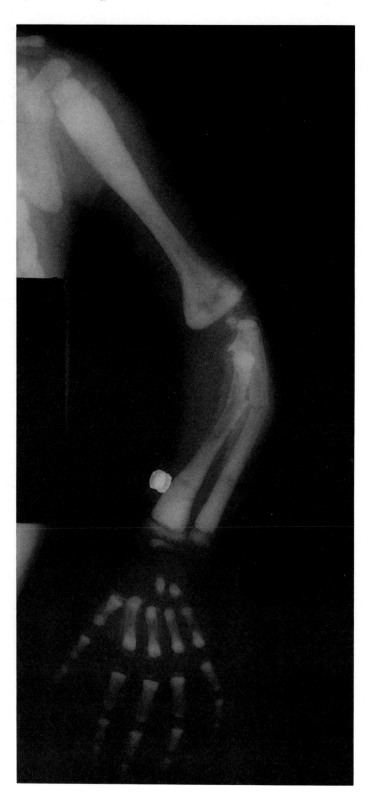

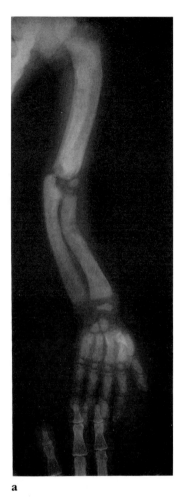

a

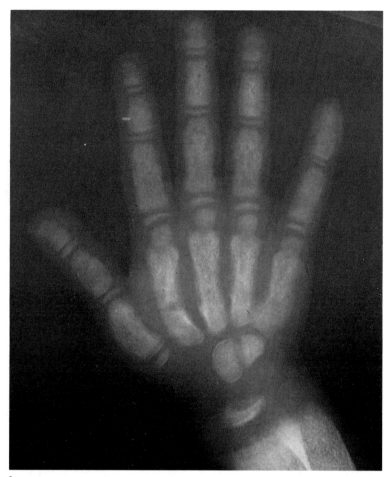

b

Figure 5.28

Hypophosphatasia. (**a,b**) There is gross metaphyseal irregularity with poor ossification and splaying affecting all the long bones. The epiphyses are also irregular. These changes are much more florid than those seen in rickets and extend further into the diaphyses.

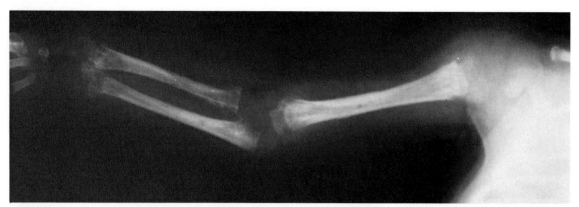

c

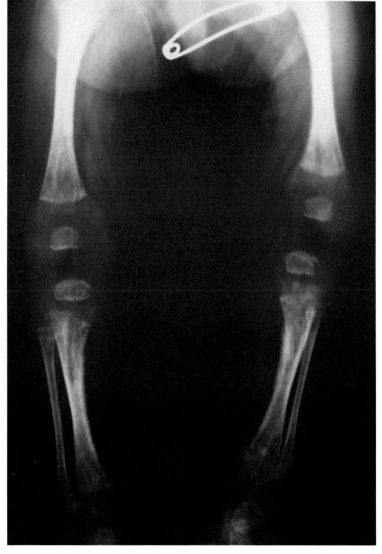

Figure 5.28 *continued*

(**c,d**) The changes are like rickets but are more gross. There is quite marked irregularity of the metaphyses but the changes extend into the shafts. The epiphyses are also irregular.

d

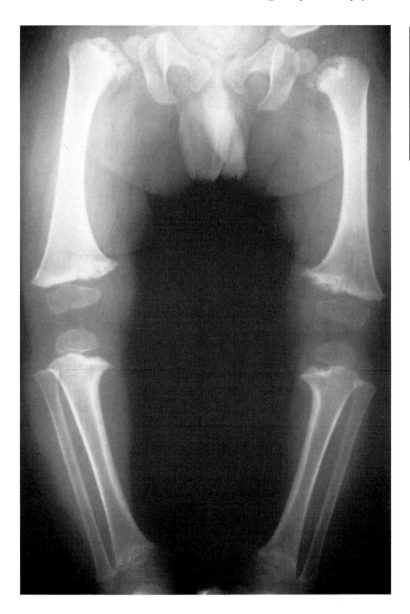

Figure 5.29

In this patient with metaphyseal dysostosis, type Schmid, there is irregularity and broadening of the metaphyses, but the epiphyseal plates are not generally widened. The bones are much more dense and sharply defined than in rickets.

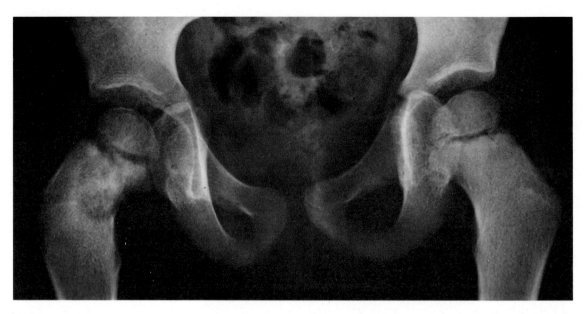

Figure 5.30

Perthes' disease. There is
irregularity of the right femoral
neck, which is broadened with
loss of cortical definition
medially and in the region of the
epiphyseal plate. The epiphysis
shows a necrotic cortex and a
subjacent crescentic lucency.

Figure 5.31

Battered baby. Metaphyseal chip
fractures are often the only
indication of acute trauma. The
flakes of bone are avulsed
because of the firm local
attachment of the underlying
periosteum.

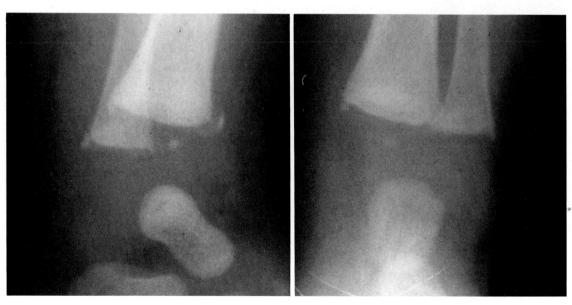

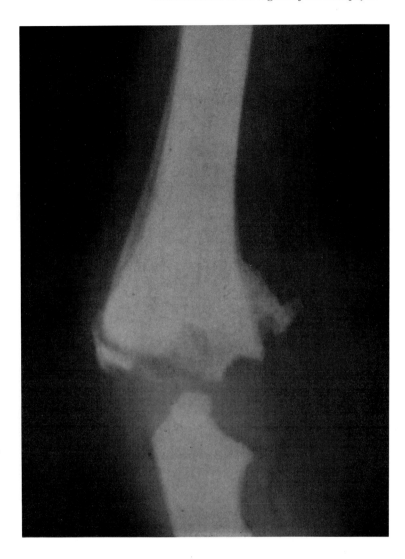

Figure 5.32

In this battered baby, further stripping of the periosteum results in subperiosteal new bone formation at the metaphysis.

childhood. Flattening and fragmentation of the epiphysis is associated with broadening and shortening of the femoral neck. The metaphysis shows cystic changes adjacent to the epiphyseal plate (Figure 5.30).

Metaphyseal trauma

Although trauma is generally not discussed in this book, two conditions involving metaphyseal trauma are of interest. In baby battering, the only indication of an acute lesion may be a chip fracture, or flake of bone, at the metaphysis, which arises because of the firm local attachment of the periosteum. The loosely applied diaphyseal periosteum is easily stripped with violent twisting of the limb (Figures 5.31 and 5.32), and this later results in gross periostitis. However, at the metaphysis, the underlying cortical bone is locally elevated. There may also be epiphyseal malalignment.

Figure 5.33

Idiopathic juvenile osteoporosis.
There is widespread loss of bone
density, and areas of increased
density at the metaphyses. These
are the result of metaphyseal
impaction fractures.

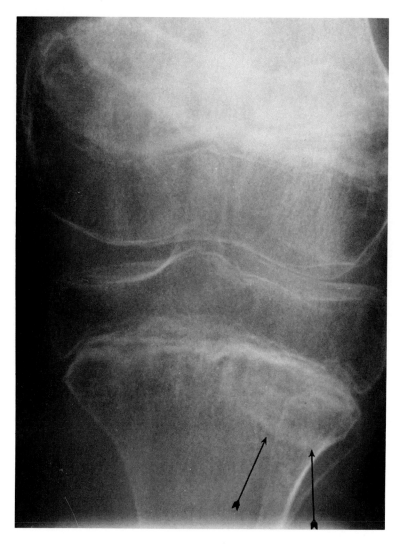

Table 5.5 Solitary tumours arising in the metaphysis.

Simple bone cyst Aneurysmal bone cyst Enchondroma Fibrous dysplasia	Benign
Chondroblastoma Giant-cell tumour	Only occasionally metaphyseal
Osteosarcoma Metastasis	Malignant

Idiopathic juvenile osteoporosis (IJO) (see
Chapter 1, page 14) is associated with metaphyseal fractures, which distinguishes this lesion
from osteogenesis imperfecta at adolescence, in
which fractures tend to be diaphyseal. The shaft
impacts into the metaphysis, where the cortex is
deficient and almost absent (Figure 5.33).

Tumours arising in the metaphyses are listed in
Table 5.5.

6 | Periosteal reactions

Elevation of the periosteum is followed by the laying down of new bone by osteoprogenitor cells. The periosteum may be elevated by malignant or benign processes but, occasionally, the cause of periosteal elevation and new bone formation is unknown. Some authors (Edeiken J, Hodes PJ, Caplan LH et al, *American Journal of Roentgenology,* (1966) **97**: 708) have attempted to demonstrate that the radiological appearance of the new bone is often an indicator of the underlying disease process.

The two main types of periosteal new bone either lie parallel to the cortex or at right angles to it (Figures 6.1 and 6.2). Edeiken et al further divide those lying parallel to the cortex into solid or lamellar types. A solid periostitis is totally applied to the underlying cortex with no intervening lucent zone (Figure 6.3). According to these authors, when the thickness of the new bone exceeds 1 mm, which it does in most solid periosteal reactions, the underlying lesion is benign. Lamellar periosteal reactions may be benign or malignant in origin.

According to Edeiken et al, a solid periostitis occurs in the following conditions:

- Eosinophilic granuloma
- Fractures
- Osteomyelitis
- Hypertrophic osteoarthropathy

- Osteoid osteoma
- Vascular and storage diseases

The contour of both solid and lamellar periostitis may be smooth, undulant or very irregular (Figures 6.4 and 6.5). Lamellar lesions may have as many as five or six layers of new bone external to the cortex. Lamellations are thought to be due to intermittent changes in growth rates in the underlying lesion. If the lesion temporarily stops growing, the elevated periosteum has time to form new bone beneath itself, which is initially woven, but then becomes more mature (Figure 6.6).

The periosteum is loosely applied to the diaphysis in children and so periostitis is often much more florid. This is particularly marked in infections resulting in a florid involucrum (Figure 6.7).

Perpendicular spiculation occurs when new bone is laid down upon stretched subperiosteal blood vessels and upon the Sharpey's fibres, which tether periosteum to bone (Figure 6.8).

Most periosteal reactions are the result of subperiosteal pathology, but soft tissue lesions can also cause new bone to be laid down by the underlying periosteum (Figure 6.9). With tumours, periosteal new bone may be present in conjunction with new bone formed within the tumour itself (Figure 6.2), while in infections,

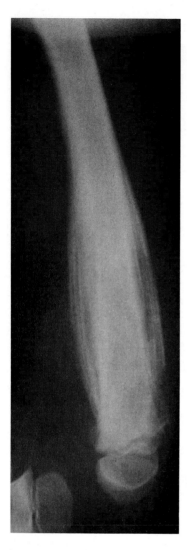

Figure 6.1

Ewing's sarcoma. A fine lamellar periosteal reaction lies parallel to the cortex.

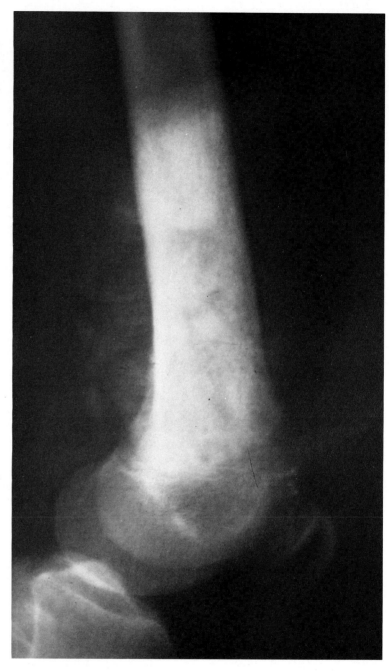

Figure 6.2

Osteogenic sarcoma. In this patient the periostitis is perpendicular to the shaft.

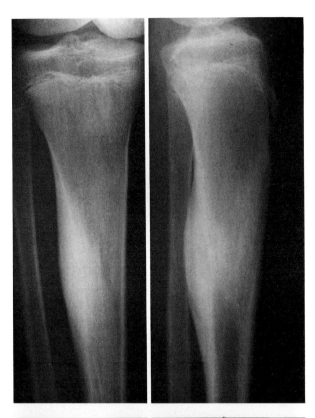

Figure 6.3

Solid periostosis—osteoid osteoma. The osteoid osteoma is not visible and is obscured by a solid layer of locally applied periosteal new bone.

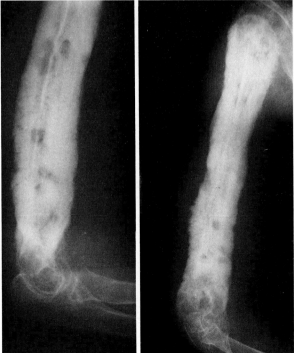

Figure 6.4

Osteomyelitis. The nature of the underlying process is evident from the extensive cortical sequestrum buried deep in the bone. The periostitis itself is undulant and irregular, but solid.

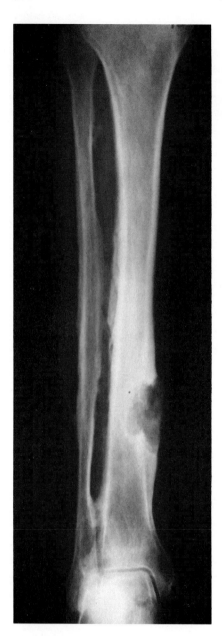

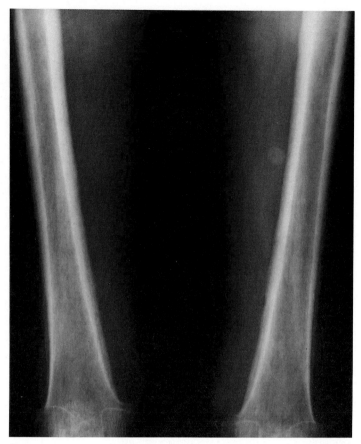

a

Figure 6.6

Hypertrophic osteoarthropathy.
(**a**) In this patient, the
new bone has united with the
underlying cortex in places.

Figure 6.5

Osteomyelitis. A shaggy lamellar
periostitis is seen on the tibia and
fibula, and bony fusion is
occurring between the two
bones. In places the periostitis is
solid.

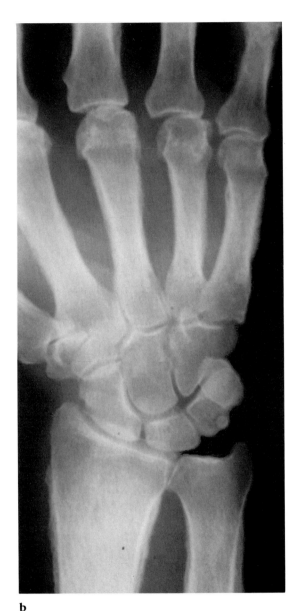

b

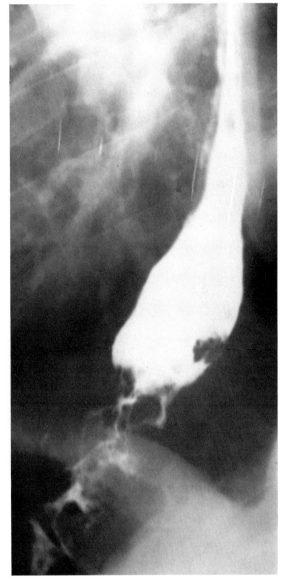

c

Figure 6.6 *continued*

(**b**,**c**) In this patient, a
more usual form of lamellar
periostitis is due to an
oesophageal carcinoma.

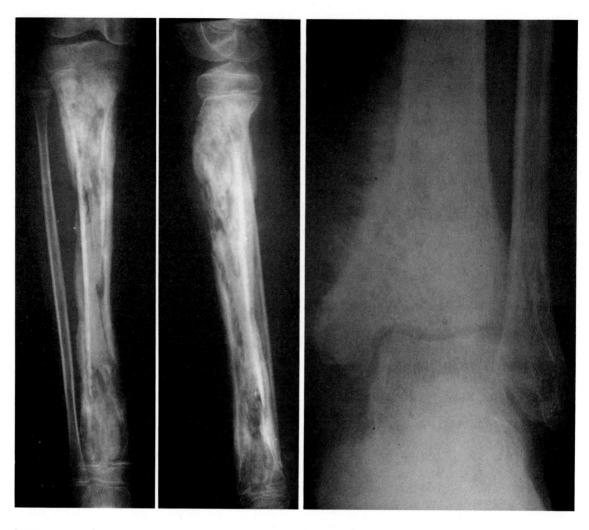

Figure 6.7

Osteomyelitis. There is a florid involucrum. The original cortex has died and now presents as a linear density lying within the involucrum. This is essentially another example of cortical splitting.

Figure 6.8

Mycetoma. Perpendicular spiculation or a hair-on-end appearance in a fungal infection which is a variety of Madura foot. The patchy defects in the region of the medial malleolus are related to osteomyelitis.

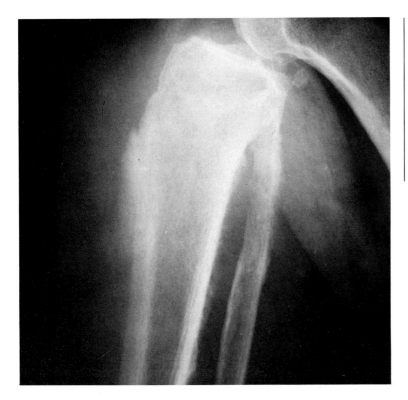

Figure 6.9

In this patient with liposarcoma, periostitis is related to an overlying tumour. The soft tissue swelling is visible although its nature is not evident. Translucency is not a feature of liposarcoma. The tumour has caused a florid hair-on-end periostitis at the proximal tibia and fibula.

Table 6.1   Causes of local periostitis.

Arthritides	Adjacent to affected synovium. Less common in rheumatoid arthritis and juvenile chronic arthritis. More common in psoriasis and Reiter's syndrome. Osteoarthritis at the hip
Fractures	Following major injury, or stress fractures
Osteomyelitis	Usually localized unless associated with immune defects. Florid in children
Following haemorrhage	
Vascular stasis	Usually in the lower limb associated with varicose veins, occasionally with lymphatic obstruction, with or without local ulceration

Tumours	1 Benign, such as osteoid osteoma
	2 Malignant:
	    Osteosarcoma—central
	                —periosteal
	                —parosteal
	    Ewing's sarcoma
	    Chondrosarcoma
	    Fibrosarcoma

sequestra may be associated with the periostitis (Figure 6.4 and Table 6.1).

Causes of local periostitis

Arthritides

Periosteal new bone is unusual in rheumatoid arthritis, but can occur along the shafts of the tubular bones of the hands and feet. Erosions may be visible locally, but often the change is associated with a synovitis in the local tendon sheath causing soft tissue swelling and osteoporosis. Fine, lamellar new bone is laid down at the metaphysis or diaphysis, as shown in Figure 4.18. A similar situation occurs in Still's disease (juvenile chronic arthritis). Seronegative arthritides in adults are associated with a much more florid and generalized form of periosteal reaction. Patients with Reiter's syndrome and psoriasis have erosions with a different distribution to those seen in rheumatoid arthritis (see Chapter 4, page 223), and bone density is usually preserved. Erosions are frequently associated with a florid, often shaggy, perpendicular periostitis in the same area, for example, around the calcaneum and malleoli (Figure 6.10), and along phalangeal shafts, resulting in an increase in bony density (Figure 6.11).

Degenerative disease is often associated with florid new bone formation at disc and joint margins, but a true periostitis is seen at the medial aspect of the femoral neck in osteoarthritis, probably due to a buttressing phenomenon following altered local stresses (Figure 4.29).

Figure 6.10

Psoriasis. Irregularity with fluffy new bone formation is present particularly on the medial malleolus, but also on the lateral.

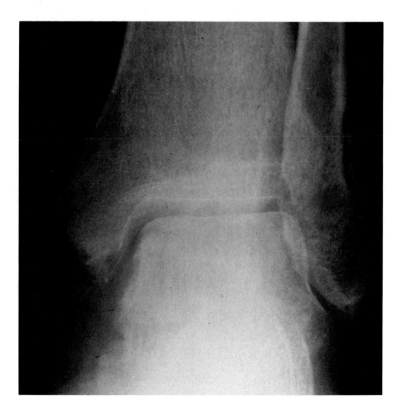

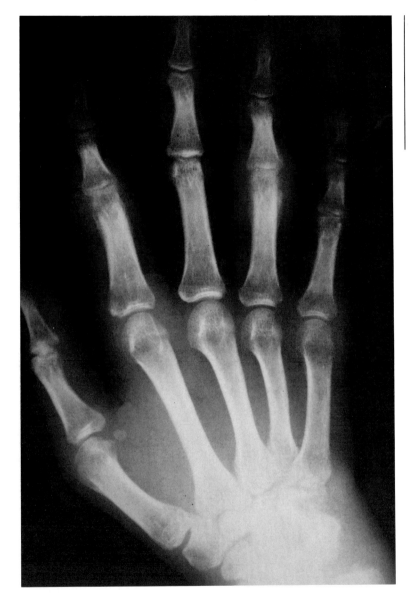

Figure 6.11

Reiter's syndrome—sausage digits. Soft tissue swelling is present over the proximal phalanges of the index and ring fingers. This is associated with an increase in bony density, largely due to an overlying, rather shaggy periostitis.

Fractures

Bleeding at a fracture elevates the periosteum, and within 7 to 14 days amorphous new bone, known as callus, begins to form. Generally, the amount of callus is greater at fractures immobilized in plaster, than at those fixed by nail or plate, where less local movement can occur. With a greenstick fracture, new bone formation at the concave surface results in a lamellar buttress, while bone is resorbed on the opposite convexity, so that the periostitis is part of a remodelling phenomenon (Figure 6.12).

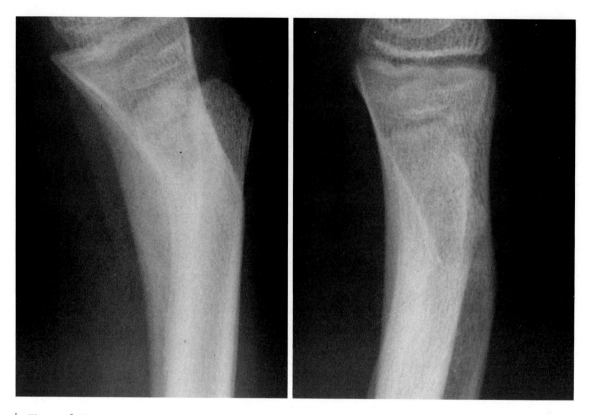

Figure 6.12

New bone formation following a fracture. A distal radial fracture has resulted in the laying down of new bone on the concavity of the fracture (*left*) resulting in eventual remodelling, even in the absence of initial reduction of the fracture (*right*).

Stress fractures

Stress fractures are the result of normal activity on abnormal bone, or regular, repeated subliminal trauma to normal bone. Particular sports or occupations produce stress lesions at characteristic sites, as shown in Table 1.7. For example, common sites for stress fractures in an athlete are the proximal tibia (Figure 6.13) and the second or third metatarsal neck (Figure 6.14). These painful lesions are often bilateral and symmetrical and initially not visible on a radiograph, but will show up on a radioisotope bone scan (Figure 6.15).

Characteristically, a stress fracture appears as a poorly defined transverse band of lucency surrounded by sclerosis extending through the

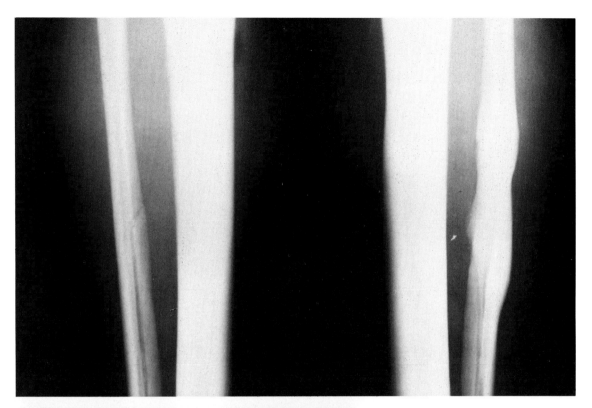

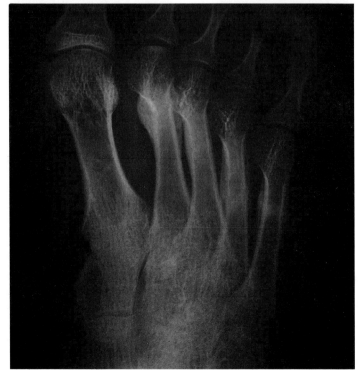

Figure 6.13

Stress fractures may be seen on the left and right tibia and fibula of a professional footballer. On the left a more longstanding lesion is associated with a solid periostitis of the midshaft of the fibula, while on the right, the more recent stress fracture is seen.

Figure 6.14

Stress fractures. Typical healing fractures of the second, third, fourth and fifth metatarsal necks are visible. Fracture lines can still be seen and are transverse. Both a lamellar and solid periostitis are present.

Figure 6.15

Stress fractures. Radioisotope
bone scan showing stress
fractures of the midshaft of the
tibia and fibula in an athlete.

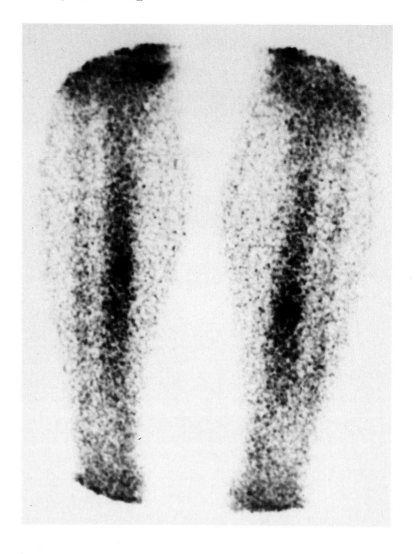

medulla to a cortical surface, which shows a
localized area of subperiosteal new bone formation (Figure 6.16), which is initially hazy and
then becomes well-defined. A smooth local mass
of bone is produced, which is eventually
resorbed into the cortex (Figure 6.17).

A similar appearance may be seen around an
osteoid osteoma (Figure 6.18), in chronic
osteomyelitis (Figure 6.19), a Looser's zone in
osteomalacia (Figure 6.20) and, occasionally,
with other bone-forming tumours including
osteosarcoma. In these lesions a small, usually
smooth, cortical exostosis formed by a localized
focus of subperiosteal new bone is associated
with a central zone of endosteal sclerosis or lysis,
which may be observed radiologically but is
often better defined with conventional or com-
puted tomography.

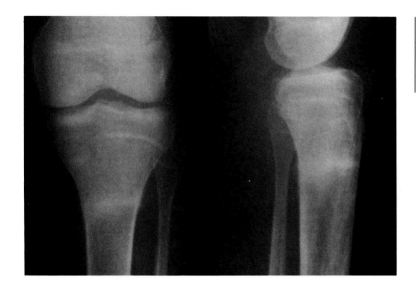

Figure 6.16

Stress fracture. A typical transverse density is seen in the proximal tibia associated with a localized lamellar periostitis.

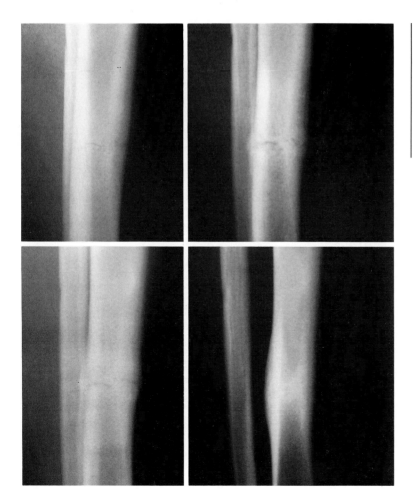

Figure 6.17

Progression of a stress fracture. The initial lesion across the midshaft of the tibia is barely visible. Progressive films show the formation of callus and finally the fracture line becomes poorly defined with a surrounding solid localized periostitis.

Figure 6.18

A subperiosteal or periosteal osteoid osteoma causes a superficial sclerotic reaction, obscuring the tumour.

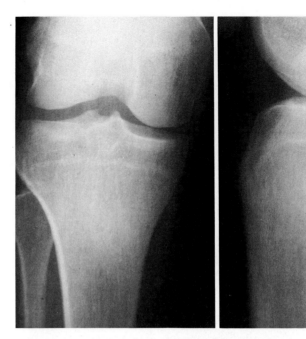

Figure 6.19

Osteomyelitis. There is thickening of the cortex, both endosteally and superficially, with obliteration of the medullary cavity. The external periosteal reaction is solid.

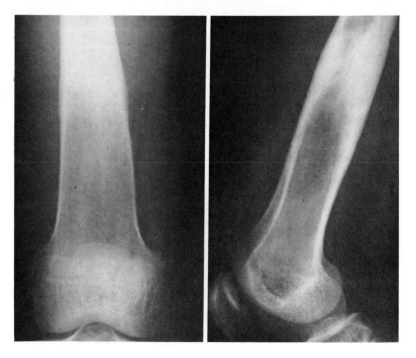

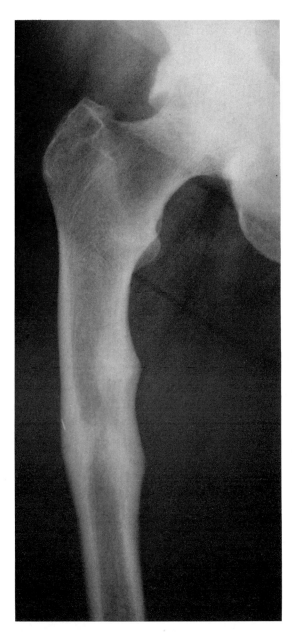

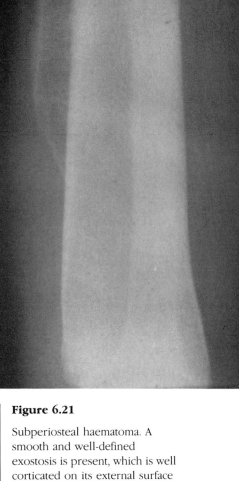

Figure 6.20

In this patient with osteomalacia there are Looser's zones which are a characteristic feature of the disease. Transverse bands of lucency are associated with local areas of solid periostitis in the healing phase.

Figure 6.21

Subperiosteal haematoma. A smooth and well-defined exostosis is present, which is well corticated on its external surface and closely applied to the underlying bone.

Subperiosteal haematoma

A subperiosteal haematoma is the result of trauma, often without a frank fracture, although a fracture line may be visible eventually. In children, the loose application of periosteum to bone can result in avulsion, for example, by a twisting motion. The elevated periosteum forms a localized bony protrusion which eventually amalgamates with the underlying cortex (Figure 6.21).

Osteomyelitis

The basic features of osteomyelitis have been described previously. Pus breaches the cortex through cloacae and elevates the periosteum. This occurs to a greater extent in children than in adults, when the entire periosteum of a long bone may be stripped off. Therefore, in infants a thick, wavy involucrum forms, which often sheaths the entire shaft of a long bone, but is clearly separated from it, as shown in Figure 6.7. The underlying sequestra and necrotic tissue become absorbed beneath the involucrum and, with growth, a normal shape of bone results. In adolescents and adults, the changes at the periosteum are more localized and bony expansion less marked (Figure 6.22).

Figure 6.22

Adult osteomyelitis. There is a solid periostitis. The underlying bony detail is obliterated, and in this patient the lesion is localized to the metaphysis.

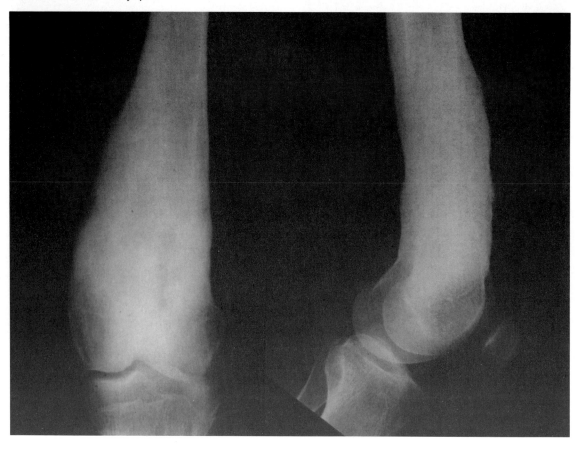

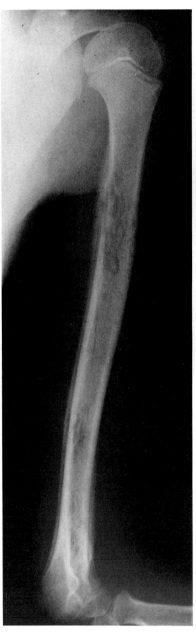

Figure 6.23

In this patient with osteomyelitis there is patchy destruction of bone associated with sequestrum formation. The cortex of the bone is breached, giving a cloaca. The periostitis in this patient is delicate and lamellar.

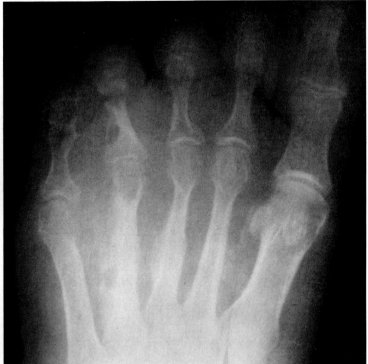

Figure 6.24

Madura foot. Fungal osteomyelitis results in a number of changes. The defects in the bone are caused by soft tissue fungus balls, and there is sunray periostitis.

In adults the tubular bones are not usually the site of blood-borne infection, which is generally confined to the spine and pelvis. Infection of the small bones of the hands and feet is usually due to direct inoculation.

There is no specific type of periostitis in osteomyelitis. A solid, perhaps wavy periostitis may be formed which is typically benign. Fine lamellar periostitis, of one or more layers, may also be seen so that the lesion may resemble Ewing's sarcoma (see below) (Figure 6.23). In addition, the periostitis may be diaphyseal and widespread along the shaft.

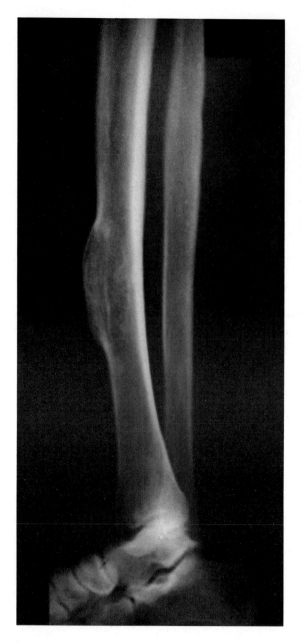

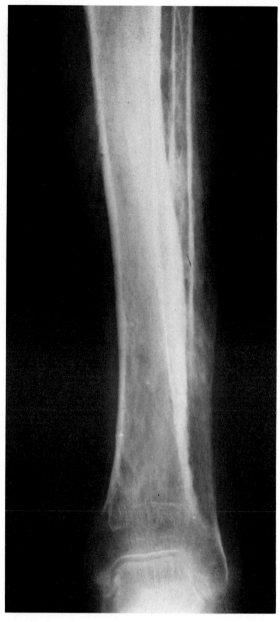

Figure 6.25

A small dome-like exostosis is produced beneath this tropical ulcer.

Figure 6.26

Vascular stasis. Patients with chronic varicose disease develop a very profuse, shaggy periostitis. In this patient, it has incorporated into the underlying bones.

With unusual infections, more bizarre patterns of periosteal new bone are seen. Brucellosis and mycetomal lesions are associated with sclerosis and coarse, vertical spiculation of the sunray type (Figure 6.24).

Soft tissue infections such as decubitus ulcers can also cause change in the underlying bone. The bone beneath varicose ulcers at the ankle may show a local lamellar or florid sunray periostitis although a periostitis occurs in varicose disease in the absence of ulceration. A small, dome-like exostosis occurs beneath tropical ulcers which is rarely seen in temperate climes (Figure 6.25).

Vascular stasis

Longstanding varicose veins in the lower limbs are associated with periosteal new bone formation along the diaphysis and metaphysis of the tibia and fibula, and in the small bones of the foot. The periostitis may be lamellar but is usually solid and applied to the cortex, with an outer irregular or undulant margin. Its presence is not dependent upon a varicose ulcer. Varicosities may be visible in subcutaneous fat and the soft tissues are generally thickened and oedematous. Phleboliths are often present (Figure 6.26). Similar changes occur with lymphatic obstruction and arterial insufficiency.

Periosteal reactions associated with tumours

The important criteria for distinguishing between benign and malignant lesions have already been listed (see Chapter 3, page 130). A solid periosteal reaction is almost always indicative of a benign lesion, while a lamellar periostitis may be due to an underlying benign or malignant lesion. Malignancy cannot be diagnosed on the basis of the periosteal pattern alone. All other features must be taken into account.

Aggressive tumours break through the cortex and elevate the periosteum beneath which new bone is laid down. Cyclical tumour activity results in a lamellar periostitis which may be fine or coarse, according to the tumour type. If further tumour growth occurs, it may exceed the ability of the periosteum to lay down new bone. The tumour bursts through the periosteum centrally, leaving an elevated triangle of new bone at the tumour margins—Codman's triangle (Figure 6.27). This is radiologically similar to the process of buttressing which occurs at the margin of the periosteal elevation with benign tumours, where new bone fills the angle between cortex and elevated periosteum. This phenomenon is seen with aneurysmal bone cysts and giant-cell tumours (Figure 6.28). Codman's triangles also occur after subperiosteal infection or haemorrhage.

Ewing's sarcoma and osteogenic sarcoma

Ewing's sarcoma classically infiltrates along the shaft, breaking through the cortex over a considerable distance (see Chapter 3, page 195). The resulting periostitis is usually lamellar, with fine parallel layers of new bone, indicating a cyclic process. The lamellae are delicate and thinner than the tumour-filled spaces between them.

A perpendicular periostitis is occasionally produced, due to new bone laid down upon stretched subperiosteal Sharpey's fibres and blood vessels. Fine, short, delicate spicules of new bone are laid down perpendicular to the eroded cortex, often over a considerable length of shaft. Again, the new bone spicules formed are often thinner than the spaces between them, producing a hair-on-end appearance (Figure 6.29).

Osteogenic sarcoma does not infiltrate along the shaft but tends to radiate from a central focus, through cortex and into soft tissues, which produces a large soft tissue mass with irregular, coarse tumour new bone formation. The periosteal lamellations are also coarse, thick and often irregular, with little clear space between them. If a hair-on-end appearance is present, it is coarse and of the sunray type, radiating from a central focus (Figure 6.30).

Parosteal osteosarcoma

This uncommon lesion occurs in patients of 25–35 years of age and has a better prognosis than

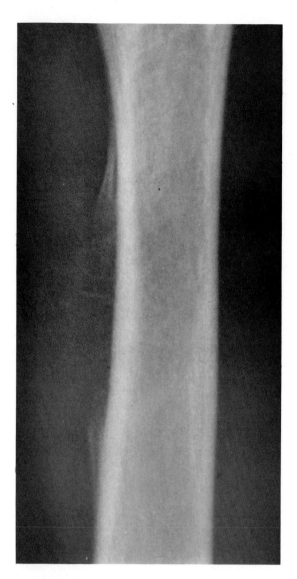

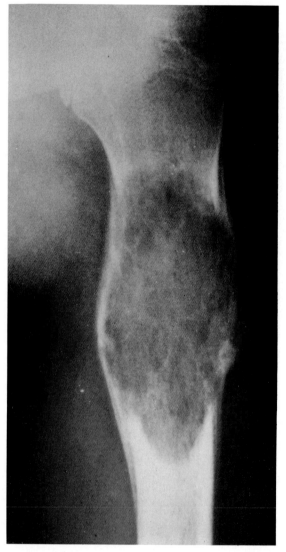

Figure 6.27

Ewing's sarcoma with a
Codman's triangle. There is a
very faint and barely perceptible
destructive process affecting the
cortex and medulla, but sunray
spiculation is associated with a
soft tissue mass and a peripheral
Codman's triangle. The delicate
nature of the new bone is typical
of Ewing's sarcoma.

Figure 6.28

Aneurysmal bone cyst. At the
margin of the cyst and the shaft,
a buttressing or lamellar
periostitis is visible. This
phenomenon does not occur
with simple bone cysts.

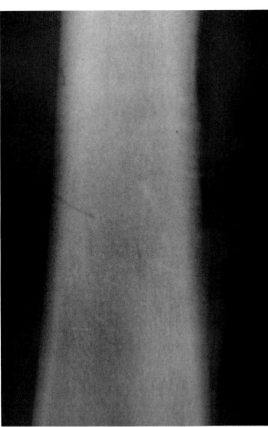

Figure 6.29

This Ewing's sarcoma is associated with a Codman's triangle and also saucerization of the cortex at the site of the soft tissue mass, a feature of malignant tumours. It also has a hair-on-end appearance.

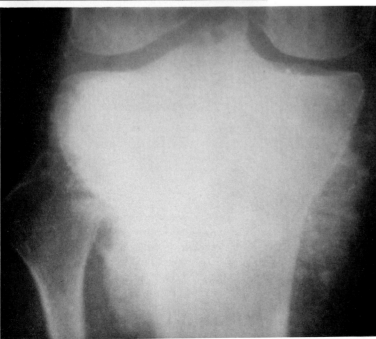

Figure 6.30

In this patient with osteogenic sarcoma, the periostitis is much more coarse than in Ewing's sarcoma. The lesion has caused much sclerosis, and sunray spiculation.

Figure 6.31

Parosteal osteosarcoma. (**a**) The
final radiograph of this patient,
taken after many years, shows a
typical parosteal osteosarcoma.
There is a well defined dense
tumour with undulant margins,
closely applied to the cortex of
the upper humerus. Because of
its close proximity to a joint and
intracapsular location, fragments
have broken off into the joint and
are separating the humeral head
from the glenoid. (**b**) This is a
chest X-ray taken eight years
previously which shows the same
shoulder, but the lesion was
missed. Its growth can thus be
accessed over eight years. (**c**)
Five years after the initial
radiograph some growth has
occurred. Again, this is part of a
chest X-ray. Therefore
maximal growth occurred in the
subsequent three years.

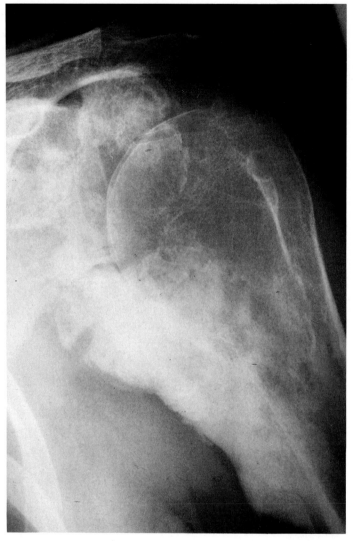

a

the central osteogenic sarcoma. Dense new bone
is laid down upon the cortex of the metaphysis
of a long bone, usually around the knee or
shoulder. The outer margin is undulant. Occasionally, lumps of ossified tumour become
detached, presumably because of muscular activity (Figure 6.31).

Characteristically, a lucent plane of cleavage
separates the cortex from the tumour. This lesion
can closely resemble traumatic myositis ossificans, in which the bony mass often blends with
the underlying bone and, occasionally, it is
difficult to differentiate between them. In the
early stage of both lesions, peripheral definition
may be poor. The haematoma ossifies much
more rapidly under observation, incorporates
into the cortex and eventually often vanishes.
Under observation, growth and ossification of the

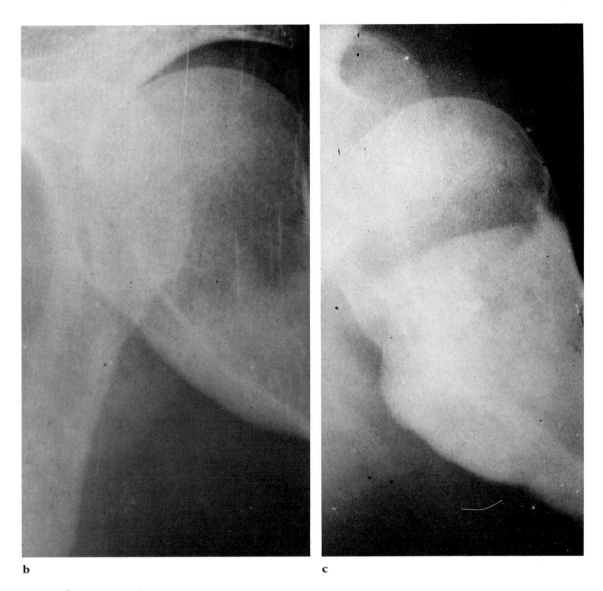

b

c

Figure 6.31 *continued*

parosteal sarcoma is slow, and years elapse before the underlying medulla is invaded; therefore this lesion metastasizes later. Prognosis following surgery is good.

Periosteal osteosarcoma

This rare variant is seen as a short 1–3 cm defect in the cortex associated with a soft tissue mass, with a slightly irregular and perpendicular hair-on-end periostitis (Figure 6.32). Its behaviour and prognosis is between that of parosteal and conventional osteogenic sarcoma.

Primary malignant tumours occurring in the fourth and fifth decades are reticulum cell sarcoma, fibrosarcoma and chondrosarcoma, whose features are discussed in more detail in Chapter 3. Reticulum cell sarcoma resembles

Figure 6.32

Periosteal osteosarcoma. (**a**) A
localized lesion is associated with
a characteristic, fine hair-on-end
periostitis. (**b**) The CT scan
shows a more extensive lesion.

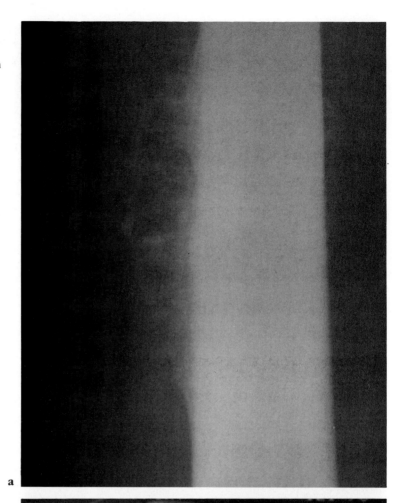

a

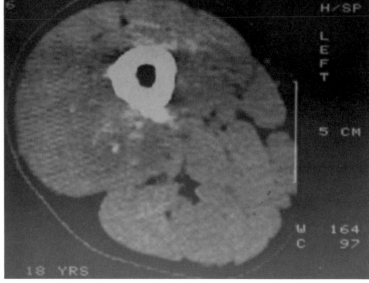

b

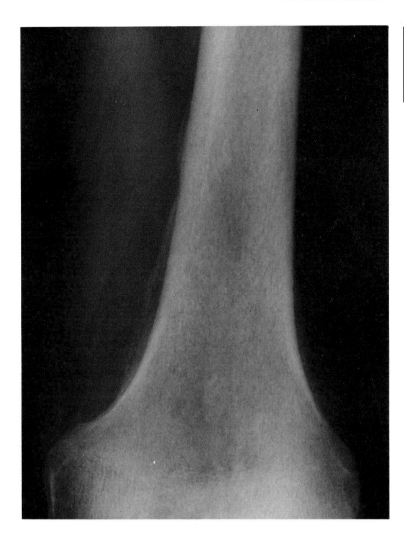

Figure 6.33

In reticulum cell sarcoma, early infiltration of the medulla is associated with a fine lamellar periostitis.

Ewing's sarcoma and can cause a lamellar periostitis (Figure 6.33). Fibrosarcoma does not cause a marked periosteal reaction but can be associated with one or two layers of irregular new bone formation (Figure 6.34). Chondrosarcoma is a relatively slowly growing malignant tumour which scallops the cortex from within but which allows a thick layer of subperiosteal new bone to form. The cortical margin of the lesion may be thicker than the normal cortex.

Generalized periostitis

Generalized periosteal new bone formation is unusual, and may occasionally be seen with widespread skeletal metastases, for example, from the prostate (Figure 6.35) or osteogenic sarcoma, and with widespread angiomatous tumours. However, metastatic disease is not commonly associated with florid or even minor periostitis (Table 6.2).

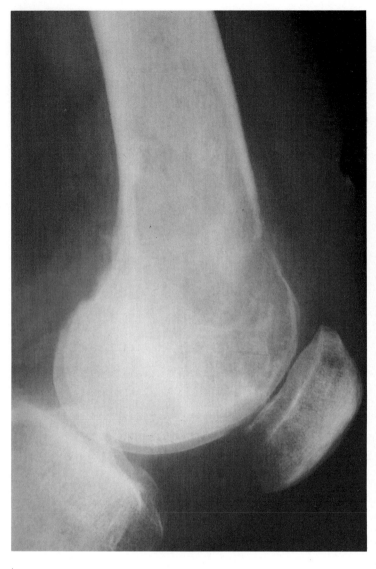

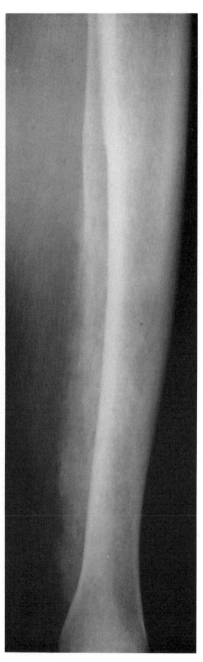

Figure 6.34

Irregular destruction of the distal
femur associated with a delicate
periostitis is visible in this
patient with fibrosarcoma.

Figure 6.35

Periostitis due to secondary
deposits is uncommon but, in
this patient, has resulted from a
carcinoma of the prostate.

Table 6.2   Generalized periostitis in adults.

Hypertrophic osteoarthropathy

Primary or idiopathic pachydermoperiostitis

Secondary to benign or malignant pulmonary and
   pleural lesions
     Chronic lung infections, tuberculosis
     Chronic liver disease
     Congenital cyanotic heart disease
     Chronic inflammatory bowel disease

Arthritides

Thyroid acropachy

Polyarteritis nodosa

Myeloma and, occasionally, secondary deposits,
   eg from the prostate

Periostitis associated with soft tissue swelling

Hypertrophic (pulmonary) osteoarthropathy

This is a painful condition in which periosteal new bone is laid down in response to lesions elsewhere, usually in the lung. The new bone is most commonly found at the distal radius and ulna, distal tibia and fibula, metatarsals, metacarpals and phalanges. The epiphyseal regions are spared. The periostitis has many forms. A common presentation is of a fine solitary layer of new bone separated from the intact, underlying cortex by a plane of lucency but, occasionally, up to six layers of lamellar new bone may be seen. The new bone may merge with the underlying cortex or may be irregular and, occasionally, hair-on-end (Figure 6.36).

The affected areas of the skeleton show a diffuse or linear peripheral increase in uptake on radioisotope scans. Although epiphyses do not

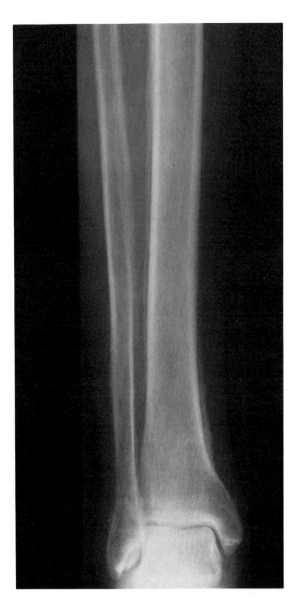

Figure 6.36

Hypertrophic osteoarthropathy. Fine lamellar periostitis is seen along the diaphysis and metaphysis of the tibia and fibula. The epiphyseal regions are not affected.

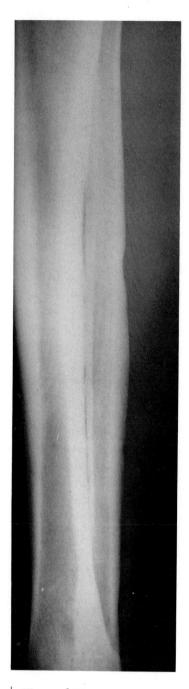

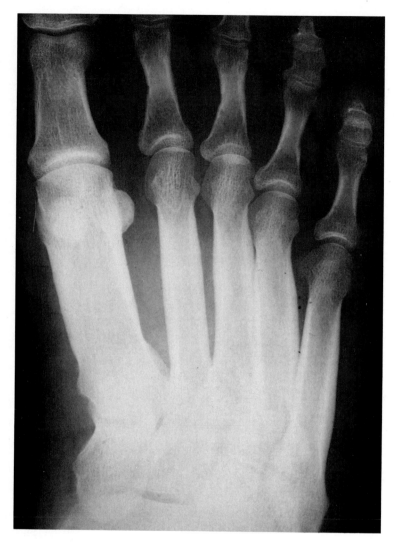

Figure 6.37

The three radiographs showing
pachydermoperiostosis illustrate
that it is radiologically similar to
hypertrophic osteoarthropathy,
but more florid and extensive.

show new bone formation, a non-erosive synovitis is often present and may be the presenting
symptom, with pain and soft tissue swelling
around joints.

The lesions regress following removal or
treatment of the underlying (usually pulmonary)
lesion, and even after vagotomy or pleural
section.

Clubbing of the fingers is often associated with

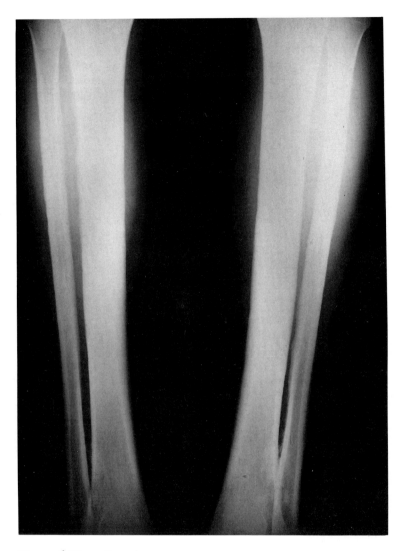

Figure 6.37 *continued*

hypertrophic osteoarthropathy but the two do not always accompany each other.

Pachydermoperiostosis

This is an idiopathic form of hypertrophic osteoarthropathy which is not associated with an underlying visceral lesion. It is associated with clubbing and gross thickening of the skin of the scalp, face, hands and feet. The disease often starts in adolescence, long before the usual age of onset of lung-related hypertrophic osteoarthropathy, most of which are associated with malignant lung or pleural disease. The periostitis is similar in distribution to hypertrophic osteoarthropathy, but extends to the epiphyses and is shaggy rather than finely lamellar. Gross thickening of the diaphysis may be seen (Figure 6.37).

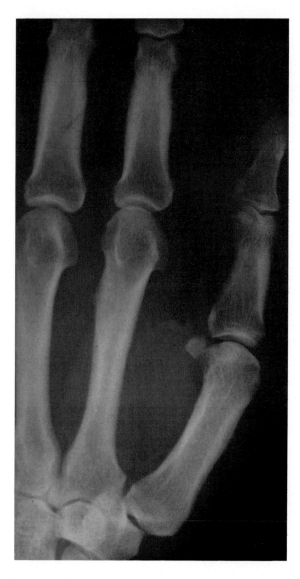

Figure 6.38

Thyroid acropachy. The extent of
periostitis in this disease can vary
greatly, but in this patient
thickening of the cortices is
demonstrated, associated with a
hair-on-end appearance at the
midshafts of the tubular bones.

Thyroid acropachy

This occurs in patients who are usually myxoede-
matous following treatment for thyrotoxicosis.
Pretibial myxoedema is present with swelling of
hands and feet, associated with a shaggy periostitis of the tubular bones in these areas and, less
commonly, the distal tibia and fibula (Figure
6.38).

Polyarteritis nodosa

This can be associated with gross, coarse,
symmetrical or velvety new bone formation on
the tibia, fibula and tubular bones of the feet. The
lesions may be due to arterial insufficiency and
therefore, possibly related to vascular stasis or
hypoxia (Figure 6.39).

Periosteal new bone in children (Table 6.3)

Caffey's infantile cortical hyperostosis

In this disease periosteal reactions appear before
five months of age. The affected children are ill

Table 6.3   Generalized periostitis in children.

Prematurity	} Normal bone density	
++Battered baby		
Idiopathic cortical hyperostosis		
++Osteogenesis imperfecta	Metaphyseal lucent bands	Reduced bone density
+Leukaemia		
+Neuroblastoma		
Congenital syphilis (rare)		
+Rickets	Widened epiphyseal plates	

+ or + + associated with fractures.

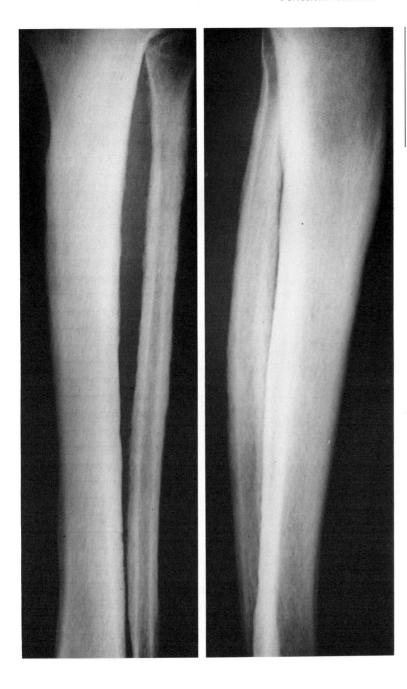

Figure 6.39

Polyarteritis nodosa. The amount of periostitis in this disease can vary greatly. In this radiograph, a solid periostitis is laid down along the midshafts of the paired long bones. Often a hair-on-end appearance results.

with fever, irritability and a raised ESR. Soft tissue masses occur, beneath which new bone formation appears. One or many bones may be involved and, as some lesions heal, others appear. Changes are usually seen in the mandible, scapula and ribs, as well as in the long bones of the limbs (Figure 6.40). A lamellar or coarse periostitis can appear, which may be even thicker than the underlying shaft, and unite the paired long bones.

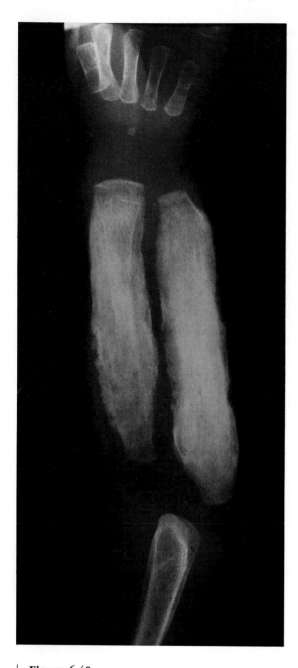

Figure 6.40

Infantile cortical hyperostosis. A
florid multilamellar periostitis
may be seen, and the underlying
bone is hardly visible.

New bone is diaphyseal and metaphyseal but
the epiphysis is spared. In the long bones, the
lesions are not generally symmetrical. The usual
tendency is towards remission but, occasionally,
the changes persist into adult life.

Baby battering

Multiple fractures of different generations are
classically found together with deformities (see
Chapter 5, page 294). The skull, ribs and lower
limbs are involved and the changes imply long-
term child abuse (Figure 1.24). In an acute case,
the only manifestation may be a metaphyseal
chip fracture, where the strongly attached
periosteum pulls off a small flake of bone. The
diaphyseal periosteum, which is not firmly
attached to the underlying cortex, is easily
stripped and large subperiosteal haematomas
may form, which are not necessarily related to
an underlying fracture of the shaft. These lesions
may be single, or multiple and asymmetrical.
Osteoporosis is not usually present (Figure
6.41).

Osteogenesis imperfecta

This can be difficult to differentiate from baby
battering (see Chapter 1, page 14). Clinically,
blue sclerae are not always present. Diaphyseal
fractures, which are usually multiple and of
different generations, are associated with deformity. Callus formation is probably more gross
than in any other disease associated with fractures (Figures 6.42 and 6.43) and, in addition,
there are features of bone softening such as
platybasia and bowing (Figure 6.44), as well as
osteoporosis. The skull vault may be extremely
thin and the sutures widened (Figure 6.45).

Scurvy

This is rare in the Western world, is associated
with vitamin C deficiency and is occasionally
seen in patients on bizarre diets. Defects in

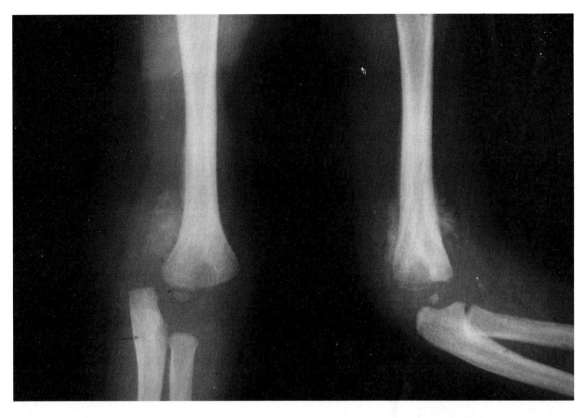

Figure 6.41

Battered baby. Amorphous new bone is laid down beneath the elevated periosteum following avulsion of a metaphyseal flake.

collagen result in capillary fragility and bleeding beneath the periosteum. This elevates, and a symmetrical lamellar periostitis is formed along the shafts of affected long bones (see Chapter 1, page 17). Metaphyseal fractures, osteoporosis and ring epiphyses are also present (Figure 6.46).

Rickets

In its healing phase this also causes periosteal new bone formation due to ossification of previously non-mineralized osteoid. There is generalized alteration of bone density and texture in epiphyses as well as shafts (Figure 6.47). The epiphyseal plates are widened, which is a feature almost unique to rickets, but they are progressively narrowed during healing (Figure 6.48).

Leukaemia and neuroblastoma

Elevation of the periosteum by malignant cells may cause a single, or lamellar, periostitis. Metaphyseal lucent bands, which are also present in scurvy and generalized osteoporosis, may also be seen but focal areas of bone destruction indicate a malignant infiltrative aetiology (Figure 6.49).

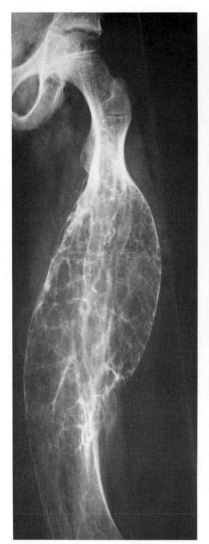

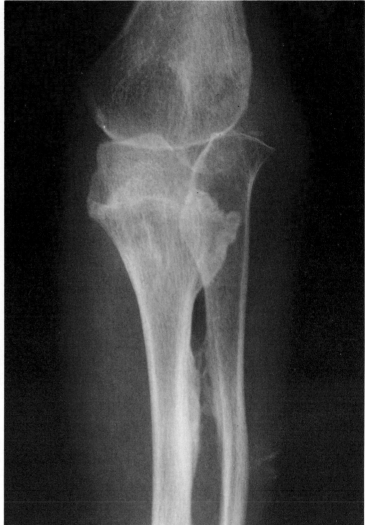

Figure 6.42

Osteogenesis imperfecta.
Hypertrophic callus has resulted
in marked expansion of the
femur following repeated
fracture.

Figure 6.43

Osteogenesis imperfecta. There
is cross-fusion across the
interosseous membrane between
the radius and ulna.
Hypertrophic callus is also visible
proximally on the ulna. The
deformity of the radial neck is
due to a previous fracture. Bone
density is decreased overall.

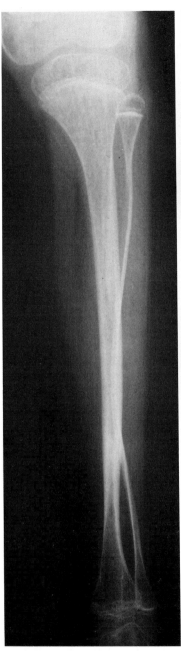

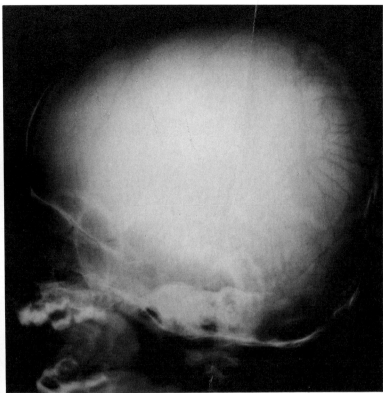

Figure 6.45

Osteogenesis imperfecta. The skull shows multiple Wormian bones.

Figure 6.44

A patient with osteogenesis imperfecta, showing thin, bowed osteoporotic long bones.

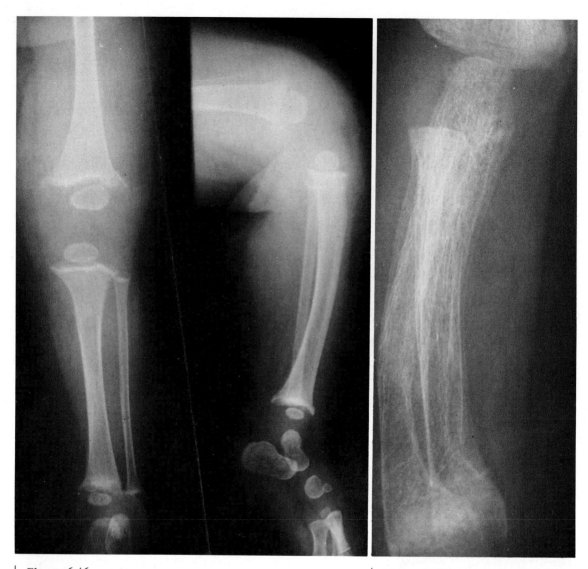

Figure 6.46

Metaphyseal fractures, ring
epiphyses and osteoporosis are
evident in this patient with
scurvy. There is also soft tissue
swelling, indicating recent
fracture.

Figure 6.47

Rickets. The presence of rickets is
shown by the broadened and
irregular metaphyses. Bone
density is reduced. There is
bowing of the radius with
evidence of a previous midshaft
fracture or Looser's zone. Quite
widespread lamellar periostitis is
present, which may follow
fracture healing, or ossification of
previously non-mineralized
osteoid when the patient is
treated.

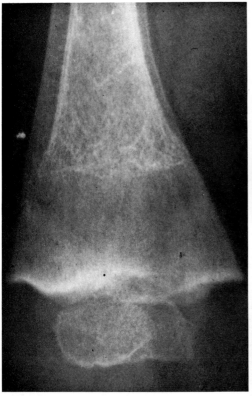

Figure 6.48

Healing rickets. A prominent bone-within-a-bone appearance is shown at the distal femur. The healing process has initiated new bone formation along the cortex and at the metaphysis, and the epiphyseal plate is now narrow.

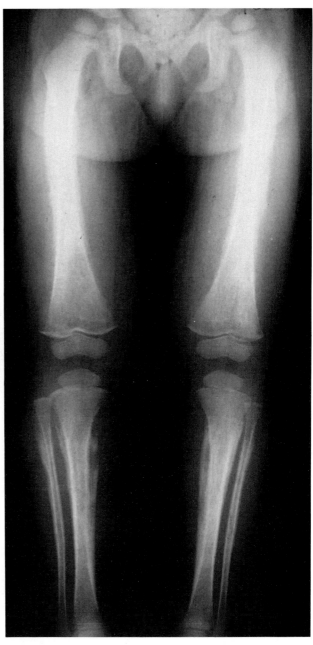

Figure 6.49

Leukaemia. Bands of metaphyseal lucency are visible which are irregular at the margins of the bone and are accompanied by lamellar periostitis around the midshafts.

Table 6.4   Causes of generalized hyperostosis.

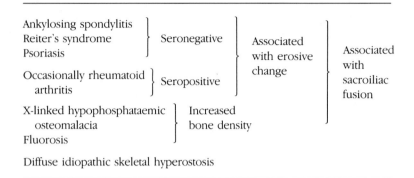

Diffuse idiopathic skeletal hyperostosis

Generalized hyperostosis

A number of conditions, some of which are related, have new bone formation at musculo-tendinous insertions as a common feature. The appearances are those of a generalized hyperostosis often affecting the pelvis, ribs and occasionally hands and feet, as well as the spine (Table 6.4).

Seronegative spondylarthropathies

The seronegative spondylarthropathies, including ankylosing spondylitis, psoriasis and Reiter's syndrome, have some distinguishing features, but also many common features.

Erosions occur initially on the lateral margins of the sacroiliac joints at the mid or lowest portions. The upper parts of the sacroiliac joints

Figure 6.50

Ankylosing spondylitis—early bilateral sacroiliitis. The lateral margins of the sacroiliac joints are indistinct and surrounded by reactive sclerosis; therefore individual erosions are not easily visible.

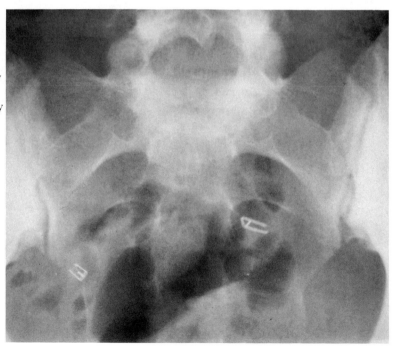

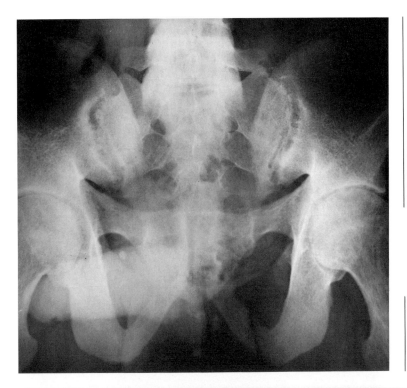

Figure 6.51

As ankylosing spondylitis progresses, erosive change is much more evident on both sides of the sacroiliac joints, symmetrically and bilaterally. The changes of an erosive arthropathy are also present at the hips, and appear more severe on the left side, where the joint space is reduced and the articular surfaces are irregular. There is little reactive sclerosis.

Figure 6.52

The CT scans show erosions and sclerosis in this fairly early case of ankylosing spondylitis to be on the lateral side of the joints.

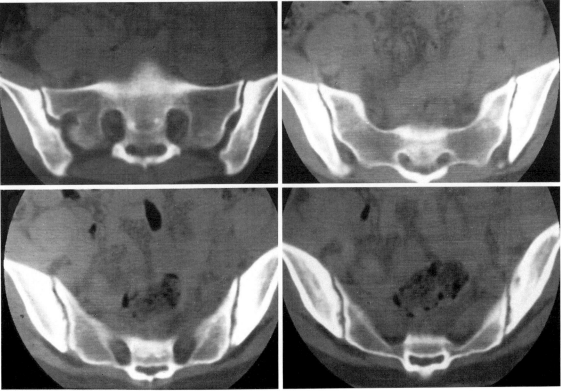

are not synovial, but bound only by ligaments. Erosions make the articular cortices indistinct (Figures 6.50, 6.51 and 6.52). This appearance may be normal in teenagers. Ankylosing spondylitis almost inevitably proceeds to symmetrical involvement of the sacroiliac joints; however, in Reiter's syndrome and psoriasis, the sacroiliac joints may remain unilaterally involved (Figure 6.53).

Eventually the medial cortices of the sacroiliac joints erode, reactive sclerosis is seen behind and between erosions, and the joints fuse (Figure 6.54). Confirmation of fusion may often be obtained by using oblique views, prone views or even CT scanning. The inferior margin of the joint at the pelvic brim shows bony continuity, confirming fusion. Isotope bone scans may be positive even before plain film changes occur, but fused sacroiliac joints may be normal as the disease is quiescent. Paravertebral syndesmophytosis and a peripheral erosive arthritis are found in varying degrees in these conditions.

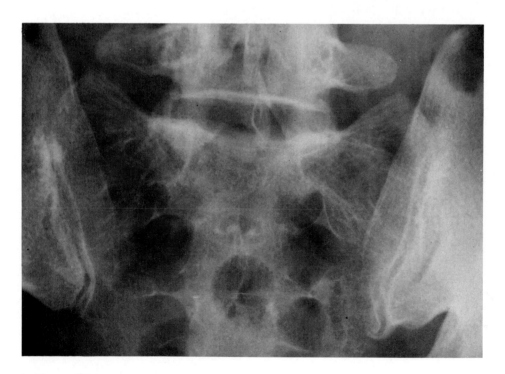

Figure 6.53

Reiter's syndrome. The three radiographs taken over a 12-year period demonstrate the progression of a unilateral sacroiliitis.

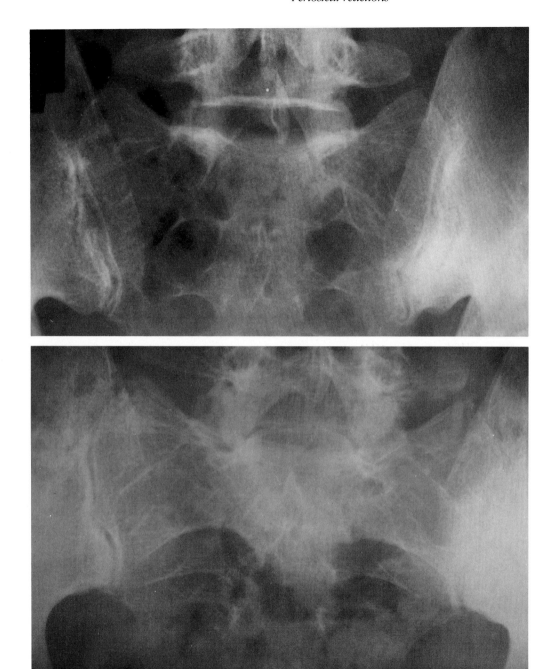

Figure 6.53 *continued*

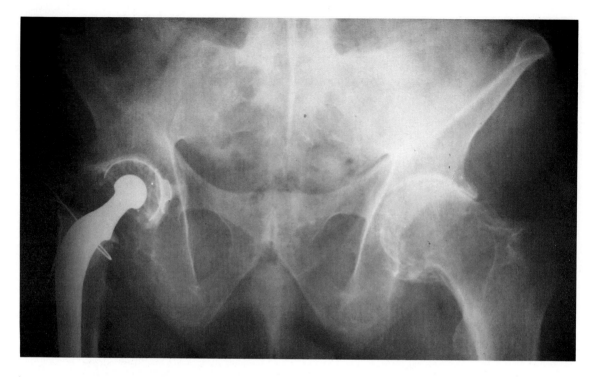

Figure 6.54

Ankylosing spondylitis. Sacroiliac
fusion is visible and the
symphysis pubis is also fused.
There is extensive new bone
formation, known as whiskering,
on the ischia.

In ankylosing spondylitis, the vertebral bodies
should be inspected for signs of erosion followed
by healing at the margins of the upper and lower
end-plates, initially at the thoracolumbar junction, but eventually throughout the spine. The
erosions at the vertebral margins initially result
in squaring of the vertebral bodies (Figure 6.55),
and this appearance may be compounded by new
bone formation on the anterior margin (Figure
6.56). Syndesmophytes form, which are vertically directed spurs of new bone in the annulus
which bridge the normal disc spaces, and eventually unite. They should be distinguished from
osteophytes, which are a feature of degeneration,
are horizontally directed and associated with
discal narrowing (Figure 6.57).

Paraspinal syndesmophyte formation also
occurs in X-linked hypophosphataemic osteomalacia (Figure 6.58) accompanied by sacroiliac
joint fusion, and without fusion in pseudohypo-

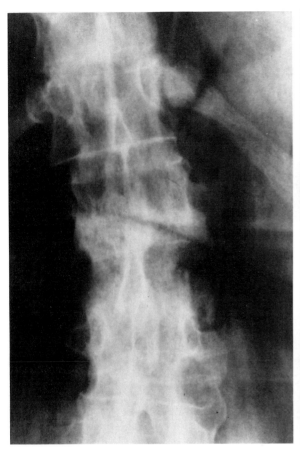
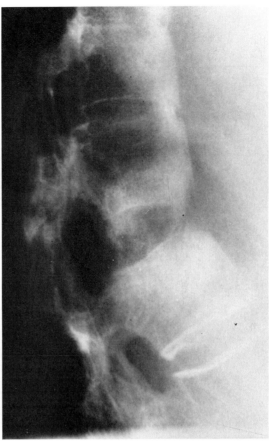

Figure 6.55

Ankylosing spondylitis. The lateral view demonstrates marked squaring of the vertebral bodies, and superior and inferior erosion of the anterior edges which is accompanied by local sclerosis. A fracture has occurred through one of the affected disc spaces, which is therefore widened. This is a relatively uncommon complication of ankylosing spondylitis and follows a fall. Patients may end up paraplegic. Hypermobility and instability occur at the level of the fracture and result in end-plate irregularity.

parathyroidism and, rarely, in hyperparathyroidism.

Erosions occur at characteristic sites in the seronegative spondylarthritides (Figure 6.59). The ischia and pubic bones (Figure 6.60), femoral trochanters, calcaneal bones (Figure 6.61) and iliac blades are eroded and heal with the formation of new bone extending perpendicularly into the soft tissues, a phenomenon which has been described as 'whiskering' (Figure 6.60).

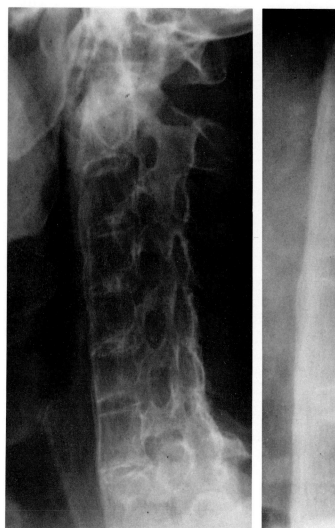

a

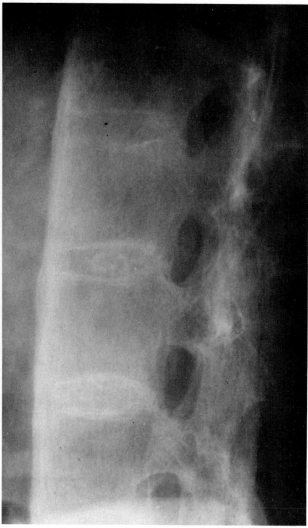

b

Figure 6.56

Ankylosing spondylitis. There is
loss of normal curvature in the
cervical (**a**) and lumbar (**b**)
regions with squaring of
vertebral bodies and ossification
of the anterior longitudinal
ligament. Discal calcification
occurs in areas of vertebral
fusion.

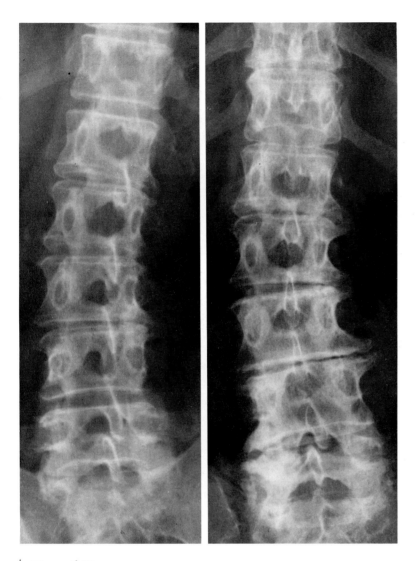

Figure 6.57

Osteophytes in osteoarthritis. A scoliosis concave to the left and buttressing osteophytes on the concavity are demonstrated in these two radiographs taken over an 11-year period. The osteophytes are well-corticated, rather thick structures which are horizontally directed. Syndesmophytes are more vertically directed.

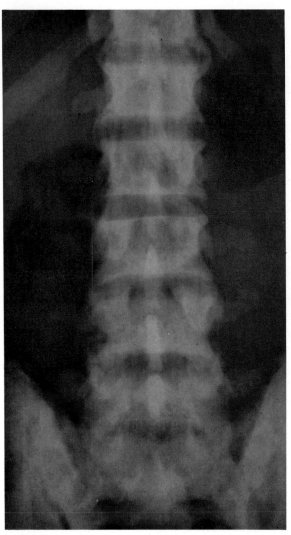

Figure 6.58

This patient has X-
linked hypophosphataemic
osteomalacia with paradiscal
syndesmophyte formation. The
sacroiliac and spinal changes
resemble those seen in
ankylosing spondylitis, but the
bones are dense, and there is
bowing of the long bones.
However, such bowing is not
present in fluorosis.

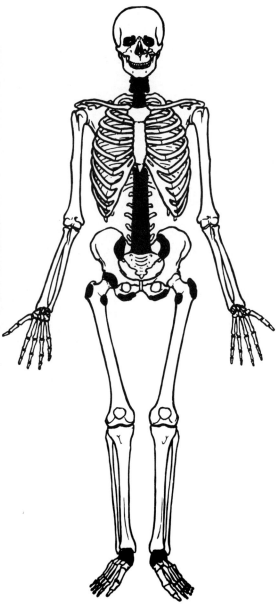

Figure 6.59

The major sites of involvement of
ankylosing spondylitis (shaded
areas).

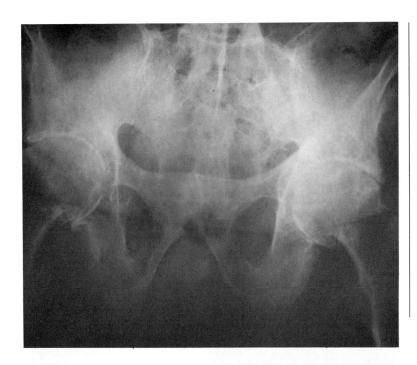

Figure 6.60

In this patient with ankylosing spondylitis, the sacroiliac joints are fused, with little or no reactive sclerosis and the disease is quiescent. Both hip joints are narrowed, showing medial migration of the femoral heads. These have a fringe of new bone around them which is another characteristic feature of ankylosing spondylitis. Much irregular new bone is laid down upon the ischia, and the original contours can still be seen. Similar fringing occurs at all the muscle attachments. The symphysis pubis is also fused and there is ossification of the interspinous ligaments.

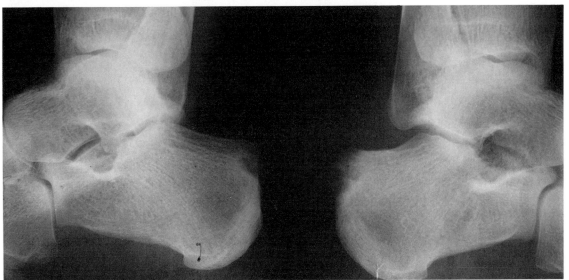

Figure 6.61

Ankylosing spondylitis. Erosions can be seen on the posterior aspects of the calcaneal bones. In this patient these are at the insertion of the Achilles tendons and also in the region of the retrocalcaneal bursa.

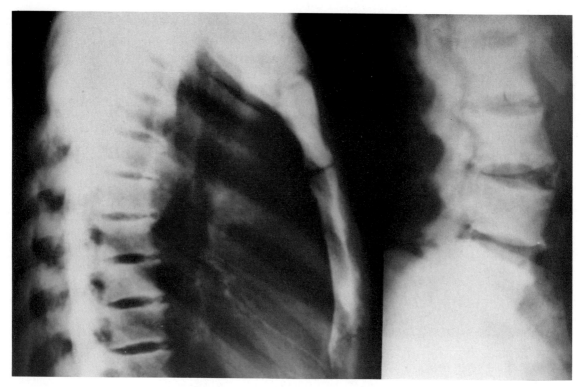

Figure 6.62

Fluorosis. An increase in bony
density is associated with
paradiscal ossification.

Rheumatoid arthritis

Rheumatoid arthritis is less commonly associated
with sacroiliac disease and spinal fusion, and
erosions only rarely heal with new bone formation.

Fluorosis

Fluorosis is usually associated with drinking
water containing more than 8 parts/million of
fluorine and therefore occurs in endemic areas.
The bones are increased in density, new bone
extends into soft tissues beneath the ribs (Figure
6.62), around the pelvis and at other muscle

insertions, and is also increased in density
(Figure 6.63). The changes of whiskering should
not be confused with an increase in bony density
and cortical thickening seen in osteopetrosis, for
example, where the bones are diffusely
expanded (see Chapter 2, page 107).

X-linked hypophosphataemic osteomalacia

The bones become thickened with increase in
density; bowing of long bones is a characteristic
feature. Looser's zones are seen, and whiskering
occurs at musculo-tendinous insertions, as well
as paraspinal ossification.

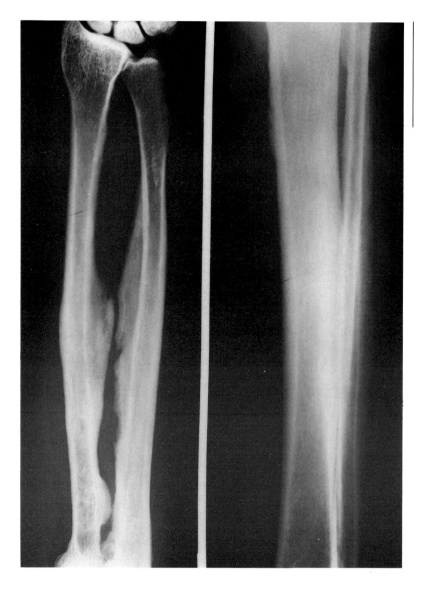

Figure 6.63

In this patient with fluorosis, there is ossification at the interosseous membrane linking the radius and ulna. This disease is another cause of cross-union between paired long bones.

Diffuse idiopathic skeletal hyperostosis (DISH)

This is also known as Forestier's disease, and is now recognized as a disease affecting much of the skeleton, not only the spine. Patients are not inevitably geriatric and usually have normal bone density, even in old age. Ossification of musculo-tendinous insertions occurs around the pelvis (Figure 6.64), trochanters, tuberosities, calcaneal and mid-tarsal bones (Figure 6.65). There is a spectrum of hyperostosis which varies from minimal to gross; the sacroiliac joints are not involved. In the spine, florid new bone is formed separately around intact discs and this later merges, often anterolaterally to the vertebral bodies, to form linked, flame-shaped excrescences extending between four or more vertebrae (Figure 6.66). In the cervical spine, these

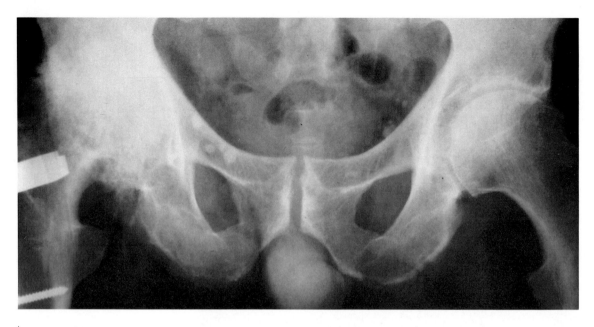

Figure 6.64

This patient with diffuse idiopathic skeletal hyperostosis has osteoarthritis of the right hip and preserved bone density. There is whiskering at the ischia, but the sacroiliac joints were patent.

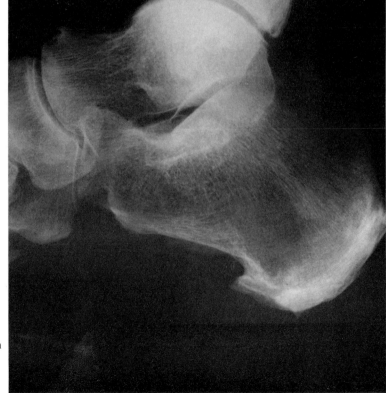

Figure 6.65

Diffuse idiopathic skeletal hyperostosis. The foot shows marked new bone formation posteriorly on the calcaneum, on the base of the fifth metatarsal, and on the superior aspects of the talus and navicular.

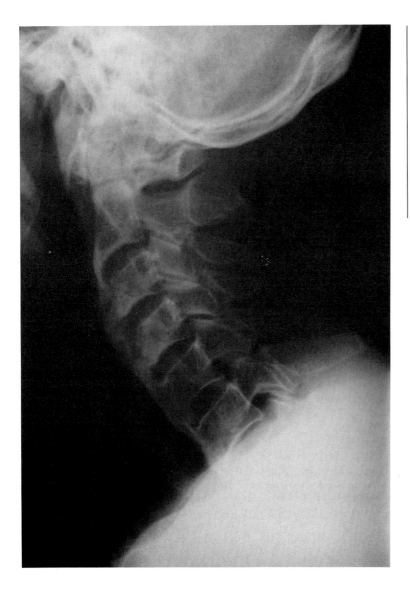

Figure 6.66

Diffuse idiopathic skeletal hyperostosis of cervical spine. Marked new bone formation anteriorly extends from C2 to C7. This is probably more florid than in any other form of skeletal ankylosis and is associated with intact disc heights. New bone extends anteriorly some distance from the vertebral bodies and affects at least four segments in continuity.

changes may result in dysphagia and, in the thoracic spine, they are mainly right-sided, possibly because the descending aorta prevents them occurring on the left. Normal discs, the contiguity and extent of the changes, as well as the vertical orientation of the new bone, distinguish the spinal changes from those seen in degeneration.

In all these conditions, therefore, spinal changes are prominent and should be assessed, together with the presence or absence of sacroiliitis.

7 | Abnormalities in size and modelling of bone

Common causes of short-limbed dwarfism

Achondroplasia

This is the commonest form of dwarfism and is predominantly due to limb shortening (Table 7.1). Recently, many conditions have been separated from achondroplasia, including hypochondroplasia and thanatophoric dwarfism. Although inherited as a dominant condition, the majority of patients are new mutants.

In the long bones, the shortening is predominantly rhizomelic. The metaphyses are grossly splayed and have a local chevron sign at the knees. This is seen as a central failure of growth resulting in a defect in which the abnormally shaped epiphysis sits. In addition, the metaphyses around the knee are narrow in the sagittal plane, causing the area to appear lucent on anteroposterior films (Figure 7.1).

The pelvis is abnormally shaped with a 'champagne glass' pelvic brim (Figure 7.2). In children, the cartilages are prominent, so that the ischiopubic synchondrosis and the triradiate cartilages are wider than normal. The iliac blades in the adult are round and squat, with little waisting above the acetabulum. The spine shows progressive narrowing of the interpedicular distance in the lumbar region. The discs further narrow the spinal canal and neurological symptoms are common. Canal stenosis is clearly demonstrated at radiculography (Figure 7.3). In addition, an exaggerated lumbar lordosis makes the buttocks prominent. The hands are 'trident' in type with short tubular bones so that the fingers all appear the same length and diverge from the midline (Figure 7.4).

The skull has a large calvarium with a short base. The narrow foramen magnum causes hydrocephalus which may further enlarge the skull.

Thanatophoric dwarfism

In the neonate thanatophoric dwarfism has in the past been confused with achondroplasia but there are marked dissimilarities between these conditions. In thanatophoric dwarfs, the extremely short limbs are curved (Figure 7.5), which is not a feature of achondroplasia, in which the diaphyses are straight. In addition, there is a severe generalized platyspondyly with more normal posterior elements, so that the vertebrae resemble the letter H. The skull shows a trefoil deformity, known as the 'clover-leaf' skull with prominent temporal bulges. This condition is usually fatal.

348

Table 7.1 Abnormalities in size and modelling of bone.

Common causes of short-limbed dwarfism

Achondroplasia

This has been confused in the past with

Hypochondroplasia

Pseudoachondroplasia

Thanatophoric dwarfism ⎫

Achondrogenesis ⎭ Often fatal

Short-trunked dwarfism

Spondyloepiphyseal dysplasia

Proportionate dwarfism

Mucopolysaccharidoses ⎫ Associated ⎫

Hypophosphataemia ⎬ with diminished ⎪

Osteogenesis imperfecta ⎭ bone density ⎪ Associated with

⎬ multiple fractures

Osteopetrosis ⎫ Associated with ⎪

Pyknodysostosis ⎭ increased bone density ⎭

Cleidocranial dysostosis ⎱ Normal bone density ⎱ Clavicular hypoplasia;

⎰ ⎰ acro-osteolysis; Wormian bones

Adapted from Wynne-Davies R, *Heritable disorders in orthopaedic practice*, (Blackwell: Oxford 1973), with permission.

Table 7.2 Common causes of localized discrepancy in length.

Overgrowth

Arteriovenous malformation ⎫ Associated with ⎫

Haemangioma ⎪ changes in local ⎪

Lymphangioma ⎬ soft tissues ⎪

Macrodystrophia lipomatosa ⎪ ⎪

Neurofibromatosis ⎭ ⎪ Associated with

⎬ overgrowth of

Melorheostosis ⎪ all or part

Dysplasia epiphysealis hemimelica ⎪ of a limb

⎪

Tuberculosis ⎫ Associated with ⎪

Juvenile rheumatoid arthritis ⎬ increased blood ⎪

Haemophilia ⎭ flow at joints ⎭

Congenital hemihypertrophy

Shortening

Infection ⎫

Trauma ⎪

Radiation ⎪ Damage to the

Sickle-cell disease ⎬ epiphyseal plate

Scurvy ⎪

Thermal injury ⎭

Polio ⎱ Congenital or acquired

Spina bifida ⎰ defects of motor function

Enchondromatosis ⎱ Growth abnormalities associated

Diaphyseal aclasia ⎰ with cartilaginous tumours

Table 7.3   Causes of undertubulation.

Sickle-cell disease
Thalassaemia
	} Due to marrow
	     hyperplasia
		} Erlenmeyer flask
		     appearance

Gaucher's disease	} Due to marrow infiltration	
Fibrous dysplasia Enchondromatosis Diaphyseal aclasia	} Associated with multiple local tumours	

Osteopetrosis
Pyknodysostosis
	} Gross sclerosis
	     and dwarfism
		} Failure of
		     remodelling at
		     metaphyses

Lead poisoning	} Metaphyseal sclerosis	
Healing rickets Healing scurvy	} Diaphyseal new bone beneath the periosteum	
Adult X-linked hypophosphataemic osteomalacia Mucopolysaccharidoses		
Trauma in children Infantile cortical hyperostosis		

Table 7.4   Causes of overtubulation.

Longstanding paralysis, eg, polio, spina bifida

Muscular dystrophy

Osteogenesis imperfecta

Neurofibromatosis

Juvenile chronic arthritis

Local extrinsic masses—soft tissue tumours,
   benign or malignant, eg, neurofibroma, angioma,
   lipoma

Achondrogenesis

This is a rare, fatal dysplasia which is similar to thanatophoric dwarfism. The long bones are extremely short and often curved, but ossification is defective in the lower spine, pelvis and lower limbs, so that often these parts can barely be seen (Figure 7.6).

Hypochondroplasia

Hypochondroplasia has also been distinguished from achondroplasia, because hypochondroplasts generally are not as short as achondroplasts and the skull is normal. The interpedicular distances in the lumbar spine become progressively narrow caudally (Figure 7.7), but limb shortening is not as pronounced and trident hands are not present. The fibula is longer than

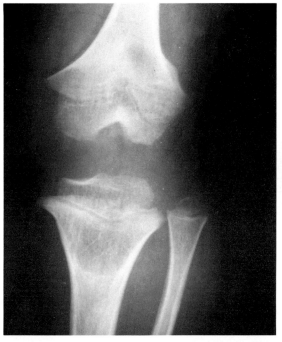

a

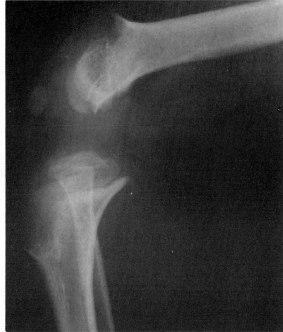

b

Figure 7.1

Achondroplasia. (**a**) Chevron deformities are present at the metaphyses, and the epiphyses fit into the metaphyseal defects. In addition, there are metaphyseal lucencies. (**b**) The lucencies are due to defects of the anterior tibial and femoral metaphyses.

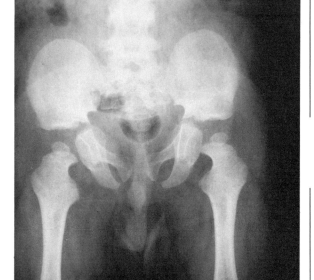

Figure 7.2

Achondroplasia. The iliac blades are squat and show no constriction above the acetabula, which have horizontal roofs. They are also slightly irregular. The pelvic inlet is shaped like a champagne glass. There is rhizomelic dwarfism. The interpedicular distances of the lower lumbar spine are narrow, and the triradiate ischiopubic cartilages are prominent.

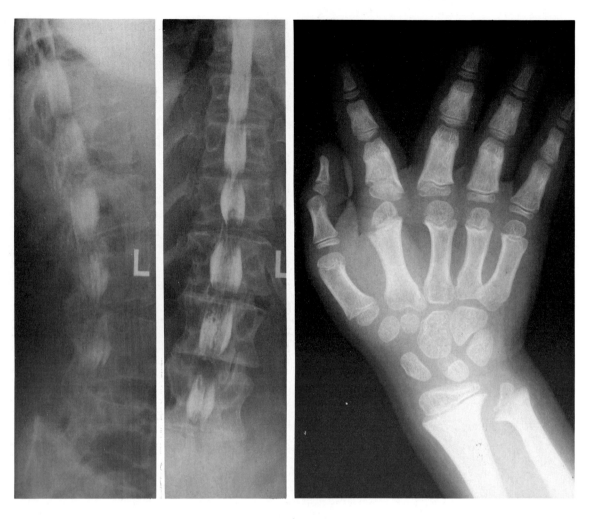

Figure 7.3

The radiculogram in this
achondroplastic patient shows
posterior scalloping of vertebral
bodies and multiple constrictions
related to the intervertebral
discs. The interpedicular
distances narrow from above
downwards in the lumbar region.

Figure 7.4

This patient with achondroplasia
has a trident hand. There is
divergence at the second and
third fingers, and all the fingers
are similar in length. There are
also multiple growth anomalies.
The distal ulna shows a minor
chevron deformity.

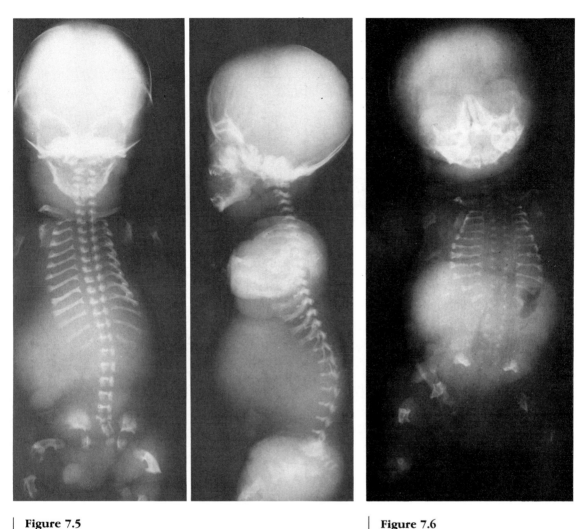

Figure 7.5

Thanatophoric dwarfism. There is a clover-leaf skull and marked platyspondyly in the lumbar spine with H-shaped vertebrae and short-limbed dwarfism. The major long bones are curved which differentiates thanatophoric dwarfism from achondroplasia, which is not fatal. This patient is stillborn.

Figure 7.6

Achondrogenesis. The skull vault is barely mineralized in this stillborn child; the ribs are hypoplastic and have suffered multiple fractures. The pedicles in the spine are mineralized but no other parts are seen. There is gross shortening of the long bones, which are curved and irregular. There is hardly any mineralization of the pelvis.

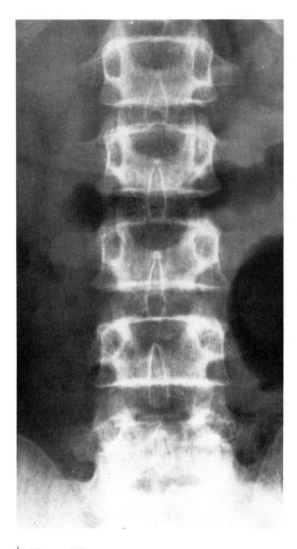

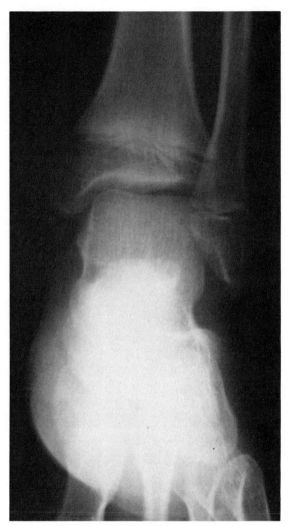

Figure 7.7

Hypochondroplasia. The
interpedicular distances narrow
in the lumbar spine from above
downwards.

Figure 7.8

Hypochondroplasia. Overgrowth
of the fibula is seen, but the
epiphyses are normal in
appearance.

the tibia at the ankle (Figure 7.8), which is also a feature of achondroplasia but the metaphyseal splaying and irregularity seen in this disease does not occur in hypochondroplasia, and the epiphyses are not irregular.

Pseudoachondroplasia

The pseudoachondroplastic forms of spondyloepiphyseal dysplasia are another group of conditions that resemble achondroplasia. It is not a single entity but a heterogenous group of diseases with rhizomelic dwarfism inherited in dominant and recessive forms of varying severity. In the most severe form, in adults, joint alignment deformities are prominent (Figure 7.9).

Unlike achondroplasia, changes are not present at birth but become apparent in childhood, and progressively more severe in adolescence. The skull is always normal, as in hypochondroplasia, but metaphyseal flaring may be more gross than in achondroplasia, and the epiphyses may be irregular (Figure 7.9). In contrast to achondroplasia, the spine shows varying degrees of platyspondyly with scoliosis (Figure 7.10), and also anterior beaking in the lumbar vertebral bodies.

Therefore, the pseudoachondroplastic forms of spondyloepiphyseal dysplasia have some features of achondroplasia, particularly rhizomelia, metaphyseal flaring and short hands, but also some features of true spondyloepiphyseal dysplasias which do not show rhizomelia, have normal skulls and which show a short-trunked, not short-limbed, dwarfism, with abnormal spines (Figure 7.11), platyspondyly and often scoliosis. Spondyloepiphyseal dysplasia tarda has already been mentioned (see page 245).

Proportionate dwarfism

Mucopolysaccharidoses

Of these uncommon disorders, only MPS I-H (Hurler's syndrome) is seen relatively frequently. Affected children are normal at birth and changes start appearing at around 1–2 years of age.

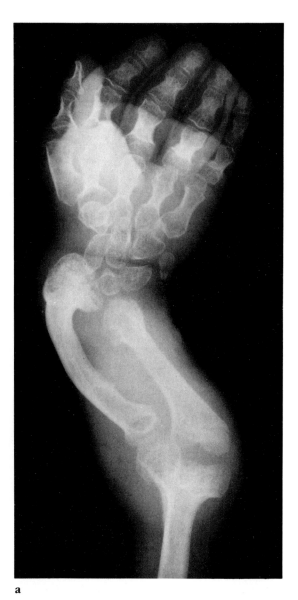

a

Figure 7.9

This patient has the severe recessive form of pseudoachondroplasia. Gross limb shortening (**a**) with irregularity of the epiphyses (**b**) can be seen. The deformities are considerable and greater than those seen in achondroplasia (**c**).

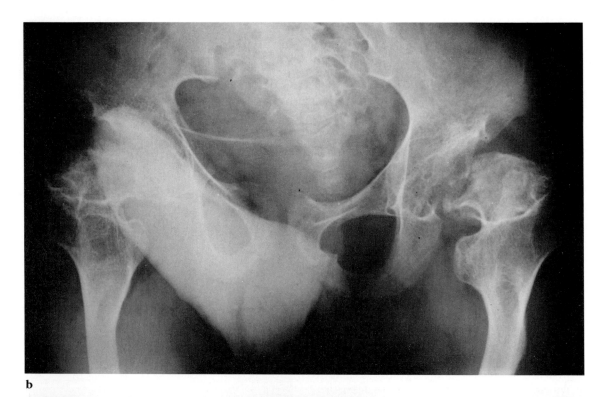

b

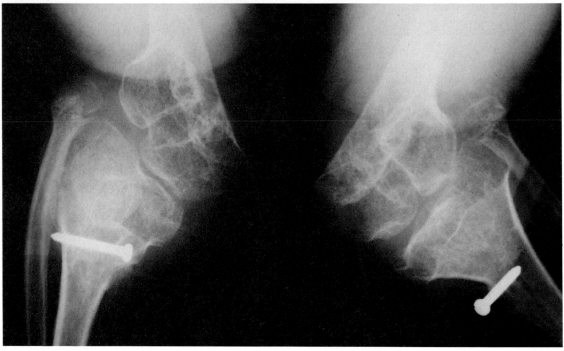

c

Figure 7.9 *continued*

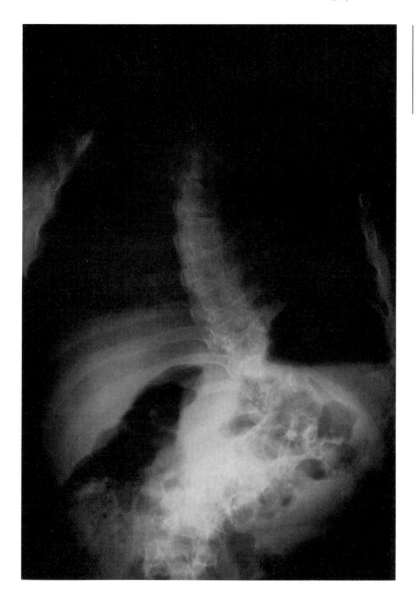

Figure 7.10

Pseudoachondroplasia. The spine of the patient shown in Figure 7.9 shows a gross kyphoscoliosis and platyspondyly.

Mental defect progresses and the coarsened face resembles that of a gargoyle. Epiphyses become progressively irregular, metaphyses broaden and the diaphyses thicken. A tibio-talar slant develops at the ankles (Figure 4.59) and a radio-ulnar tilt deformity at the wrists (Figure 4.57).

In the hands, the phalanges become bullet-shaped and the metacarpals broaden with proximal pointing (Figure 4.57), which is a characteristic appearance. The skull shows a J-shaped sella, scaphocephaly, odontoid hypoplasia and irregular condyles at the temporomandibular joints

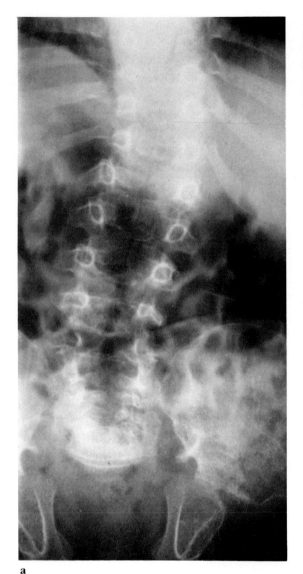

a

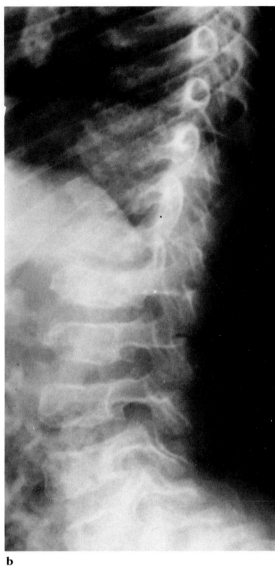

b

Figure 7.11

Spondyloepiphyseal dysplasia congenita. (**a,b**) There is gross platyspondyly with a scoliosis. Some of the vertebral bodies also show anterior beaking. The congenita form does not have the posterior vertebral body humps seen in the tarda type of spondyloepiphyseal dysplasia. (**c**) The acetabular roofs are flat and irregular. The femoral heads are displaced, the metaphyses broad and irregular, and the medial acetabular walls thickened.

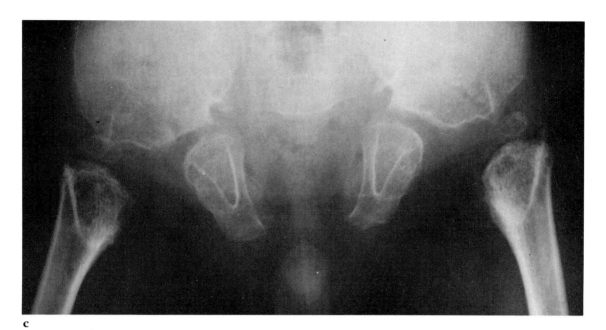

c

Figure 7.11 *continued*

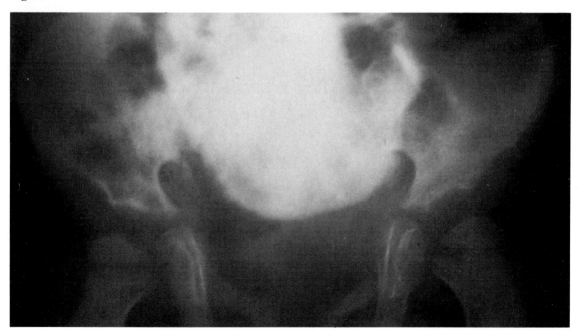

Figure 7.12

MPS I-H. There is quite marked enlargement of the liver and a large umbilical hernia, with coxa valga and hypoplasia of the ilium in the supra-acetabular region.

Figure 7.13

MPS IV. There is an acute kyphos at L1 which shows a prominent anterior beak and hypoplasia of the superior surface. Multiple areas of stenosis are present on the radiculogram. There is platyspondyly with end-plate irregularity and the ribs are abnormal in shape.

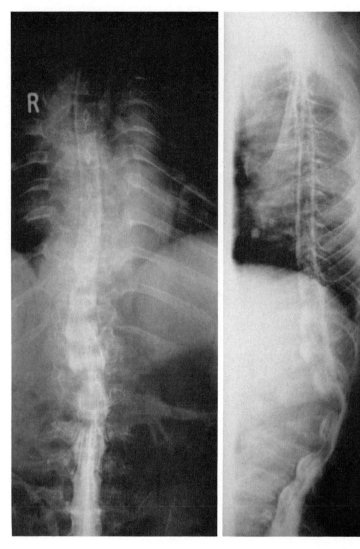

(Figure 4.58). In the spine, one or more vertebral bodies in the thoracolumbar region show an anterior beak with an associated kyphos (Figure 7.14). The pelvis is abnormally shaped with coxa valga and acetabular dysplasia. In the abdomen, the liver and spleen are grossly enlarged (Figure 7.12).

MPS IV

MPS IV (Morquio–Brailsford disease) is a well recognized, but extremely rare, disease which

unlike MPS I-H is not associated with mental defect, and in which the skull is normal, although odontoid hypoplasia is present. Throughout the spine there is irregular platyspondyly with central anterior beaking (Figure 7.13), whereas the beak in MPS I-H tends to be antero-inferior (Figure 7.14). The pelvis shows progressive acetabular dysplasia and the flattened, fragmented epiphyses lie in pseudo-acetabula beneath the iliac blades, which are prominent (Figure 7.15) unlike those seen in achondroplasia. In general, the metaphyses are flared, the

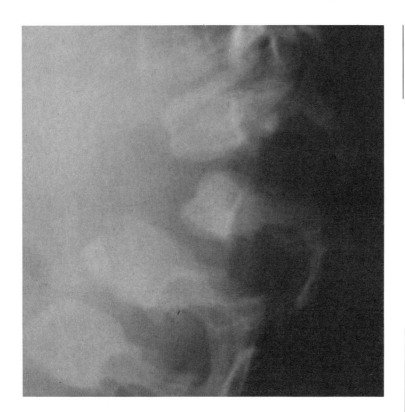

Figure 7.14

MPS I-H. There is a hypoplastic vertebral body at the thoraco-lumbar junction with a central anterior defect.

Figure 7.15

MPS IV. There are very prominent iliac blades with deepened acetabula. The femoral heads are broad and flat, and articulate laterally.

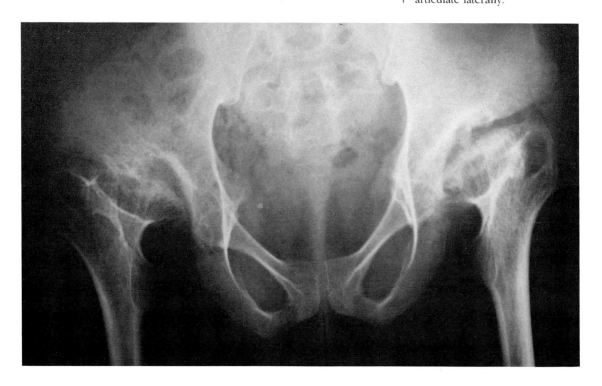

Figure 7.16

MPS IV. The appearances are those of a mucopolysaccharidosis, with bullet-shaped phalanges and pointed metacarpals in the feet and hands.

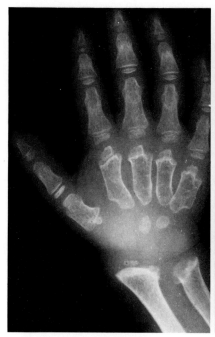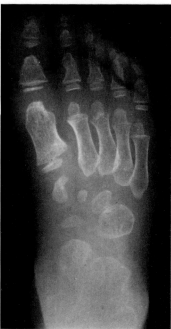

epiphyses irregular, the phalanges bullet-shaped, and the metacarpals show proximal pointing (Figure 7.16).

Osteogenesis imperfecta

Osteogenesis imperfecta is described in Chapter 1 as showing osteopenia, multiple fractures which heal with hyperplastic callus, Wormian bones in the skull (Table 4.2) and platyspondyly, resulting from bone softening. Limb shortening and bowing also result from softening and pathological fractures (see Figure 1.15). Thin, gracile, bowed, demineralized long bones are also a feature of this disease; they are also occasionally seen in juvenile chronic arthritis and rickets but, in osteogenesis imperfecta, the

metaphyses and epiphyses are more normal in appearance. Often fractures are of different generations and tend to be diaphyseal, unlike those seen in idiopathic juvenile osteoporosis which are characteristically metaphyseal in adolescents (see Figure 1.22).

Osteopetrosis (Albers–Schoenberg disease)

This causes limb deformity due to multiple fractures, with shortening. In the recessively inherited congenital form, dwarfism can be severe but, in the dominant, tarda form, it may not be readily apparent. The vertebral bodies do not seem to show collapse (see Chapter 2, page 107).

Pyknodysostosis

This rare condition is characterized by severe symmetrical dwarfism, osteosclerosis and pathological fractures, so that it resembles osteopetrosis. However it differs from osteopetrosis because increased density is diffuse rather than in alternating bands. It has many features in common with cleidocranial dysostosis (see Chapter 2, page 109).

Cleidocranial dysostosis

This may be associated with slight shortening, but bone density and the spine are normal. The skull shows Wormian bones and often numerous supernumerary teeth (Figure 7.17). In childhood, there are typically midline defects at the symphysis pubis (Figure 7.18) and symphysis mentis (Figure 7.19), and clavicular aplasia or hypoplasia (Figure 7.20). In the hands, acro-osteolysis may be present, as well as an accessory epiphysis at the base of the second metacarpal (Figure 7.21).

Further conditions causing shortening of bone

Enchondromatosis

Masses of immature cartilage remain at the metaphyses, resulting in tumours which have the characteristic features of cartilaginous lesions. They are mainly lucent, ossifying centrally, and have a narrow zone of reactive sclerosis. This produces expansion of the metaphysis with shortening of the shaft.

A characteristic change is seen in the radius and ulna (Figure 7.22). The ulna is short, broad and deformed by an enchondromal mass distally,

Figure 7.17

Cleidocranial dysostosis. The orthopantomograph shows failure of shedding of deciduous teeth, failure of eruption of the secondary dentition and numerous supernumerary teeth leading to a crowded dentition. The maxilla is hypoplastic.

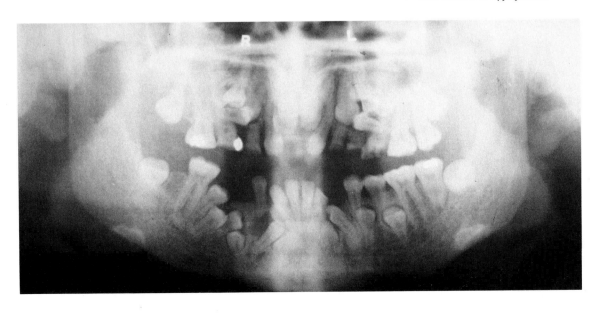

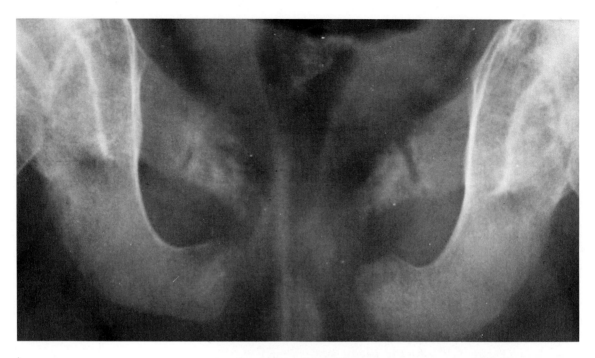

Figure 7.18

Cleidocranial dysostosis. There is failure of ossification of the symphysis pubis, resulting in an appearance similar to osteomalacia.

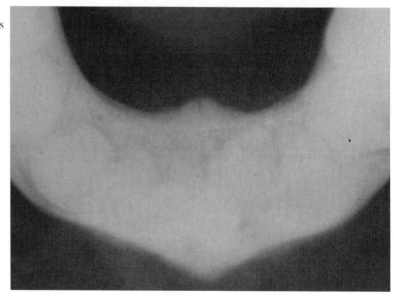

Figure 7.19

In this patient with cleidocranial dysostosis, a midline defect is seen at the symphysis mentis.

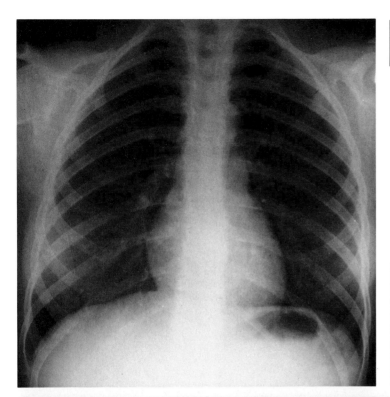

Figure 7.20

Cleidocranial dysostosis. In this patient the clavicles are absent.

Figure 7.21

Cleidocranial dysostosis. Abnormalities of length and modelling of the metacarpals and phalanges are prominent; secondary ossification centre is seen at the base of the second metacarpal.

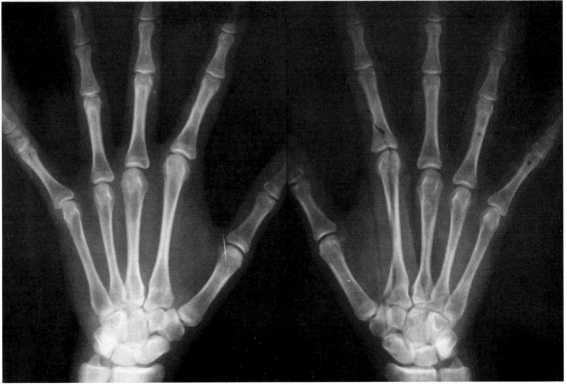

Figure 7.22

This patient with enchondromatosis has hypoplasia of the ulna with overgrowth of the radius. Islands of cartilage are visible at the distal radial and ulnar metaphyses. In the tibia, ray-like strands of cartilaginous lucencies stream backwards from the epiphyseal plate.

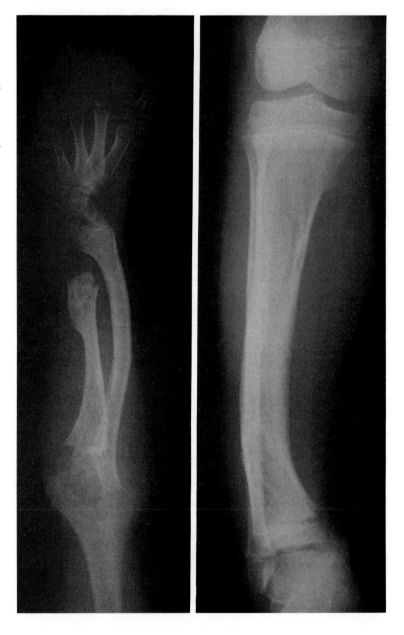

and the radius may then overgrow at the wrist and dislocate proximally. The hands become particularly deformed because of the large expansile, medullary cartilaginous masses (Figure 7.23), and function may be severely impaired. Malignant change is rare, but is more common in Maffucci's syndrome (enchondromatosis and haemangiomas) (Figure 7.23).

Diaphyseal aclasia (multiple exostoses)

Progressive, eventually gross, metaphyseal expansion with superimposed cartilage-capped exostoses affects major joints as well as the spine and pelvis (Figure 7.24). Exostoses also arise

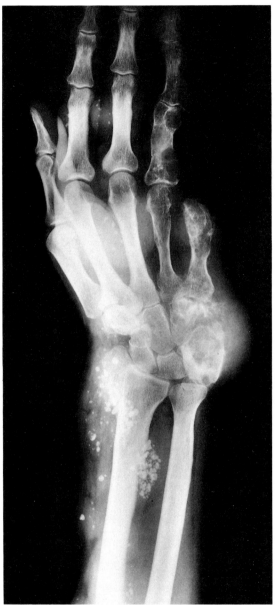

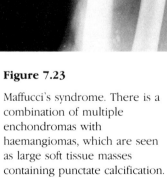

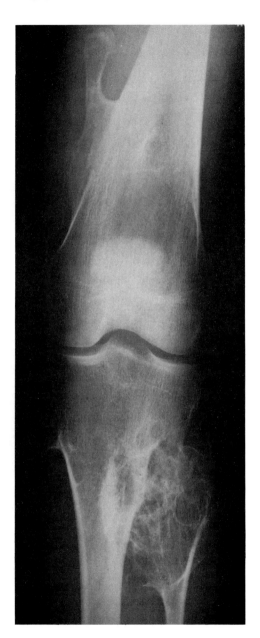

Figure 7.23

Maffucci's syndrome. There is a combination of multiple enchondromas with haemangiomas, which are seen as large soft tissue masses containing punctate calcification.

Figure 7.24

Diaphyseal aclasia. Broadening of the metaphyses is associated with 'coat-hanger' exostoses at the distal femur, while the gross expansion of the fibula has resulted in proximal tibio-fibular fusion.

Figure 7.25

Diaphyseal aclasia. Shortening of
the fourth and fifth metacarpals
results from a growth anomaly,
while the distal radius and ulna
show local expansion with
exostoses.

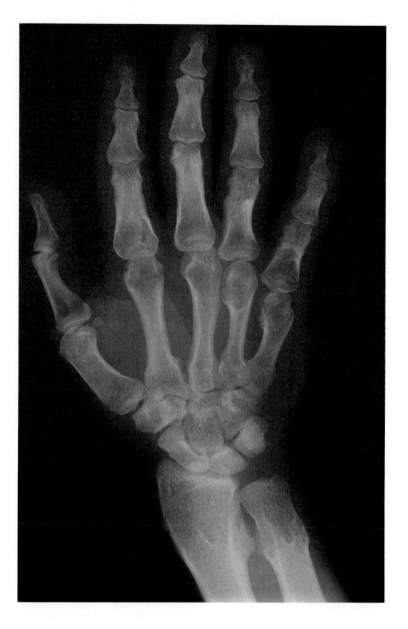

characteristically on the scapula, which is best
seen on axial views (Figure 5.25). This produces
limb shortening and shortening of phalanges,
metacarpals and metatarsals.

A characteristic lesion affects the radius and
ulna, which is similar in appearance to that seen
in enchondromatosis. Shortening and deformity
of the distal ulna results in overgrowth and

deformity of the distal radius and dislocation of
the proximal radius (Figure 7.25) (see Chapter
5, page 282).

For lesions of the epiphyseal plate causing
shortening, see page 215. For abnormalities of
motor function, see Table 7.2.

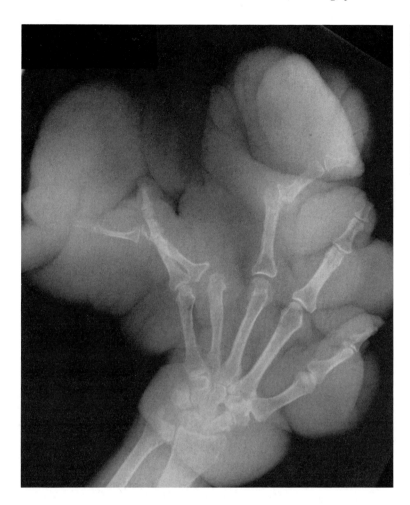

Figure 7.26

Neurofibromatosis. Gross soft tissue abnormality is seen, and some of the bones are overgrown. The proximal phalanges are as long as the metacarpals. Many of the bones are scalloped due to soft tissue masses causing extrinsic erosion of bone.

Overgrowth of bone

Neurofibromatosis

Overgrowth of all or part of a limb is a feature of this disease. The overgrowth is often related to a plexiform neurofibroma and hyperplasia of local blood vessels and lymphatics supplying the enlarged part of the limb. The changes in long bones, including the ribs, may be (1) overgrowth, with an increase in length and breadth of an affected bone (Figure 7.26), (2) bone thinning, as in the thin, twisted 'ribbon ribs', which is a dysplastic change (Figure 7.27) and (3) defects due to extrinsic pressure by localized neurofibromas, such as those seen on the undersides of ribs (Figure 7.28). Defects due to neurofibromas also enlarge spinal exit foramina, thin pedicles and laminae and may be seen as soft tissue masses at radiculography and CT scanning. Often these spinal changes as well as posterior scalloping of vertebral bodies (Figure 7.29) are

Figure 7.27

Neurofibromatosis. There is an
acute-angled kyphos associated
with thin, twisted ribbon ribs.
The local pedicles are thinned
and the neural canal widened.

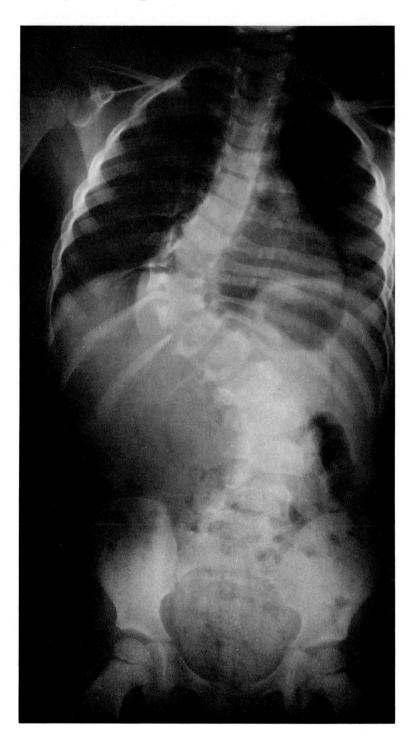

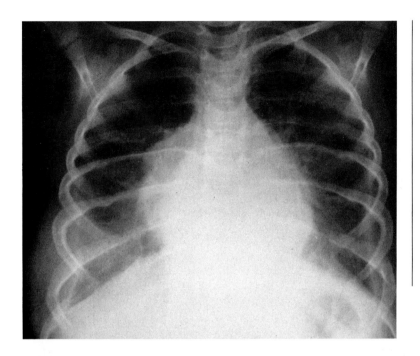

Figure 7.28

In this patient with neurofibromatosis, thin, twisted, ribbon ribs are associated with defects due to neurofibromas on the intercostal nerves. However, there is also a rather dense shadow behind the heart, caused by a large plexiform neurofibroma, associated with pedicular destruction and expansion of the spinal canal in the thoracic region. There are also neurofibromas related to the pleura and the chest wall in the axillae on both sides.

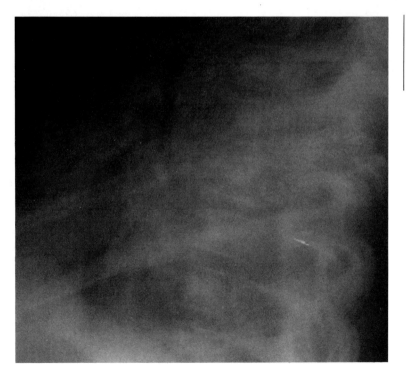

Figure 7.29

Posterior scalloping of the vertebral bodies may be seen in this patient with neurofibromatosis.

Figure 7.30

Neurofibromatosis. The radiculogram shows marked widening of the spinal canal in the thoracic region and associated intradural extramedullary neurofibromas displacing the spinal cord. In addition, there are sacular dilatations of the meninges, known as dural ectasia. There is a kyphoscoliosis, and the ribs differ in shape.

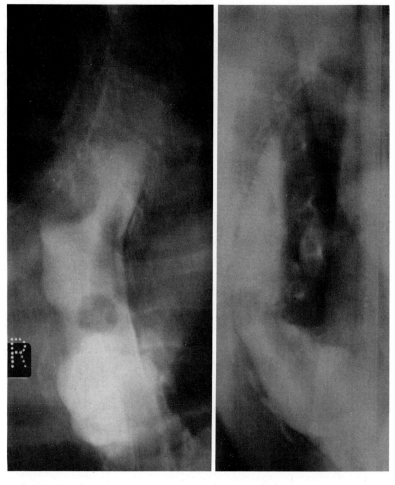

Table 7.5   Causes of posterior vertebral scalloping.

Normal variant

Achondroplasia

Neurofibromatosis

Intraspinal tumour

Acromegaly

Marfan's syndrome

Syringomyelia

Mucopolysaccharidoses

Pyknodysostosis

not due to tumours but are caused by dural ectasia and meningocoeles (Table 7.5). In the spine, the characteristic deformity is an acute kyphosis or scoliosis, which is not necessarily associated with a local tumour (Figure 7.30), but is a dysplastic change.

In the skull, there are orbital and occipital defects which are not necessarily associated with local tumours, but are true manifestations of a local dysplasia (Figure 7.31).

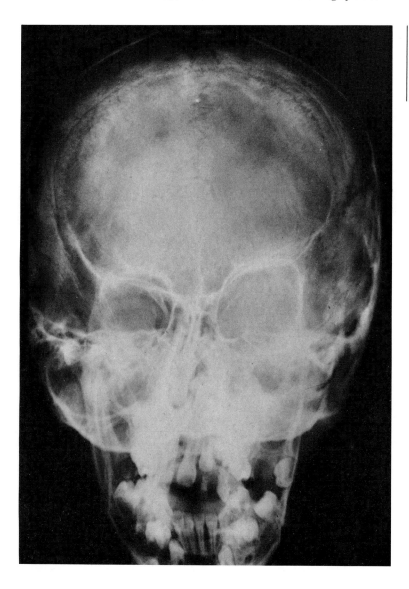

Figure 7.31

Neurofibromatosis. The left orbit is expanded and no markings are visible within it. This is the 'empty orbit' sign.

The paired bones, usually of the lower limbs, show abnormalities of texture in childhood which result in softening and bowing deformities and, finally fractures which do not heal, producing pseudarthrosis and shortening (Figure 7.32). A similar change is described in fibrous dysplasia. The two diseases have other common features, including skin pigmentation, associated endocrine anomalies, sarcomatous degeneration of tumours and tumoural osteomalacia; (see Chapter 1, page 48). Interestingly, these two conditions were described simultaneously by von Recklinghausen.

Macrodystrophia lipomatosa

Marked overgrowth of the digits is associated with gross proliferation of new bone around the

Figure 7.32

Pseudarthroses in
neurofibromatosis. Fractures are
followed by resorption of bone.
In this patient both ulnae are
affected, the radii have dislocated
proximally and are bowed.
There appears to be fusion
between the distal humerus and
the proximal ulna.

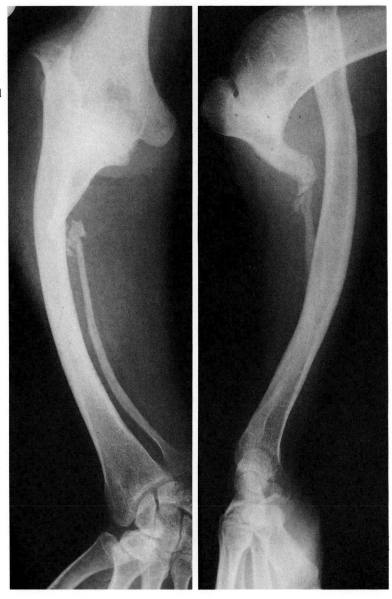

affected joints and accumulation of fat in local
soft tissues (Figure 7.33).

Melorheostosis

The areas of increased bone density which lie in
the distribution of the sclerotomes are also
increased in length in this condition resulting in,

for example, curvature of digits (Figure 7.34)
(see Chapter 2, page 96).

Dysplasia epiphysealis hemimelica

In this condition the affected epiphyses are
overgrown *in toto*, not just in the region from
which the osteochondroma originates. Also,
other bones locally may be enlarged.

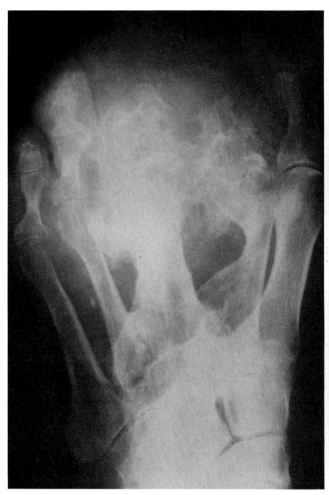

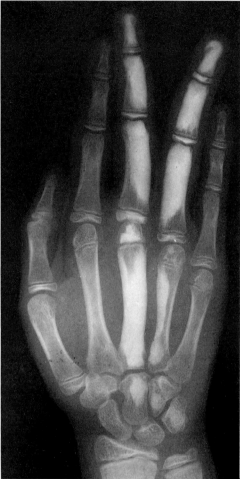

Figure 7.33

Macrodystrophia lipomatosa. It is difficult to see the radiolucent fat in the soft tissues but there is obvious abnormality of growth of many of the metatarsals and phalanges, and huge osseous excrescences resulting in deformity.

Figure 7.34

In this patient with melorheostosis, the abnormal bone shows an increase in size which expands the bone cortically and obliterates the medulla. The third and fourth fingers are separated because of the position of the new bone and these fingers are probably elongated.

Appendix

Suggestions for further reading

Major textbooks on bone disorders

Greenfield GB, *Radiology of bone diseases*, 4th edn, (Lippincott: Philadelphia 1986).

Murray RO, Jacobson HG, *The radiology of skeletal disorders*, 2nd edn., (Churchill Livingstone: Edinburgh 1977).

Resnick D, Niwayama G (eds), *Diagnosis of bone and joint disorders*, 2nd edn., (WB Saunders: Philadelphia 1981).

General radiological textbooks with good chapters on orthopaedics

Grainger RG, Allison D (eds.), *Diagnostic radiology: a textbook of organ imaging*, (Churchill Livingstone: Edinburgh 1986).

Sutton D (ed.), *A textbook of radiology and imaging*, 4th edn., (Churchill Livingstone: Edinburgh 1987).

Specialist monographs

Aitken M, *Osteoporosis in clinical practice*, (J Wright & Sons: Bristol 1984).

Davidson JK (ed.), *Aseptic necrosis of bone*, (Excerpta Medica: Amsterdam 1976).

Galasko CSP, *Skeletal metastases*, (Butterworths: London 1986).

Hamdy RC, *Paget's disease of bone*, (Prager: New York 1981).

Lodwick GS, *The bones and joints*, (Year Book Medical Publishers: Chicago 1971).

Simon G, *Principles of X-ray diagnosis*, (Butterworths: London 1960).

Sissons HA, Murray RO, Kemp HBS, *Orthopaedic diagnosis*, (Springer Verlag: Berlin 1984).

Weiss L, Gilbert HA, (eds.), *Bone metastasis*, (GK Hall Medical Publishers: Boston 1981).

Rheumatology

Arden GP, Ansell BM, (eds), *Surgical management of juvenile chronic arthritis*, (Academic Press: London 1978).

Forester DM, Brown JC, *The radiology of joint disease*, 3rd edn., (WB Saunders: Philadelphia 1987).

Scott JT, (ed.), *Copeman's textbook of the rheumatic diseases*, 6th edn., (Churchill Livingstone: Edinburgh 1986).

Inherited disorders

Beighton P, *Inherited disorders of the skeleton*, (Churchill Livingstone: Edinburgh 1978).

Kozlowski K, Beighton P, *Gamut index of skeletal dysplasias*, (Springer Verlag: Berlin 1984).

Taybi H, *The radiology of syndromes and metabolic disorders*, 2nd edn., (Year Book Medical Publishers: Chicago 1983).

Wynne-Davies R, *Heritable disorders in orthopaedic practice*, (Blackwell: Oxford 1973).

Normal variants

Keats TE, *Atlas of radiological variants*, 3rd edn., (Year Book Medical Publishers: Chicago 1984).

Kohler A, Zimmer E, *Borderlands of the normal and early pathologic in skeletal roentgenology*, 3rd American edn., (arranged by Stefan P Wilk) (Grune & Stratton: New York 1968).

Nuclear medicine

Galasko CSB, Webber DA (eds.), *Radionuclide scintigraphy in orthopaedics*, (Churchill Livingstone: Edinburgh 1984).

Fogelman I, Maisey M, *An atlas of clinical nuclear medicine,* (Martin Dunitz: London 1988).

Growth and development

Greulich WW, Pyle SI, *Radiographic atlas of skeletal development of the hand and wrist*, 2nd edn., (Stamford University Press: Stamford, California 1959).

Tanner JM, Whitehouse RH, Cameron N et al, *Assessment of skeletal maturity and prediction of adult height*, (Academic Press, London 1983).

Index